Hypoparathyroidism

Editor

MICHAEL A. LEVINE

ENDOCRINOLOGY AND METABOLISM CLINICS OF NORTH AMERICA

www.endo.theclinics.com

Consulting Editor
ADRIANA G. IOACHIMESCU

December 2018 • Volume 47 • Number 4

ELSEVIER

1600 John F. Kennedy Boulevard ● Suite 1800 ● Philadelphia, Pennsylvania, 19103-2899

http://www.theclinics.com

ENDOCRINOLOGY AND METABOLISM CLINICS OF NORTH AMERICA Volume 47, Number 4
December 2018 ISSN 0889-8529, ISBN 13: 978-0-323-64218-7

Editor: Stacy Eastman
Developmental Editor: Meredith Madeira

Endocrinology and Metabolism Clinics of North America (ISSN 0889-8529) is published quarterly by Elsevier Inc., 360 Park Avenue South, New York, NY 10010-1710. Months of issue are March, June, September, and December. Periodicals postage paid at New York, NY and additional mailing offices. Subscription prices are USD 357.00 per year for US individuals, USD 721.00 per year for US institutions, USD 100.00 per year for US students and residents, USD 447.00 per year for Canadian individuals, USD 893.00 per year for Canadian institutions, USD 490.00 per year for international individuals, USD 893.00 per year for international institutions, and USD 245.00 per year for international and Canadian and foreign students/residents. To receive student/resident rate, orders must be accompanied by name of affiliated institution, date of term, and the signature of program/residency coordinator on institution letterhead. Orders will be billed at individual rate until proof of status is received. Foreign air speed delivery is included in all *Clinics* subscription prices. All prices are subject to change without notice. **POSTMASTER:** Send address changes to *Endocrinology and Metabolism Clinics of North America*, Elsevier Health Sciences Division, Subscription Customer Service, 3251 Riverport Lane, Maryland Heights, MO 63043. **Customer Service: Telephone: 1-800-654-2452** (U.S. and Canada); **1-314-447-8871** (outside U.S. and Canada). **Fax: 1-314-447-8029. E-mail: journalscustomerservice-usa@elsevier.com (for print support); journalsonlinesupport-usa@elsevier.com (for online support).**

Reprints. For copies of 100 or more, of articles in this publication, please contact the Commercial Rights Department, Elsevier Inc., 360 Park Avenue South, New York, NY 10010-1710; phone: +1-212-633-3874; fax: +1-212-633-3820; E-mail: reprints@elsevier.com.

Endocrinology and Metabolism Clinics of North America is covered in *MEDLINE/PubMed (Index Medicus)*, *EMBASE/Excerpta Medica, Current Contents/Clinical Medicine, Current Contents/Life Sciences, Science Citation Index, ISI/BIOMED, BIOSIS,* and *Chemical Abstracts.*

Contributors

CONSULTING EDITOR

ADRIANA G. IOACHIMESCU, MD, PhD, FACE
Professor of Medicine (Endocrinology) and Neurosurgery, Emory University School of Medicine, Atlanta, Georgia, USA

EDITOR

MICHAEL A. LEVINE, MD, MACE, FACP, FAAP
Professor of Pediatrics and Medicine, University of Pennsylvania Perelman School of Medicine, Chief Emeritus, Division of Endocrinology and Diabetes, Center for Bone Health, The Children's Hospital of Philadelphia, Philadelphia, Pennsylvania, USA

AUTHORS

MURIEL BABEY, MD
Attending Physician, Department of Medicine, Highland Hospital, Oakland, California, USA

JOHN P. BILEZIKIAN, MD, PhD (hon)
Dorothy L. and Daniel H. Silberberg Professor of Medicine, Professor of Pharmacology, Vice Chair for International Education and Research, Chief, Emeritus, Division of Endocrinology, Department of Medicine, Columbia University Vagelos College of Physicians and Surgeons, New York, New York, USA

MARIA-LUISA BRANDI, MD, PhD
Department of Surgery and Translational Medicine, University of Florence, Florence, Italy

BART L. CLARKE, MD
Professor of Medicine, Division of Endocrinology, Diabetes, Metabolism, and Nutrition, Mayo Clinic, Rochester, Minnesota, USA

BRIAN G. CONDIE, PhD
Associate Professor, Department of Genetics, University of Georgia, Athens, Georgia, USA

NATALIE E. CUSANO, MD, MS
Assistant Professor, Department of Medicine, Director, Bone Metabolism Program, Lenox Hill Hospital, Donald and Barbara Zucker School of Medicine at Hofstra/Northwell, New York, New York, USA

DAVID GOLTZMAN, MD
Professor, Departments of Medicine and Physiology, McGill University, Research Institute of the McGill University Health Centre, Montreal, Quebec, Canada

REBECCA J. GORDON, MD
Division of Endocrinology and Diabetes, Center for Bone Health, The Children's Hospital of Philadelphia, Department of Pediatrics, University of Pennsylvania Perelman School of Medicine, Philadelphia, Pennsylvania, USA

YASSER HAKAMI, MD, FRCPC
Calcium Disorders Clinic, McMaster University, Hamilton, Ontario, Canada

HARALD JÜPPNER, MD
Endocrine Unit and Pediatric Nephrology Unit, Massachusetts General Hospital, Harvard Medical School, Boston, Massachusetts, USA

HADIZA S. KAZAURE, MD
Fellow, Section of Endocrine Surgery, Department of Surgery, Duke Cancer Institute, Duke University Medical Center, Durham, North Carolina, USA

ALIYA KHAN, MD, FRCPC, FACP, FACE
Clinical Professor of Medicine, Director Calcium Disorders Clinic, McMaster University, Hamilton, Ontario, Canada

MICHAEL A. LEVINE, MD, MACE, FACP, FAAP
Professor of Pediatrics and Medicine, University of Pennsylvania Perelman School of Medicine, Chief Emeritus, Division of Endocrinology and Diabetes, Center for Bone Health, The Children's Hospital of Philadelphia, Philadelphia, Pennsylvania, USA

AGNÈS LINGLART, MD, PhD
INSERM U1185, Paris Sud Paris-Saclay University, APHP, Reference Center for Rare Disorders of the Calcium and Phosphate Metabolism, filière OSCAR and Plateforme d'Expertise Maladies Rares Paris-Sud, APHP, Endocrinology and Diabetes for Children, Bicêtre Paris Sud Hospital, Le Kremlin Bicêtre, France

NANCY R. MANLEY, PhD
Professor, Department of Genetics, University of Georgia, Athens, Georgia, USA

MUNRO PEACOCK, DSc, FRCP
Professor, Department of Medicine, Division of Endocrinology, Indiana University School of Medicine, Indianapolis, Indiana, USA

KRISTEN PEISSIG, MS
Graduate Student, Department of Genetics, University of Georgia, Athens, Georgia, USA

MISHAELA R. RUBIN, MD, MS
Associate Professor of Medicine, Columbia University Irving Medical Center, Metabolic Bone Disease Unit, Columbia University Vagelos College of Physicians and Surgeons, New York, New York, USA

DOLORES SHOBACK, MD
Endocrine Research Unit, Professor, Department of Medicine, San Francisco VA Medical Center, University of California, San Francisco, San Francisco, California, USA

NAMRAH SIRAJ, MBBS
Bone Research and Education Centre, Affiliated with McMaster University, Hamilton, Ontario, Canada

JULIE ANN SOSA, MD, MA, FACS
Leon Goldman, MD Distinguished Professor of Surgery, Chair, Department of Surgery, Professor, Department of Medicine, University of California, San Francisco, San Francisco, California, USA

GAIA TABACCO, MD
Division of Endocrinology, Department of Medicine, Columbia University Vagelos College of Physicians and Surgeons, New York, New York, USA; Unit of Endocrinology and Diabetes, Department of Medicine, Campus Bio-Medico University of Rome, Rome, Italy

TAMARA J. VOKES, MD
Professor, Section of Endocrinology, Department of Medicine, University of Chicago, Chicago, Illinois, USA

Contents

> The parathyroid glands are essential for regulating calcium homeostasis in the body. The genetic programs that control parathyroid fate specification, morphogenesis, differentiation, and survival are only beginning to be delineated, but are all centered around a key transcription factor, GCM2. Mutations in the *Gcm2* gene as well as in several other genes involved in parathyroid organogenesis have been found to cause parathyroid disorders in humans. Therefore, understanding the normal development of the parathyroid will provide insight into the origins of parathyroid disorders.

> Parathyroid hormone (PTH) is the major secretory product of the parathyroid glands, and in hypocalcemic conditions, can enhance renal calcium reabsorption, increase active vitamin D production to increase intestinal calcium absorption, and mobilize calcium from bone by increasing turnover, mainly but not exclusively in cortical bone. PTH has therefore found clinical use as replacement therapy in hypoparathyroidism. PTH also may have a physiologic role in augmenting bone formation, particularly in trabecular and to some extent in cortical bone. This action has been applied to the clinic to provide anabolic therapy for osteoporosis.

> Hypoparathyroidism is associated with a spectrum of clinical manifestations in the acute and chronic settings, from mild to debilitating. Although the acute symptoms of hypocalcemia are primarily due to neuromuscular irritability, the chronic manifestations of hypoparathyroidism may be due to the disease itself or to complications of therapy or to both. The chronic complications of hypoparathyroidism can affect multiple organ systems, including the renal, neurologic, neuropsychiatric, skeletal, and immune systems. Further research is needed to determine the pathophysiology of complications in hypoparathyroidism and whether interventions can decrease the risk of these complications.

impaired formation of the parathyroid glands, disordered synthesis or secretion of parathyroid hormone, or postnatal destruction of the parathyroid glands.

Chronic parathyroid hormone (PTH) deficiency has a marked effect on the skeleton, leading to characteristic decreases in bone remodeling and increases in bone mass. Numerous lines of evidence using biochemical, imaging, and histomorphometric methodologies have demonstrated that the skeleton is altered when PTH is absent and that these abnormalities might be reversed with PTH treatment. More evidence is needed to determine whether fracture risk is altered in hypoparathyroidism.

Hypocalcemia and hyperphosphatemia are the pathognomonic biochemical features of hypoparathyroidism, and result directly from lack of parathyroid hormone (PTH) action on the kidney. In the absence of PTH action, the renal mechanisms transporting calcium and phosphate reabsorption deregulate, resulting in hypocalcemia and hyperphosphatemia. Circulating calcium negatively regulates PTH secretion. Hypocalcemia causes neuromuscular disturbances ranging from epilepsy and tetany to mild paresthesia. Circulating phosphate concentration does not directly regulate PTH secretion. Hyperphosphatemia is subclinical, but chronically promotes ectopic mineralization disease. Vitamin D–thiazide treatment leads to ectopic mineralization and renal damage. PTH treatment has the potential for fewer side effects.

Patients with hypoparathyroidism have a multitude of physical, emotional, and cognitive complaints consistent with reduced quality of life (QOL). Impaired QOL in patients treated with conventional therapy with calcium and active vitamin D has been documented in epidemiologic (registry) studies, case-controlled studies, and surveys, and at baseline in clinical trials of parathyroid hormone (PTH). Treatment with PTH has been shown to improve QOL in some but not all studies.

Pseudohypoparathyroidism (PHP) refers to a heterogeneous group of uncommon, yet related metabolic disorders that are characterized by impaired activation of the Gsα/cAMP/PKA signaling pathway by parathyroid hormone (PTH) and other hormones that interact with Gsa-coupled receptors. Proximal renal tubular resistance to PTH and thus hypocalcemia and hyperphosphatemia, frequently in presence of brachydactyly, ectopic ossification, early-onset obesity, or short stature are common features of PHP. Registries and large cohorts of patients are needed to conduct

ENDOCRINOLOGY AND METABOLISM CLINICS OF NORTH AMERICA

ISSUE OF RELATED INTEREST

Atlas of Oral & Maxillofacial Surgery Clinics, September 2017 (Vol. 25, Issue 2)
Oral Manifestations of Systemic Diseases
Joel J. Napeñas, *Editor*

VISIT THE CLINICS ONLINE!
Access your subscription at:
www.theclinics.com

Foreword

Hypoparathyroidism

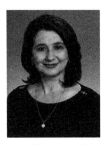

Adriana G. Ioachimescu, MD, PhD, FACE
Consulting Editor

The "Hypoparathyroidism" issue of the *Endocrinology and Metabolism Clinics of North America* is a state-of-the-art review of conditions characterized by functional deficiency of the parathyroid hormone. The guest editor is Dr Michael A. Levine, MD, MACE, FACP, FAAP, Professor of Pediatrics and Medicine at University of Pennsylvania in Philadelphia, a distinguished researcher and expert in the field of bone and mineral metabolism disorders. Dr Levine is an author of the first international Consensus Statement on diagnosis and management of pseudohypoparathyroidism released in 2018.

We dedicated the current issue to hypoparathyroidism because of recent scientific discoveries and changes in the therapeutic landscape. In this issue, renowned scientists highlight novel information that pertains to development, genetics, and molecular actions of PTH. Clinical researchers present updates on epidemiology, clinical manifestations, natural history, and management of hypoparathyroidism and pseudohypoparathyroidism. The authors share with us their insights on medical and surgical hypoparathyroidism, and the impact these disorders have on bones, kidneys, and quality of life. Last but not least, the issue contains updates regarding conventional treatment with calcium supplements and active forms of vitamin D, and an overview of recently approved therapy with full-length recombinant human parathyroid hormone therapy.

We hope you will find this issue of the *Endocrinology and Metabolism Clinics of North America* stimulating in your research and helpful in your practice. We thank Dr Levine for guest-editing this thought-provoking issue and the authors for their excellent contributions. We recognize the Elsevier editorial staff for their support that allowed us to review this important topic.

Adriana G. Ioachimescu, MD, PhD, FACE
Emory University School of Medicine
1365 B Clifton Road, Northeast, B6209
Atlanta, GA 30322, USA

E-mail address:
aioachi@emory.edu

Endocrinol Metab Clin N Am 47 (2018) xiii
https://doi.org/10.1016/j.ecl.2018.09.002
0889-8529/18/© 2018 Published by Elsevier Inc.

Preface

The Coming of Age of Hypoparathyroidism: Novel Insights into Causation, Innovative Options for Management

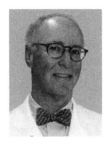

Michael A. Levine, MD, MACE, FACP, FAAP
Editor

This issue of the *Endocrinology and Metabolism Clinics of North America* provides a collection of articles that describes our current understanding of the basis and management of hypoparathyroidism, an endocrine disorder characterized by functional deficiency of parathyroid hormone (PTH). The term "hormone" comes from the Greek homzas, meaning to excite or arouse, and was introduced by Ernest Henry Starling in his Croonian lecture in 1905 on "The Clinical Correlation of the Functions of the Body" to describe those newly discovered substances that traveled through the bloodstream to stimulate other organs. It is my hope that these articles will, like hormones, stimulate new action, and in this case, focused on hypoparathyroidism!

The publication of this issue is timely. Clinicians and scientists both will benefit from the new insights into development and physiology of the parathyroid glands, the biological processing and actions of PTH, and the consequences of PTH deficiency. Up-to-date articles detail our growing knowledge of the genes that are associated with hypoparathyroidism, including defects that affect parathyroid gland development or sustenance, impair production of PTH, or reduce secretion of PTH. Moreover, no exposition of hypoparathyroidism would be complete without an acknowledgment of the pathophysiologic counterpart, pseudohypoparathyroidism, in which resistance to PTH action rather than deficiency of PTH secretion accounts for hypocalcemia and hyperphosphatemia. Here, we present a comprehensive description of the clinical, biochemical, and molecular features of pseudohypoparathyroidism and summarize

Endocrinol Metab Clin N Am 47 (2018) xv–xvi
https://doi.org/10.1016/j.ecl.2018.09.001
0889-8529/18/© 2018 Published by Elsevier Inc.

endo.theclinics.com

the role that genomic imprinting of *GNAS* plays in the phenotypic variability of this disorder.

Finally, this issue concludes with detailed recommendations for optimization of conventional treatment of hypoparathyroidism with active forms of vitamin D plus supplemental calcium as well as insights and guidelines for the use of recombinant human PTH 1-84 as hormone replacement therapy in selected patients.

Although the recognition and study of the parathyroid glands represent a relatively new subspecialty in the field of endocrinology, there has been an explosion of information over the past few years that now offers many exciting opportunities for investigators, clinicians, and patients. I would therefore like to thank all the contributing authors for their thorough and scholarly reviews and for sharing their wisdom. I hope you will enjoy their perspectives and incorporate the information into your research and practice.

Michael A. Levine, MD, MACE, FACP, FAAP
Division of Endocrinology and Diabetes
University of Pennsylvania
The Children's Hospital of Philadelphia
Abramson Research Building, 510A
3615 Civic Center Boulevard
Philadelphia, PA 19104, USA

E-mail address:
levinem@chop.edu

Embryology of the Parathyroid Glands

Kristen Peissig, MS, Brian G. Condie, PhD, Nancy R. Manley, PhD*

KEYWORDS

- Parathyroid • Organogenesis • GCM2 • PTH • SHH

KEY POINTS

- Parathyroid cell fate specification in the endodermal pharyngeal pouches is dependent on signaling from the Sonic hedgehog (SHH) pathway and modulated by fibroblast growth factor signaling, leading to initiation of *Gcm2* gene expression.
- Gcm2 upregulation is dependent on the HOXA3 transcription factor, working with a suite of other transcriptional regulators. In the absence of *Gcm2* upregulation, parathyroid cells undergo early and coordinated apoptosis.
- GCM2 also regulates parathyroid cell differentiation, regulating the expression of key functional genes including parathyroid hormone (PTH). GCM2, with another transcription factor MAFB, directly regulate *Pth* gene expression.

INTRODUCTION

Maintaining a stable level of serum calcium is important for proper muscle function, neurotransmission, and enzyme and hormone secretion, among many other functions.[1] Calcium homeostasis in terrestrial vertebrates is regulated by the parathyroid glands, endocrine organs located in the neck near the thyroid gland. Parathyroid glands express calcium-sensing receptors (CaSRs) that monitor serum calcium levels.[2] When these receptors detect low levels of calcium, the parathyroids secrete parathyroid hormone (PTH), which interacts with G-protein-coupled receptors on bone cells to release calcium from long bones into the bloodstream. In the kidney, PTH increases resorption of calcium in the ascending limb of the loop of Henle and in the distal tube as well as increasing excretion of inorganic phosphate into the urine.[3] When the parathyroids do not function properly, calcium/phosphorus homeostasis is disrupted. This results in 1 of 2 parathyroid disorders: hyperparathyroidism or hypoparathyroidism. Hyperparathyroidism is usually caused by parathyroid adenomas, which are benign parathyroid tumors that cause an excess of PTH to be produced

Disclosure Statement: The authors have nothing to disclose.
Department of Genetics, University of Georgia, 500 DW Brooks Drive, Coverdell Building Suite 270, Athens, GA 30602, USA
* Corresponding author.
E-mail address: nmanley@uga.edu

and secreted. For hyperparathyroidism, the current treatment option is to surgically remove the affected parathyroid, and the patient is cured following this procedure. Hypoparathyroidism is observed much less frequently in the clinic and has a number of causes, including mutations in genes required for proper parathyroid development.[4] There is currently no permanent cure for hypoparathyroidism, and patients are managed by daily use of activated forms of vitamin D, calcium supplements, and/or recombinant PTH to help regulate their calcium levels (please see Muriel Babey and colleagues' article, "Conventional Treatment of Hypoparathyroidism," and Gaia Tabacco and John P. Bilezikian's article "New Directions in Treatment of Hypoparathyroidism," in this issue.)

Understanding the normal process of parathyroid development can provide important information about how and why parathyroid disorders manifest. Much of the research in this area has been done in mice. Embryonic development of the parathyroid is a topic that has been studied since the 1930s, and the findings up to the present will be summarized in this review.

MAJOR EVENTS DURING PARATHYROID ORGANOGENESIS AND MORPHOGENESIS IN MICE

Beginning at approximately embryonic day 9 (E9.0) in mouse development, bilateral endodermal outpocketings called pharyngeal pouches form on the lateral aspects of the pharynx. These pouches are epithelial structures surrounded by neural-crest–derived mesenchymal cells (NCC). Both pharyngeal endoderm and NCC provide signals that play an important role in initial pouch patterning. In mice, the parathyroid glands develop in the third pharyngeal pouches, yielding 1 set of bilateral parathyroid glands.[5] Humans have 2 pairs of parathyroid glands, developing from both the third and fourth pouches.[6–8] In mice, the anterior-dorsal region of each third pharyngeal pouch forms a parathyroid gland, whereas the posterior-ventral region develops into 1 lobe of the thymus, the organ responsible for T-cell development.[9] Early parathyroid organogenesis initiates by specifying parathyroid and thymus cell fates, and by E11.5, essentially all cells in the developing primordium have assumed either glial cells missing (GCM)2+ parathyroid or FOXN1+ thymus fates (**Fig. 1**). This stage is followed

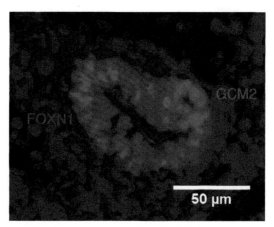

Fig. 1. Third pharyngeal pouch–derived primordium from an E11.5 mouse embryo. Dorsal parathyroid-fated cells marked with anti-GCM2 antibody shown in magenta; ventral thymus-fated cells marked with anti-FOXN1 antibody shown in purple.

by separation of the combined parathyroid-thymus primordia from the pharynx, which occurs by coordinated apoptosis[10] and is regulated in part by fibroblast growth factor[11] and bone morphogenetic protein 4 (BMP4)[12] signaling, and possibly other signals from the neighboring mesenchyme.

Once separated from the pharynx, the combined parathyroid-thymus primordia begin to migrate ventrally and posteriorly, mediated by Ephrin signaling between NCC and thymic epithelium.[13] During this migration at approximately E12.5, the parathyroid and thymus primordia begin to separate from each other. Unlike the separation from the pharynx, this separation event does not involve apoptosis, but rather occurs via a combination of differential cell adhesion mediated by higher levels of E-cadherin expression on thymus cells compared with parathyroid cells.[12] BMP4 signaling in particular modulates formation of a "wedge" of mesenchyme expressing F-actin filaments,[14] implying that physical forces are also involved in this separation event. Separation is complete between E12 and E13, during the migration period. After separation is complete, the thymic lobes continue in their migration to the anterior mediastinum above the heart, while the parathyroids do not continue to migrate. Variability in the timing of this separation leads to a somewhat variable location of the parathyroids in the neck region, usually lateral to the thyroid lateral lobes.[15]

The physical separation of the thymus and parathyroids, coupled with the low expression of homotypic adhesion molecules on parathyroid cells, leads to the generation of a "trail" of small clusters of parathyroid cells between the 2 organs along the migratory path of the thymus.[8] These small clusters of cells can either maintain their parathyroid differentiation state or, at a low frequency, can downregulate the parathyroid gene expression program and undergo spontaneous transdifferentiation to a thymic epithelial cell fate, resulting in parathyroid-derived cervical thymi.[16] The data from mice suggest that fetal parathyroid cell fate is unstable, but is stabilized postnatally,[16] although the mechanism behind this instability and subsequent fate switch is unclear.

The common embryonic origin and process of thymus-parathyroid separation has also led to the idea that the thymus itself makes physiologically relevant levels of PTH.[17] PTH was first detected in the thymus in the original analysis of *Gcm2* null mutants, which lack parathyroid glands. However, subsequent investigation revealed that thymus PTH originated from 2 sources: (1) parathyroid cells that were "trapped" underneath the thymic capsule during the separation of the parathyroid and thymus during embryonic development, and (2) medullary thymic epithelial cells that express PTH as a self-antigen and do not have any endocrine function.[8] Therefore, the sole source of endocrine-active PTH is the parathyroid.

GCM2: THE KEY REGULATOR OF PARATHYROID DEVELOPMENT

GCM was first discovered in *Drosophila* as a transcription factor that acts as a binary switch for neural cells to become either neurons or glial cells.[18,19] Characterization of the mammalian homologs of *Drosophila* GCM called *Gcm1* and *Gcm2* revealed high expression of *Gcm2* in parathyroid glands in developing mice, suggesting a non-neuronal function for this transcription factor.[20] *Gcm2* is expressed at very low levels in the dorsal second and third pharyngeal pouches at E9.5, and by E10.5 its expression is upregulated in and restricted to approximately the dorsal-anterior third of the third pouch endoderm.[9] *Gcm2* null mice fail to develop parathyroid glands, leading to primary hypoparathyroidism.[17] In humans, *GCM2* mutations are associated with hypoparathyroidism and hyperparathyroidism (OMIM 603716). In mice, *Gcm2* is required for both parathyroid cell differentiation and survival. In *Gcm2* null mice, and in *Hoxa3* mutants in which *Gcm2* fails to be upregulated, the parathyroid domain is specified, but these cells undergo rapid and coordinated programmed cell death.[21] The *Pth* gene is a direct target of GCM2, and its expression is never activated in parathyroid-fated cells in *Gcm2* null mice.

PATTERNING IN THE THIRD PHARYNGEAL POUCH AND INITIATION OF GCM2 EXPRESSION

Initial patterning of the third pharyngeal pouch at E9.5 determines the cell fate of the endodermal cells within it, with cells being fated to either parathyroid or thymus lineages. Parathyroid development occurs at the dorsal end marked by *Gcm2* and thymus development at the ventral end marked by *Foxn1*. These domains are specified and subsequent differentiation determined by a network of signaling pathways and transcription factors (**Fig. 2**). One of the earliest genes that affects third pharyngeal pouch patterning encodes the signaling molecule Sonic Hedgehog (SHH), which is expressed throughout the pharyngeal endoderm but is excluded from the third pharyngeal pouch[22,23] In *Shh* null mutants, the parathyroid domain is not specified and Gcm2 is never activated.[22,24] SHH signaling occurs in both the dorsal endoderm and the adjacent NCC mesenchyme, and recent evidence using tissue-specific deletion or activation of SHH signaling showed that signaling from either location is sufficient to specify parathyroid fate and activate *Gcm2* expression.[25] In addition to its role in initiating parathyroid differentiation, SHH has been shown to prevent parathyroid-specific genes such as *Gcm2* from being activated in other pharyngeal pouches,[23] suggesting that its role in *Gcm2* expression could be dosage-sensitive.

SHH signaling may act in part through activation of the T-box transcription factor TBX1 in the parathyroid domain. *Tbx1* is expressed throughout the pharyngeal pouches at their earliest stages of development, and is required for pouch outgrowth[26,27]; however, in the third pharyngeal pouch, *Tbx1* is downregulated in the ventral pouch during outgrowth, resulting in its restriction to the parathyroid

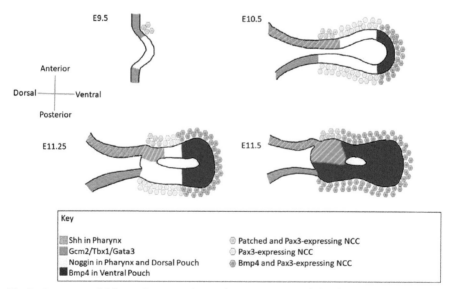

Key

▨ Shh in Pharynx	◉ Patched and Pax3-expressing NCC
▨ Gcm2/Tbx1/Gata3	◯ Pax3-expressing NCC
Noggin in Pharynx and Dorsal Pouch	◍ Bmp4 and Pax3-expressing NCC
■ Bmp4 in Ventral Pouch	

Fig. 2. Current model for early patterning and organogenesis of the third pharyngeal pouch in mice.

domain.[28] This restriction may be necessary for specification of thymus fate, as ectopic *Tbx1* is sufficient to block thymic epithelial cell differentiation.[29] However, neither ectopic SHH signaling nor ectopic TBX1 is sufficient to expand *Gcm2* expression into the ventral region,[25,29] indicating that either additional positive regulators are present in the dorsal domain, or that negative regulators are present in the ventral domain that block parathyroid fate and/or *Gcm2* expression.

Another transcription factor that is required for *Gcm2* activation is the transcription factor GATA3. In *Gata3* null mice, *Gcm2* is never activated, and *Gata3* heterozygotes have fewer *Gcm2*-expressing cells during embryonic development and have hypoparathyroidism.[30] This regulation is via *GATA3* binding sites in the *Gcm2* promoter. Furthermore, human mutations in *GATA3* cause hypoparathyroidism, indicating that this aspect of *Gcm2* regulation is conserved in humans and mice.[31] As SHH signaling induces *Gata3* expression in the brain in mice,[32] it is possible that *Gata3* is also acting downstream of SHH signaling during early parathyroid development, although this possibility has not been experimentally tested.

From E10.5 to E11.5, the signaling molecule BMP4 is expressed in both NCC and endoderm at the ventral end of the third pharyngeal pouch where the thymus will develop,[22,33] and multiple lines of evidence suggest that BMP signaling is a positive regulator of thymus differentiation.[12,24,34–36] As opposing gradients of SHH and BMP4 signaling are antagonistic during neural tube patterning, a similar model has been proposed to operate during third pharyngeal pouch patterning.[12,22,25] This model was supported by expansion of *Bmp4* expression into the pharynx in *Shh* null mutants,[22] and by the expression of the BMP inhibitor NOGGIN in the dorsal domain during pouch patterning and early organogenesis.[33] However, little functional evidence has supported the possibility that BMP4 signaling suppresses parathyroid fate or *Gcm2* expression.

GCM2 IS UPREGULATED BY HOXA3 AND INTERACTING TRANSCRIPTION FACTORS

Gcm2 is initially expressed at a low level at the dorsal end of the E9.5 third pharyngeal pouch, but by E10.5 is upregulated dramatically. Failure to upregulate *Gcm2* leads to coordinated apoptosis in the parathyroid-fated cells, emphasizing the importance of *Gcm2* upregulation in parathyroid cells. *Hoxa3* was the first *Hox* gene to be knocked out in mice via homologous recombination, and has been shown to play a role in the development of multiple pharyngeal organs, and is required for both parathyroid and thymus organogenesis.[15,37,38] Although there is overlapping function between the group 3 HOX paralogs, only *Hoxa3* has a specific role in the development of the parathyroid and thymus.[15] The formation of the third pharyngeal pouch is normal in *Hoxa3* null mice; however, by E12, the parathyroids are absent, and the thymus rudiments are severely hypoplastic. By E12.5 in *Hoxa3* mutants, all of the third pharyngeal pouch derivatives have disappeared due to coordinated apoptosis.[38–40]

Detailed analysis of global and tissue-specific null alleles for *Hoxa3* showed that *Hoxa3* is not required to specify the parathyroid domain or for initial *Gcm2* expression. In *Hoxa3* null mice, *Gcm2* expression is initiated, but fails to be upregulated at E10.5, and by E11.5 *Gcm2* expression is undetectable.[40,41] Analysis of inefficient *Hoxa3* deletion in endoderm via tamoxifen-inducible Cre recombinase showed that HOXA3 upregulation of *Gcm2* expression at E10.5 is cell-autonomous,[40,42] although it remains to be shown that *Gcm2* is a direct HOXA3 target.

HOXA3 has been shown to work in concert with a network of PAX, EYA, and SIX family transcriptional regulators to regulate many of its downstream functions, including thymus and parathyroid organogenesis.[43] *Pax1* null mutants show decreased *Gcm2* expression at E11.5 and parathyroid hypoplasia.[44] *Pax1* expression is reduced in the third pharyngeal pouch in *Hoxa3* null mutants,[38] and *Gcm2* expression is further reduced or absent by E11.5 in *HoxA3$^{+/-}$Pax1$^{-/-}$* compound mutants,[44] suggesting that *Pax1* may be downstream of *Hoxa3*. *Pax1* expression is also dependent on the expression of *Eya1* and *Six1* in the third pharyngeal pouch. In *Six1* null mutants, *Gcm2* is initiated but cannot be maintained,[45] and the cells subsequently undergo apoptosis consistent with loss of *Gcm2* expression. These results suggest that a HOX-PAX-EYA-SIX network interacts to upregulate *Gcm2* expression.

HOXA3 may also interact with PBX1, a TALE-class transcription factor. *Pbx1* null mutants have parathyroid and thymic hypoplasia, and reduced *Gcm2* expression.[28] As HOX and PBX proteins are known to act together to regulate multiple developmental processes, these data suggest that PBX1 is also a member of the transcriptional network regulating early *Gcm2* expression.[43,46]

DIFFERENTIATION OF PARATHYROID CELLS

After upregulation of *Gcm2*, downstream parathyroid genes are activated. including those encoding PTH and CaSR. In addition, the chemokine ligand 21 (CCL21) is expressed in the early parathyroid domain at E11.5, and plays a role in initial attraction of lymphoid progenitors to the thymus domain, although this expression is transient and does not have a known role in parathyroid biology.[47] The initiation of *Casr* and *Ccl21* expression in the parathyroid domain is *Gcm2*-independent, but maintenance of their expression is *Gcm2*-dependent.[21] In contrast, *Pth* expression is initiated later, at E12, and is dependent on *GCM2* for both initiation and maintenance.[21]

The transcriptional activator MAFB was also found to be important for the activation of PTH.[48] *MafB* is expressed in the parathyroid after E11.5 and its expression is *Gcm2*-dependent. In *MafB* null mutants, PTH expression and secretion are greatly reduced. MAFB was shown to physically associate with GCM2 to interact with the *Pth* promoter via a MAF-recognition element and a GCM2 binding site to turn on its expression.[48] GATA3 also physically interacts with MAFB and GCM2 together with the ubiquitous transcription factor, SP1, to activate *Pth* expression.[49]

PARATHYROID DEVELOPMENT IN HUMANS

Current evidence suggests that parathyroid development in humans occurs in a similar manner as in mice. In humans, the parathyroid glands develop in tandem with the thymus in the third pharyngeal pouch and with the ultimobranchial bodies in the fourth pharyngeal pouch, yielding 2 sets of bilateral parathyroid glands.[6,7,50,51] This was further strengthened when expression of the parathyroid marker, *GCM2*, was shown in both the third and fourth pharyngeal pouches in human embryos.[8] This study also showed the presence of "trailing" *GCM2*-positive parathyroid cells, similar to those seen during mouse parathyroid organogenesis; these small clusters of parathyroid cells were proposed to be the source of many parathyroid adenomas in humans.[8] Several genes known to be important in mouse parathyroid development have also been shown to be associated with human parathyroid disease. Loss-of-function mutations in *GCMB*, *GATA3*, and *TBX1* have all been shown to cause hypoparathyroidism in humans,[4] consistent with data from mouse studies.

SUMMARY

The field of parathyroid organogenesis is small, and there is still much to be discovered. The framework of the regulatory network controlling the establishment of parathyroid cell fate, and the central role of GCM2/GCMB in parathyroid survival and differentiation are now established. For the genes that have already been identified as playing a role in parathyroid development, the precise pathways and mechanisms of action need to be elucidated. For example, TBX1 has been implicated in the regulation of *Gcm2* expression, but further evidence is required to confirm this hypothesis. The interaction between HOXA3, PAX1, and PBX1 also needs to be clarified in terms of their role in *Gcm2* upregulation.

It will be important to identify all of the transcription factors and signaling pathways that play a role in parathyroid cell differentiation during embryonic development. With –omics techniques, researchers will be able identify all of the genes that are being expressed, which genes are in areas of open chromatin, and thus the structure of the network controlling parathyroid organogenesis. Elucidation of the transcriptional network controlling parathyroid differentiation could enable the generation of parathyroid cells from pluripotent cells in culture. The lack of an in vitro system for studying parathyroid cells remains a challenge. The only cell lines available are from human adenomas, likely because of the tight proliferation control in parathyroid cells. The question of parathyroid cell fate stability still needs to be addressed, as parathyroid cell fate has been shown to be unstable, with some parathyroid cells switching to a thymus cell fate.[16] The mechanism of this fate switch will need to be elucidated in order for cell therapy to become a viable treatment option. Solving these problems in basic parathyroid biology could lead to the development of new in vitro systems, which would have both research and therapeutic benefits.

REFERENCES

1. Ramasamy I. Recent advances in physiological calcium homeostasis. Clin Chem Lab Med 2006;44(3):237–73.
2. Chen RA, Goodman WG. Role of the calcium-sensing receptor in parathyroid gland physiology. Am J Physiol Ren Physiol 2004;286(6):F1005–11.
3. Houillier P, Nicolet-Barousse L, Maruani G, et al. What keeps serum calcium levels stable? Joint Bone Spine 2003;70(6):407–13.
4. Grigorieva IV, Thakker RV. Transcription factors in parathyroid development: lessons from hypoparathyroid disorders. Ann N Y Acad Sci 2011;1237:24–38.
5. Cordier A, Haumont S. Development of thymus, parathyroids, and ultimobranchial bodies in NMRI and nude mice. Am J Anat 1980;157:227–63.
6. Gilmour J. The embryology of the parathyroid glands, the thymus, and certain associated rudiments. J Pathol 1937;45:507–22.
7. Weller G. Development of the thyroid, parathyroid and thymus glands in man. Contrib Embryol 1933;24:93–142.
8. Liu Z, Farley A, Chen L, et al. Thymus-associated parathyroid hormone has two cellular origins with distinct endocrine and immunological functions. PLoS Genet 2010;6(12):e1001251.
9. Gordon J, Bennett AR, Blackburn CC, et al. Gcm2 and Foxn1 mark early parathyroid- and thymus-specific domains in the developing third pharyngeal pouch. Mech Dev 2001;103(1–2):141–3.
10. Gordon J, Wilson VA, Blair NF, et al. Functional evidence for a single endodermal origin for the thymic epithelium. Nat Immunol 2004;5(5):546–53.
11. Gardiner JR, Jackson AL, Gordon J, et al. Localised inhibition of FGF signalling in the third pharyngeal pouch is required for normal thymus and parathyroid organogenesis. Development 2012;139(18):3456–66.

12. Gordon J, Patel SR, Mishina Y, et al. Evidence for an early role for BMP4 signaling in thymus and parathyroid morphogenesis. Dev Biol 2010;339(1):141–54.

13. Foster KE, Gordon J, Cardenas K, et al. EphB-ephrin-B2 interactions are required for thymus migration during organogenesis. Proc Natl Acad Sci U S A 2010; 107(30):13414–9.

14. Gordon J, Manley NR. Mechanisms of thymus organogenesis and morphogenesis. Development 2011;138(18):3865–78.

15. Manley NR, Capecchi MR. Hox group 3 paralogs regulate the development and migration of the thymus, thyroid, and parathyroid glands. Dev Biol 1998; 195(1):1–15.

16. Li J, Liu Z, Xiao S, et al. Transdifferentiation of parathyroid cells into cervical thymi promotes atypical T-cell development. Nat Commun 2013;4:2959.

17. Gunther T, Chen ZF, Kim J, et al. Genetic ablation of parathyroid glands reveals another source of parathyroid hormone. Nature 2000;406(6792):199–203.

18. Hosoya T, Takizawa K, Nitta K, et al. Glial cells missing: a binary switch between neuronal and glial determination in *Drosophila*. Cell 1995;82(6): 1025–36.

19. Jones BW, Fetter RD, Tear G, et al. Glial cells missing: a genetic switch that controls glial versus neuronal fate. Cell 1995;82(6):1013–23.

20. Kim J, Jones BW, Zock C, et al. Isolation and characterization of mammalian homologs of the *Drosophila* gene glial cells missing. Proc Natl Acad Sci U S A 1998; 95(21):12364–9.

21. Liu Z, Yu S, Manley NR. Gcm2 is required for the differentiation and survival of parathyroid precursor cells in the parathyroid/thymus primordia. Dev Biol 2007; 305(1):333–46.

22. Moore-Scott BA, Manley NR. Differential expression of Sonic hedgehog along the anterior-posterior axis regulates patterning of pharyngeal pouch endoderm and pharyngeal endoderm-derived organs. Dev Biol 2005;278(2): 323–35.

23. Grevellec A, Graham A, Tucker AS. Shh signalling restricts the expression of Gcm2 and controls the position of the developing parathyroids. Developmental Biol 2011;353(2):194–205.

24. Figueiredo M, Silva JC, Santos AS, et al. Notch and Hedgehog in the thymus/ parathyroid common primordium: crosstalk in organ formation. Dev Biol 2016; 418(2):268–82.

25. Bain VE, Gordon J, O'Neil JD, et al. Tissue-specific roles for sonic hedgehog signaling in establishing thymus and parathyroid organ fate. Development 2016;143(21):4027–37.

26. Jerome LA, Papaioannou VE. DiGeorge syndrome phenotype in mice mutant for the T-box gene, Tbx1. Nat Genet 2001;27(3):286–91.

27. Xu H, Cerrato F, Baldini A. Timed mutation and cell-fate mapping reveal reiterated roles of Tbx1 during embryogenesis, and a crucial function during segmentation of the pharyngeal system via regulation of endoderm expansion. Development 2005;132(19):4387–95.

28. Manley NR, Selleri L, Brendolan A, et al. Abnormalities of caudal pharyngeal pouch development in Pbx1 knockout mice mimic loss of Hox3 paralogs. Dev Biol 2004;276(2):301–12.

29. Reeh KA, Cardenas KT, Bain VE, et al. Ectopic TBX1 suppresses thymic epithelial cell differentiation and proliferation during thymus organogenesis. Development 2014;141(15):2950–8.

30. Grigorieva IV, Mirczuk S, Gaynor KU, et al. Gata3-deficient mice develop parathyroid abnormalities due to dysregulation of the parathyroid-specific transcription factor Gcm2. J Clin Invest 2010;120(6):2144–55.
31. Van Esch H, Groenen P, Nesbit MA, et al. GATA3 haplo-insufficiency causes human HDR syndrome. Nature 2000;406(6794):419–22.
32. Liu J, Wang X, Li J, et al. Reconstruction of the gene regulatory network involved in the sonic hedgehog pathway with a potential role in early development of the mouse brain. PLoS Comput Biol 2014;10(10):e1003884.
33. Patel SR, Gordon J, Mahbub F, et al. Bmp4 and Noggin expression during early thymus and parathyroid organogenesis. Gene Expr Patterns 2006;6(8):794–9.
34. Bleul CC, Boehm T. BMP signaling is required for normal thymus development. J Immunol 2005;175(8):5213–21.
35. Tsai PT, Lee RA, Wu H. BMP4 acts upstream of FGF in modulating thymic stroma and regulating thymopoiesis. Blood 2003;102(12):3947–53.
36. Neves H, Dupin E, Parreira L, et al. Modulation of Bmp4 signalling in the epithelial-mesenchymal interactions that take place in early thymus and parathyroid development in avian embryos. Developmental Biol 2012;361(2):208–19.
37. Chisaka O, Capecchi MR. Regionally restricted developmental defects resulting from targeted disruption of the mouse homeobox gene hox-1.5. Nature 1991;350(6318):473–9.
38. Manley NR, Capecchi MR. The role of Hoxa-3 in mouse thymus and thyroid development. Development 1995;121(7):1989–2003.
39. Kameda Y, Arai Y, Nishimaki T, et al. The role of Hoxa3 gene in parathyroid gland organogenesis of the mouse. J Histochem Cytochem 2004;52(5):641–51.
40. Chojnowski JL, Masuda K, Trau HA, et al. Multiple roles for HOXA3 in regulating thymus and parathyroid differentiation and morphogenesis in mouse. Development 2014;141(19):3697–708.
41. Chen L, Zhao P, Wells L, et al. Mouse and zebrafish Hoxa3 orthologues have nonequivalent in vivo protein function. Proc Natl Acad Sci U S A 2010;107(23):10555–60.
42. Chojnowski JL, Trau HA, Masuda K, et al. Temporal and spatial requirements for Hoxa3 in mouse embryonic development. Dev Biol 2016;415(1):33–45.
43. Manley NR, Condie BG. Transcriptional regulation of thymus organogenesis and thymic epithelial cell differentiation. Prog Mol Biol Transl Sci 2010;92:103–20.
44. Su D, Ellis S, Napier A, et al. Hoxa3 and pax1 regulate epithelial cell death and proliferation during thymus and parathyroid organogenesis. Dev Biol 2001;236(2):316–29.
45. Zou D, Silvius D, Davenport J, et al. Patterning of the third pharyngeal pouch into thymus/parathyroid by Six and Eya1. Dev Biol 2006;293(2):499–512.
46. Moens CB, Selleri L. Hox cofactors in vertebrate development. Developmental Biol 2006;291(2):193–206.
47. Liu C, Saito F, Liu Z, et al. Coordination between CCR7- and CCR9-mediated chemokine signals in prevascular fetal thymus colonization. Blood 2006;108(8):2531–9.
48. Kamitani-Kawamoto A, Hamada M, Moriguchi T, et al. MafB interacts with Gcm2 and regulates parathyroid hormone expression and parathyroid development. J Bone Miner Res 2011;26(10):2463–72.
49. Han SI, Tsunekage Y, Kataoka K. Gata3 cooperates with Gcm2 and MafB to activate parathyroid hormone gene expression by interacting with SP1. Mol Cell Endocrinol 2015;411:113–20.

50. Phitayakorn R, McHenry CR. Incidence and location of ectopic abnormal parathyroid glands. Am J Surg 2006;191(3):418–23.
51. Norris E. The morphogenesis and histogenesis of the thymus gland in man: in which the origin of the Hassall's corpuscles of the human thymus is discovered. Contrib Embryol 1938;27:193.

Physiology of Parathyroid Hormone

David Goltzman, MD[a,b,]*

KEYWORDS

- Parathyroid hormone • Calcium • Phosphate • Bone turnover • Anabolic actions
- Catabolic actions

KEY POINTS

- Parathyroid hormone (PTH) is essential in the regulation of extracellular calcium and phosphate metabolism.
- PTH enhances calcium reabsorption and inhibits phosphate reabsorption in the renal tubule.
- PTH augments the renal synthesis of 1,25-dihydroxyvitamin D, which then increases intestinal calcium absorption.
- PTH can increase bone remodeling to exert a catabolic effect on cortical and to some extent trabecular bone.
- PTH can have an anabolic effect on bone mainly in trabecular bone but to some extent in cortical bone.

SYNTHESIS, SECRETION, AND METABOLISM OF PARATHYROID HORMONE

Parathyroid hormone (PTH) is the major secretory product of the chief cells of the parathyroid glands, and the human gene encoding PTH is located on chromosome 11.[1] The translation product, preproPTH, is a 115-amino acid precursor peptide, that is extended at the amino (NH_2)-terminus by a leader (signal) or "pre" sequence that facilitates its entry into the secretory apparatus of the cell, and by a short prohormone sequence. Both the leader sequence and pro sequence are cleaved within the cell, generating a straight chain peptide containing 84 amino acids, PTH(1–84), which is the major glandular form and major bioactive secreted and circulating form of the hormone. Extracellular fluid (ECF) ionized calcium, Ca^{++}, appears to be the predominant regulator of the production of PTH (**Fig. 1**). Thus, Ca^{++} binding to the calcium

Disclosure Statement: The author has nothing to disclose.
[a] Department of Medicine and Research Institute of the McGill University Health Centre, 1001 Decarie Boulevard, Montreal, Quebec H4A 3J1, Canada; [b] Departments of Medicine and of Physiology, McGill University, 845 Sherbrooke St West, Montreal, Quebec H3A 0B9, Canada
* Research Institute of the McGill University Health Centre—Glen Site, 1001 Decarie Boulevard, Room EM1.3220, Montreal, Quebec H4A 3J1, Canada.
E-mail address: david.goltzman@mcgill.ca

Endocrinol Metab Clin N Am 47 (2018) 743–758
https://doi.org/10.1016/j.ecl.2018.07.003
0889-8529/18/© 2018 Elsevier Inc. All rights reserved.

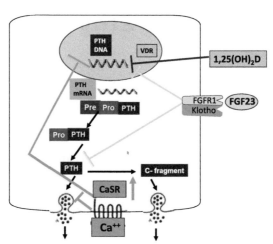

Fig. 1. Action of calcium, 1,25(OH)$_2$D and FGF23 on PTH production in the parathyroid cell. When elevated calcium (Ca^{++}) binds to the CaSR, it can inhibit PTH secretion from the parathyroid cell, and PTH gene expression. High Ca^{++} can also enhance PTH degradation to C-terminal fragments. When Ca^{++} is reduced PTH gene expression is increased, PreproPTH is synthesized. PreproPTH is converted to ProPTH and then to PTH, and PTH is secreted. 1,25(OH)$_2$D can bind to the vitamin D receptor (VDR) and also inhibit *PTH* gene expression. FGF23 can bind to the FGF receptor (FGFR1) and then to Klotho, also leading to decreased PTH synthesis, but also secretion.

sensing receptor (CaSR) results in signaling in the parathyroid gland, which inhibits PTH secretion. This inhibition occurs in a curvilinear fashion, characterized by a steep inverse sigmoidal curve. Half-maximal inhibition of PTH secretion, termed the setpoint, may occur at a Ca^{++} concentration of approximately 1 mmol/L. In human parathyroid tissue in vitro, maximal Ca^{++}-induced inhibition of PTH secretion, with continued nonsuppressible PTH secretion, generally occurs at concentrations of Ca^{++} approximately 2 mmol/L or higher and maximal secretion of PTH generally occurs at Ca^{++} concentrations of approximately 0.5 mmol/L or lower. However, the actual Ca^{++} concentrations regulating these parameters of secretion vary dependent on both physiologic and pathologic circumstances.[2] The rate at which Ca^{++} falls may also determine the magnitude of the secretory response, with a rapid fall in ECF Ca^{++} stimulating a more robust response.

Increased Ca^{++} concentrations may also increase degradation of bioactive PTH within the parathyroid cell, and lead to release of biologically inactive carboxyl (COOH)-terminal fragments,[3–5] most being PTH(34–84) and PTH(37–84).[6,7] Biologically inactive PTH fragments, which can also be generated in the liver, are cleared by the kidney.[8] Although the plasma half-life of intact PTH(1–84) is only a few minutes, renal clearance of PTH fragments is slower. Therefore, under normocalcemic conditions, up to 80% of circulating PTH is inactive fragments, whereas only approximately 20% is intact, biologically active PTH(1–84).[9]

Increased Ca^{++} may also inhibit *PTH* gene transcription and stability, although this regulatory mechanism is considerably slower than others,[9–11] and reduced Ca^{++} concentrations have also been shown to increase parathyroid cell proliferation.[12] Thus, sustained hypocalcemia can eventually lead to an increase in the total secretory capacity of the parathyroid gland. In contrast, although sustained hypercalcemia can reduce parathyroid gland size, hypercalcemia appears less effective in diminishing the number of parathyroid chief cells, once a prolonged stimulus to hyperplasia has occurred.

The active form of vitamin D, 1,25 dihydroxyvitamin D (calcitriol/1,25[OH]$_2$D) inhibits *PTH* gene transcription,[13] and also inhibits parathyroid cell proliferation in part at least by its regulation of the myc gene complex.[12,14] Modulation of *PTH* gene transcription by both Ca^{++} and 1,25(OH)$_2$D may involve the parathyroid transcription factor, GCMB (GCM2).[12] CaSR gene transcription may also be upregulated by 1,25(OH)$_2$D. Consequently Ca^{++} and 1,25(OH)$_2$D appear to act in concert to regulate parathyroid cell growth and function.

Additional modulators of PTH secretion have been reported, including cations, such as lithium,[15] transforming growth factor alpha (TGFα),[16] prostaglandins,[17] and inorganic phosphate (Pi) per se.[18] Recently evidence has been presented for a regulatory role for the phosphaturic factor, fibroblast growth factor 23 (FGF23), which appears to decrease both PTH messenger RNA (mRNA) expression and PTH secretion.[19]

MECHANISMS OF PARATHYROID HORMONE ACTION

Although the major circulating bioactive form of PTH is an 84 amino acid peptide, virtually all of the biological activity resides within its amino (NH$_2$)-terminal domain such that a synthetic peptide composed of the NH$_2$-terminal 34 residues (PTH[1–34]) appears to recapitulate all of the biologic activity of the entire molecule.[20,21] The NH$_2$–terminal domain in target tissue interacts with a classic G-protein–coupled receptor (GPCR) of the B family (class II) termed the PTH/PTHrP receptor type 1, or PTH1R.[22,23] This receptor also transduces signaling of a genetic relative of PTH termed PTH-related protein (PTHrP), which exhibits considerable homology to PTH in its NH$_2$–terminal region. PTH1R is highly expressed in bone and kidney, in which the major physiologic ligand appears to be circulating PTH, but is also expressed in many other tissues, where the endogenous ligand is likely to be PTHrP acting in a paracrine/autocrine manner. The NH$_2$-terminal domain of PTH interacts with both the extracellular domain of the receptor and with juxtamembrane regions.[24] Binding of the receptor by PTH induces conformational change in the receptor, which promotes coupling with heterotrimeric G proteins (Gαβγ), and catalyzes the exchange of guanosine diphosphate (GDP) for guanosine triphosphate (GTP) on the α-subunit of the G proteins. This exchange triggers conformational and/or dissociation events between the α and βγ subunits. PTH1R couples to several G protein subclasses, including Gs, Gq/11, and G12/13, resulting in the activation of many pathways, although the best studied are the adenylate cyclase and phospholipase C pathways. Thus, Gαs, of Gs, activates adenylate cyclase (AC), resulting in cyclic AMP (cAMP) synthesis; cAMP then activates protein kinase A (PKA). Gαq, of Gq, activates phospholipase C (PLC), which cleaves phosphatidylinositol (4,5)-bisphosphate (PIP2) into diacylglycerol (DAG) and inositol (1,4,5)-trisphosphate (IP3). IP3 then diffuses through the cytoplasm and activates IP3-gated Ca^{++} channels in the membranes of the endoplasmic reticulum, causing the release of stored Ca^{++} into the cytoplasm. This increase of cytosolic Ca^{++} promotes protein kinase C (PKC) translocation to the plasma membrane and with subsequent activation by DAG.[25] Gα12/Gα13 activates phospholipase D.[26,27]

PTH binding to PTH1R is also followed by phosphorylation of serines on the COOH-terminal intracellular tail of PTH1R by G protein–coupled receptor kinases (GRKs), a process that initiates desensitization–internalization of the receptor.[28] Thus, binding of β-arrestins to these phosphorylated sites uncouples receptors from heterotrimeric G proteins and terminates PTH-mediated G protein signaling. The

PTH–receptor complex is internalized first into clathrin-coated pits to which β-arrestin binds and then into early endocytic vesicles. At least some of the internalized receptor can undergo rapid recycling back to the cell surface. β-arrestins may also serve as multifunctional scaffolding proteins linking PTH1R to signaling molecules independent of the classic G protein–coupled second messenger-dependent pathways.[28,29] Thus β-arrestins also serve as adaptors that assemble intracellular complexes between internalized PTH1R and signaling proteins to activate MAPK pathways, among others. Alternatively AC and Gs may be internalized with the PTH/PTH1R/β-arrestin complex. Within early endosomes, functional interactions between PTH1R, Gs, and AC may then allow sustained cAMP production within the cell.

PTH1R may also interact with other cytoplasmic adaptor proteins, such as the Na/H exchanger regulatory protein factors (NHERFs), which bind to the intracellular tail of PTH1R.[30] NHERF1 inhibits β-arrestin binding to PTH1R. NHERF1 may therefore protect against PTH resistance or PTH1R downregulation. NHERFs also modulate the PTH1R coupling to different G proteins. PTH1R signaling to PLC is increased in cells expressing NHERF1. Association with NHERF1 allows PTH1R to stimulate Gq and thereby PLC without compromising its ability to stimulate Gs and AC.[31] NHERF2 promotes coupling of PTH1R to Gq and Gi, while compromising its interaction with Gs.[32] NHERF2 can thereby switch PTH1R from activating AC to activating PLC. Different patterns of expression of NHERFs among cells that express PTH1R are likely to contribute to the diversity of signaling pathways activated by PTH. Thus, in some cells, stimulation of PTH1R activates AC without activating PLC[33]; in others, it activates PLC and not AC, whereas in other cell types, notably osteoblasts and kidney tubules, stimulation of PTH1R activates both pathways. Even within the same renal proximal tubule cell, PTH may activate PLC from the apical surface and AC from the basolateral surface.[34]

Different PTH analogs stabilize different active conformations of PTH1R that may then interact selectively with either different G proteins or β-arrestins. Therefore, the intensity of the PTH stimulus, stimulus trafficking, and association with scaffold proteins may all contribute to determining the interactions of PTH1R with intracellular signaling proteins.

CONTRIBUTIONS OF PARATHYROID HORMONE TO PLASMA CALCIUM AND PHOSPHATE HOMEOSTASIS

PTH plays a central role in regulating extracellular fluid Ca^{++} and phosphate (Pi) homoeostasis. Thus, when a reduction in ECF Ca^{++} (potentially caused by an increase in ECF Pi) stimulates release of PTH from the parathyroid glands, this hormone can then act to enhance Ca^{++} reabsorption in the kidney, while at the same time inhibiting Pi reabsorption and producing phosphaturia. In the kidney, PTH (and hypocalcemia) can also stimulate the conversion of inactive 25-hydroxyvitamin D (25[OH]D), to the active metabolite $1,25(OH)_2D$ by transcriptional activation of the gene coding for the 25-hydroxyvitamin D-1α hydroxylase (CYP27B1) enzyme, apparently by the AC/PKA pathway.[35] $1,25(OH)_2D$ can then exert endocrine activities to increase intestinal absorption of Ca^{++} and to a lesser extent Pi. PTH can also increase bone turnover, leading to enhanced bone resorption and release of both Ca^{++} and Pi from the skeleton. The PTH-mediated renal effects to maintain Ca^{++} homeostasis appear more rapid than the skeletal effects. The net effect of the increased stimulation of PTH release in response to hypocalcemia, therefore, is to increase reabsorption of renal Ca^{++} (a direct effect), to mobilize Ca^{++} from bone (a direct effect) and to increase absorption of Ca^{++} from the gut (an indirect effect) restoring ECF Ca^{++} to normal and thereby inhibiting further production of PTH and $1,25(OH)_2D$.

PARATHYROID HORMONE ACTIONS IN KIDNEY IN REGULATING ION TRANSPORT

PTH promotes the absorption of calcium and magnesium, while inhibiting absorption of phosphate and bicarbonate.

Effects on Phosphate

A prominent action of PTH in the kidney is the inhibition of Pi reabsorption. Renal Pi transport is essentially restricted to proximal tubules, where 2 sodium-dependent cotransporters, NaPi-IIa (NPT2a, SLC34A1) and NaPi-IIc (NPT2c SLC34A3), are exclusively expressed in the brush border membrane[36] and mediate uptake of Pi from luminal fluid. Proximal tubules express the PTH1R at both apical and basolateral membranes[37,38] and PTH activation of apical PTH1R leads to PLC-PKC stimulation mediated by NHERF,[39] whereas activation of basolateral PTH1R uses the AC and PKA pathway.[40] PTH binding at either site results in the downregulation of brush border membrane NaPi-IIa and NaPi-IIc in which the transporter is removed from the brush border membrane via clathrin-coated pits.[41,42] Following endocytosis, NaPi-II is transported to the lysosomes for degradation.[41] The PTH-mediated formation of cAMP escapes from the cells, and much of it appears in urine.[43] Thus, urinary, or nephrogenous, cAMP is a reflection of PTH1R action in proximal tubules, and nephrogenous cAMP is considered to be a reliable index of PTH function.

Calcium

Calcium is absorbed by most nephron segments, but most calcium recovery (approximately 65%) occurs in proximal tubules coupled to the bulk transport of solutes, such as sodium and water. By creating an osmotic driving force for water absorption, active sodium transport drives paracellular calcium movement either by generating a concentration gradient for calcium diffusion or by convection/solvent drag.[44] The hormonal regulation of calcium absorption by PTH is, however, restricted to distal nephron sites, including cortical thick ascending limbs of the loop of Henle (CTAL), distal convoluted tubules, and possibly connecting tubules.

Approximately 20% of filtered Ca^{++} is reabsorbed in the CTAL. In the CTAL, PTH binds to the PTH1R, and enhances Ca^{++} reabsorption by increasing the activity of the Na/K/2Cl cotransporter that drives NaCl reabsorption and stimulates paracellular Ca^{++} and magnesium (Mg^{++}) reabsorption (**Fig. 2**). The CaSR is also present in the CTAL,[45] and increased ECF Ca^{++} via CaSR, can upregulate claudin 14 and thereby diminish paracellular Ca^{++} reabsorption.[46,47] Consequently, a raised ECF Ca^{++} antagonizes the effect of PTH in this nephron segment and ECF Ca^{++} can in fact participate in this way as a hormone in the regulation of its own homeostasis.

Approximately 15% of filtered Ca^{++} is reabsorbed in the distal convoluted tubule (DCT) and connecting tubules. Cellular Ca^{++} entry across apical membranes of late distal DCTs and connecting tubules is mediated by transient receptor potential cation channel subfamily V member 5 (TRPV5), a highly selective Ca^{++} channel. Calcium ions cross the apical membrane from the tubular lumen via TRPV5, are translocated across the cell from apical to basolateral surface by proteins, such as calbindin-D28 K, and then transported across the basolateral membrane into the blood mainly by the sodium/calcium exchanger 1 (NCX1). PTH stimulates Ca^{++} absorption through this active transcellular transport by regulating expression of TRPV5 and NCX1, as well as their activity[48] (see **Fig. 2**). The PTH regulation of at least TRPV5 appears to occur through PKC.[49] TRPV5 is also regulated through the PKC-signaling pathway by CaSR.[50]

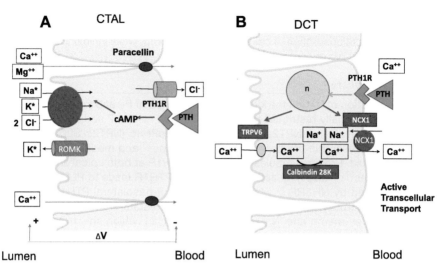

Fig. 2. PTH regulation of calcium transport in kidney. (*A*) In the cortical thick ascending limb (CTAL) of the loop of Henle, sodium (Na$^+$), potassium (K$^+$), and chloride (Cl$^-$) ions are reabsorbed from urine through the Na-K-2Cl transporter. K$^+$, which can be stimulated by PTH-induced production of cAMP via the PTH1R, and returns into the tubule lumen through the renal outer medullary potassium channel (ROMK). The recycling of K$^+$ generates a lumen-positive transepithelial potential (ΔV) that drives calcium and magnesium paracellular transport. Cl$^-$ leaves the cells at the basolateral membrane via a Cl$^-$ channel. Selective reabsorption of Ca^{++} and Mg^{++} is due to paracellin expression in the tight junction complex. Ca^{++} reabsorption is also controlled by CaSR, which can stimulate ROMK and inhibit PTH-induced Na-K-2Cl activities. Inhibition of NaCl reabsorption by Ca^{++} action via CaSR decreases the transepithelial voltage and the reabsorption of Ca^{++}. (*B*) In the DCT, PTH stimulates Ca^{++} absorption through active transcellular transport by regulating expression of TRPV5 and NCX1, as well as their activity.

Bicarbonate

Most proximal tubule bicarbonate (HCO$_3^-$) absorption is due to the type 3 Na$^+$/H$^+$ Na/H isoform NHE3, SLC9A3, which is the most abundant form of Na$^+$/H$^+$ exchanger in proximal tubule apical membranes. PTH suppresses HCO$_3^-$ transport by a PKA-mediated inhibitory action on NHE3. PTH inhibition of proximal Na$^+$/H$^+$ exchange results in diminished Na$^+$ as well as HCO$_3^-$ absorption; however, whereas the rejected Na$^+$ is recovered at downstream nephron sites, the HCO$_3$ is ultimately absorbed by terminal nephron segments as part of urinary acidification.[51]

PARATHYROID HORMONE ACTIONS IN BONE
Introduction

PTH binds to PTH1R on cells of the osteoblastic lineage,[52] including osteoprogenitor cells, lining cells, immature osteoblasts, mature osteoblasts, and osteocytes, and can stimulate a variety of factors ultimately leading to increased proliferation of mesenchymal stem cells, such that these cells are committed into the osteoblast lineage, and to enhanced osteoblast differentiation and activity with new bone matrix production and ultimately mineralization of bone tissue (**Fig. 3**). However, osteoblastic cells also produce the tumor necrosis factor–related cytokine, receptor activator of nuclear factor κ-B (RANK) ligand (RANKL), a critical stimulator of osteoclast production and action, as well as the soluble RANKL decoy receptor, osteoprotegerin (OPG).[53] PTH

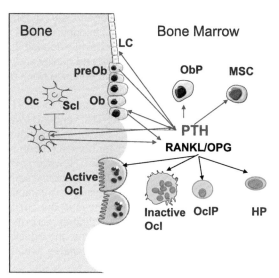

Fig. 3. Role of PTH in modulating bone remodeling. PTH can stimulate mesenchymal stem cells (MSCs) in bone marrow to commit to osteoblast progenitors (ObP) and can stimulate lining cells and marrow ObP to form preosteoblasts and then mature osteoblasts. Mature osteoblasts can then be stimulated by PTH to lay down new bone matrix. PTH can act on osteocytes (Oc), entrapped within bone matrix, to inhibit release of sclerostin an inhibitor of the Wnt pathway. This allows activation of this osteoblast-stimulatory pathway. Consequently new bone can be produced. Mature Ob and Oc stimulated by PTH, can also increase production of the cytokine RANKL and decrease production of the inhibitor, osteoprotegerin. RANKL can then stimulate the commitment of hematopoietic precursors (HP) to osteoclast precursors (OclP) and the differentiation of osteoclast precursors to inactive osteoclasts (inactive Ocl) and thence to active osteoclasts, which resorb bone. The balance between the effects of PTH on new bone formation versus bone resorption determines whether it will have an anabolic or catabolic effect.

enhances production of RANKL and inhibits production of OPG leading to increased osteoclastic bone resorption (see **Fig. 3**). Bone resorption leads to the release of Ca^{++} and Pi as a result of the degradation of hydroxyapatite, the major mineral component of bone. Consequently PTH can stimulate bone turnover leading to either a net increase in bone formation or a net increase in bone resorption. PTH seems to primarily use the PKA pathway in exerting both its catabolic and anabolic effects on osteoblasts[54,55]; however, PKC activation by PTH and intracellular Ca^{++} signaling pathways may play an important role in bone as well.[56]

Anabolic Effects

Studies of mice with genetically targeted deletion of PTH (PTH "knockout" mice) have demonstrated that the lack of PTH leads to a decrease in metaphyseal osteoblasts and a reduction in trabecular bone in fetal and neonatal mice. These observations are consistent with an important physiologic role for PTH in promoting development of the fetal and newborn skeleton, and therefore in bone anabolism.[57] This anabolic role in early development may be recapitulated later in life, as demonstrated by the fact that endogenous PTH also appears necessary for optimal fracture healing in mice[58]; however, this has still not been demonstrated beyond a reasonable doubt in humans.

Overall, both animal and human studies of endogenous PTH deficiency (hypoparathyroidism) or excess (hyperparathyroidism), or of exogenous PTH administration (as an anabolic agent in osteoporosis), provide compelling evidence that PTH is particularly important for normal trabecular bone quantity and quality and that significant increases in periosteal apposition may occur, which enhance bone modeling and may also be beneficial notably for cortical bone.

Although PTHrP was initially discovered in the search for a PTH-like factor that causes hypercalcemia of malignancy, and both PTHrP and PTH were both assumed to be osteolytic calcium-modulating hormones, further studies have shown that both also may be anabolic, with PTHrP being critical for normal growth plate development and PTH playing an essential role in bone anabolism. However, circulating PTH may cooperate with PTHrP in carrying out physiologic anabolic bone activity.[59,60] Although PTH and PTHrP are both believed to elicit cell signaling via interaction of their homologous N-terminal domains with PTH1R,[25] differences in the timing and location of expression of PTH and PTHrP during development, differences in the duration of binding of each hormone to its receptor, and additional intracrine signaling by PTHrP have been described, all of which may contribute to the variable actions of the 2 related hormones.[61,62]

Mechanistically, PTH appears to increase the active osteoblast pool both directly via increasing gene expression of a number of factors that may act intracellularly within osteoblastic cells, and by modulating production and/or secretion of factors from cells of the osteoblastic lineage that can act on osteoblastic cells in an intracrine/paracrine mechanism. It is likely that not all cellular events leading to an increased active osteoblast pool are equally activated by PTH at every stage of skeletal development, growth, and repair.

PTH-induced proliferation and/or differentiation may involve cAMP-induced expression of the transcription factor c-fos in stromal cells and osteoblasts,[63] and stimulation of the MAPK pathway resulting in increasing osteoblastic proliferation.[64,65] PTH-stimulated cyclic AMP generation may also lead to activation of the promoter of runx2 (Cbfa1), an essential and early transcriptional regulator of osteoblast differentiation, leading to increased runx2 mRNA and protein in osteoblasts.[66] Furthermore, PTH may augment the Smad3-related factor, Tmem119, which interacts with the bone morphogenetic protein (BMP)-Runx2 pathway, to promote osteoblast differentiation.[67] PTH-induced stimulation of osteoblastic differentiation may also occur via increasing exit from the cell cycle, both by attenuating the expression of cyclin D1, a protein required for cell cycle progression, and by an increasing the expression of the cell cycle inhibitors p27Kip1 and p21Cip1.[68–70] PTH may also exert an antiapoptotic effect on osteoblastic cells via a cAMP mechanism resulting in phosphorylation and inactivation of the proapoptotic factor Bad, but an increase in the expression of the survival factor Bcl.[71] PTH may also augment DNA repair.[72]

In addition, PTH may modulate the production of osteoblastic factors that act extracellularly on osteoblastic cells in a paracrine/autocrine manner, leading to increased anabolic activity. Thus, PTH has been shown to decrease production of the osteocytic factor sclerostin. Sclerostin is a secreted glycoprotein and an important negative regulator of the canonical Wnt/β-catenin signaling pathway, a critical pathway in bone formation.[73] It is assumed that sclerostin would normally pass through the osteocytic canaliculi to access osteoblasts on the bone surface, where it would inhibit and act as a negative regulator of bone accrual.[74] This PTH-induced inhibition appears to be a cAMP-mediated effect to inhibit a long-range enhancer, MEF2, of the *Sost* gene encoding sclerostin.[75] PTH-induced interference with the capacity of sclerostin to act is generally believed to lead to enhanced osteoblast differentiation and inhibition of osteoblast apoptosis. Nevertheless, although suppression of sclerostin facilitates PTH-induced bone gain, anabolic effects of PTH are not completely absent in *Sost*-null mice, suggesting that other mechanisms of PTH action may exist.[76,77]

PTH can increase gene expression and release of osteoblastic insulin-like growth factor 1 (IGF1),[78] which can then act through the osteoblast IGF1 receptor to increase osteoprogenitor proliferation and differentiation; additionally, PTH-induced release of FGF-2, leading to proliferative and antiapoptotic effects on osteoblast progenitors has also been described, and the anabolic effects of intermittent PTH were attenuated in mice with deletion of FGF-2.[79]

Therefore, in terms of its anabolic activity, PTH appears to exert pleiotropic effects on cells of the osteoblastic lineage in multiple stages of proliferation, differentiation, and apoptosis; different mechanisms may predominate, however, at different stages of skeletal growth and development.

Parathyroid Hormone Actions in Modeling and Remodeling to Enhance Bone Formation

In response to intermittent administration of PTH in osteoporosis in humans, where it has clear therapeutic efficacy, there is an early phase of stimulation of bone formation without resorption, which is followed subsequently by stimulation of bone resorption.[80–83] Excess formation may proceed for a time after remodeling has been initiated in response to PTH, so that a smaller amount of bone may still be accrued, but the increase in bone accrual is ultimately limited by enhanced osteoclastic resorption, and a plateau effect occurs. The period during which the effects of PTH on bone formation relative to resorption are maximal has been termed the "anabolic window." PTH may also stimulate bone formation without prior resorption,[84,85] and it has been estimated that in early phases of treatment with intermittent PTH(1–34), such modeling-based bone formation may account for more than 20% of the new formation in trabecular and endocortical bone; the periosteal new bone formation that has been observed after intermittent PTH administration in humans with osteoporosis likely reflects predominantly modeling effects with prolonged treatment. As bone remodeling is stimulated, modeling may account for less than 10% of new bone formation. The PTH-induced bone formation can therefore occur not only on quiescent bone surfaces, but also in areas of remodeling in which there is overfilling of bone resorption cavities due to increased formation relative to resorption[86–88] (see **Fig. 3**). Thus, PTH-induced increases in the activation frequency of remodeling units may enhance its bone-forming effect. The skeletal anabolic actions of PTH has therefore found utility in the clinic in the anabolic treatment of osteoporosis.

Catabolic Effects of Parathyroid Hormone

PTH defends against a decrease in serum calcium by increasing bone resorption more than formation. PTH appears to have discrete effects on trabecular and cortical bone compartments in its resorptive action, sparing trabecular bone and diminishing cortical bone, at least until very high concentrations of circulating PTH are attained when more generalized bone resorption may occur to release calcium from skeletal stores.

Cells of the osteoblastic lineage, including osteocytes, produce several growth factors and cytokines (such as macrophage-colony-stimulating factor, which stimulates osteoclasts), but one of the most important of these is RANKL.[89] The RANKL/RANK system is known to facilitate all aspects of osteoclastogenesis, including proliferation of hematopoietic mononuclear precursors, differentiation of osteoclast progenitor cells, fusion of such cells, and activation of multinucleated osteoclasts[53] (see **Fig. 3**). While stimulating cells of the osteoblastic lineage, PTH also enhances production of RANKL and inhibits production of its naturally occurring antagonist OPG, leading to increased osteoclastic bone resorption.[90,91] Bone resorption leads to the release of Ca^{++} and Pi but can also release a variety of matrix components into the circulation, which are useful as bone markers in monitoring PTH-induced bone resorption. Furthermore, osteoblast growth factors, such as TGFβ, BMPs, FGFs, and IGFs are laid down along with collagen during bone formation, and can be released when matrix degradation occurs, and stimulate osteoblasts, thus increasing the active osteoblast pool.[92,93] Direct signaling from osteoclastic cells to osteoblasts also appears to occur. For example, it has been reported that Ephrin B2 binding to Eph4 on osteoblastic cells stimulates osteoblast precursor differentiation by inhibiting the small GTPase, RhoA,[94] and clastokines, such as the chemokine sphingosine-1-phosphate and BMP6 may be produced by osteoclasts and directly recruit osteoblasts to the resorption site.[95,96] Although many questions remain about the molecular nature of the moieties released by osteoclasts that increase osteoblast coupling, the consequences of PTH-enhanced osteoclastic activation would be stimulation of the bone-remodeling process; that is, the formation of a resorption cavity that would be linked to a further increase in the active osteoblast pool, and influx of active osteoblasts to the resorption cavity to initiate bone formation.

The increased bone remodeling caused by PTH and its renal action on mineral metabolism also have made it an attractive agent to use in replacement therapy for hypoparathyroidism.

SUMMARY

Clear evidence exists as to the central role of the renal calcium-retaining effect of PTH, its renal phosphaturic action, and its bone resorptive role in maintaining mineral homeostasis and carrying this out when necessary at the expense of skeletal integrity. Increasing evidence also exists for an important physiologic role for PTH in promoting bone formation. Much progress has been made in understanding the molecular and cellular mechanisms that mediate and coordinate these processes, but much still remains to be discovered. Nevertheless, knowledge of the anabolic efficacy of PTH has already been translated into the clinic and as newer understanding of the interactions of PTH anabolism with osteoclastic activity and of molecular factors, which may alter this interaction, become clarified and newer PTH analogs are developed, the physiology will undoubtedly be even more successfully translated to improve patient care.

REFERENCES

1. Naylor SL, Sakaguchi AY, Szoka P, et al. Human parathyroid hormone gene (PTH) is on short arm of chromosome 11. Somatic Cell Genet 1983;9:609–16.
2. Brown EM. Four-parameter model of the sigmoidal relationship between parathyroid hormone release and extracellular calcium concentration in normal and abnormal parathyroid tissue. J Clin Endocrinol Metab 1983;56:572–81.
3. Mayer GP, Keaton JA, Hurst JG, et al. Effects of plasma calcium concentration on the relative proportion of hormone and carboxyl fragments in parathyroid venous blood. Endocrinology 1979;104:1778.
4. Hanley DA, Ayer LM. Calcium-dependent release of carboxyl-terminal fragments of parathyroid hormone by hyperplastic human parathyroid tissue in vitro. J Clin Endocrinol Metab 1986;63:1075.

5. D'Amour P, Palardy J, Bahsali G, et al. The modulation of circulating parathyroid hormone immunoheterogeneity in man by ionized calcium concentration. J Clin Endocrinol Metab 1992;74:525–32.
6. Segre BV, D'Amour P, Potts JT. Metabolism of radioiodinated bovine parathyroid hormone in the rat. Endocrinology 1976;99:1645–52.
7. Zhang CX, Weber BV, Thammavong J, et al. Identification of carboxyl-terminal peptide fragments of parathyroid hormone in human plasma at low-picomolar levels by mass spectrometry. Anal Chem 2006;78:1636–43.
8. Segre GV, D'Amour P, Hultman A, et al. Effects of hepatectomy, nephrectomy, and nephrectomy/uremia on the metabolism of parathyroid hormone in the rat. J Clin Invest 1981;67:439–48.
9. Yamamoto M, Igarishi T, Muramatsu M, et al. Hypocalcemia increases and hyper-calcemia decreases the steady state level of parathyroid hormone messenger RNA in the rat. J Clin Invest 1989;83:1053–6.
10. Naveh-Many T, Silver J. Regulation of parathyroid hormone gene expression by hypocalcemia, hypercalcemia, and vitamin D in the rat. J Clin Invest 1990;86: 1313–9.
11. Kilav R, Silver J, Naveh-Many T. A conserved cis-acting element in the parathy-roid hormone 3'-untranslated region is sufficient for regulation of RNA stability by calcium and phosphate. J Biol Chem 2001;276:8727–33.
12. Kremer R, Bolivar I, Goltzman D, et al. Influence of calcium and 1,25-dihydroxy-cholecalciferol on proliferation and proto-oncogene expression in primary cul-tures of bovine parathyroid cells. Endocrinology 1989;125:935–41.
13. Russell J, Lettieri D, Sherwood LM. Suppression by 1,25(OH)2D3 of transcription of the pre-proparathyroid hormone gene. Endocrinology 1986;119:2864–6.
14. Salehi-Tabar R, Nguyen-Yamamoto L, Tavera-Mendoza LE, et al. Vitamin D recep-tor as a master regulator of the c-MYC/MXD1 network. Proc Natl Acad Sci U S A 2012;109:18827–32.
15. Wallace J, Scarpa A. Similarities of Li+ and low Ca2+ in the modulation of secre-tion by parathyroid cells in vitro. J Biol Chem 1983;258:6288–92.
16. Dusso A, Cozzolino M, Lu Y, et al. 1,25-Dihydroxyvitamin D downregulation of TGF alpha/EGFR expression and growth signaling: a mechanism for the antipro-liferative actions of the sterol in parathyroid hyperplasia of renal failure. J Steroid Biochem Mol Biol 2004;89-90:507–11.
17. Xu M, Choudhary S, Goltzman D, et al. Do cycloxygenase-2 knockout mice have primary hyperparathyroidism? Endocrinology 2005;146:1843–53.
18. Nakajima K, Umino K, Azuma Y, et al. Stimulating parathyroid cell proliferation and PTH release with phosphate in organ cultures obtained from patients with pri-mary and secondary hyperparathyroidism for a prolonged period. J Bone Miner Metab 2009;27:224–335.
19. Silver J, Naveh-Many T. FGF23 and the parathyroid. Adv Exp Med Biol 2012;728: 92–9.
20. Tregear GW, Van Rietschoten J, Greene E, et al. Bovine parathyroid hormone: minimum chain length of synthetic peptide required for biological activity. Endo-crinology 1973;93.1349–53.
21. Goltzman D, Peytremann A, Callahan E, et al. Analysis of the requirements for parathyroid hormone action in renal membranes with the use of inhibiting ana-logues. J Biol Chem 1975;250:3199–203.
22. Jüppner H, Abou-Samra AB, Freeman M, et al. A G protein-linked receptor for parathyroid hormone and parathyroid hormone-related peptide. Science 1991; 254:1024–6.

23. Abou-Samra AB, Jüppner H, Force T, et al. Expression cloning of a common receptor for parathyroid hormone and parathyroid hormone-related peptide from rat osteoblast-like cells: a single receptor stimulates intracellular accumulation of both cAMP and inositol trisphosphates and increases intracellular free calcium. Proc Natl Acad Sci U S A 1992;89:2732–6.
24. Vilardaga JP, Romero G, Friedman PA, et al. Molecular basis of parathyroid hormone receptor signaling and trafficking: a family B GPCR paradigm. Cell Mol Life Sci 2011;68:1–13.
25. Datta NS, Abou-Samra AB. PTH and PTHrP signaling in osteoblasts. Cell Signal 2009;21:1245–54.
26. Singh AT, Gilchrist A, Voyno-Yasenetskaya T, et al. G alpha12/G alpha13 subunits of heterotrimeric G proteins mediate parathyroid hormone activation of phospholipase D in UMR-106 osteoblastic cells. Endocrinology 2005;146:2171–5.
27. Radeff JM, Nagy Z, Stern PH. Rho and Rho kinase are involved in parathyroid hormone-stimulated protein kinase C alpha translocation and IL-6 promoter activity in osteoblastic cells. J Bone Miner Res 2004;19:1882–91.
28. Ferrari SL, Behar V, Chorev M, et al. Endocytosis of ligand-human parathyroid hormone receptor 1 complexes is protein kinase C-dependent and involves beta- arrestin 2. Real-time monitoring by fluorescence microscopy. J Biol Chem 1999;274:29968–75.
29. Bohinc BN, Gesty-Palmer D. β-arrestin-biased agonism at the parathyroid hormone receptor uncouples bone formation from bone resorption. Endocr Metab Immune Disord Drug Targets 2011;11:112–9.
30. Sneddon WB, Syme CA, Bisello A, et al. Activation-independent parathyroid hormone receptor internalization is regulated by NHERF1 (EBP50). J Biol Chem 2003;278:43787–96.
31. Wang B, Ardura JA, Romero G, et al. Na/H exchanger regulatory factors control parathyroid hormone receptor signaling by facilitating differential activation of Gα protein subunits. J Biol Chem 2010;285:26976–86.
32. Mahon MJ, Donowitz M, Yun CC, et al. Na+/H+ exchanger regulatory factor 2 directs parathyroid hormone 1 receptor signalling. Nature 2002;417:858–86.
33. Maeda S, Wu S, Jüppner H, et al. Cell-specific signal transduction of parathyroid hormone (PTH)-related protein through stably expressed recombinant PTH/PTHrP receptors in vascular smooth muscle cells. Endocrinology 1996;137:3154–62.
34. Murer H, Hernando N, Forster I, et al. Regulation of Na/Pi transporter in the proximal tubule. Annu Rev Physiol 2003;65:531–42.
35. Brenza HL, Kimmel-Jehan C, Jehan F, et al. Parathyroid hormone activation of the 25-hydroxyvitamin D3-1alpha-hydroxylase gene promoter. Proc Natl Acad Sci U S A 1998;95:1387–91.
36. Custer M, Lotscher M, Biber J, et al. Expression of Na-P(i) cotransport in rat kidney: localization by RT-PCR and immunohistochemistry. Am J Physiol 1994;266:F767–74.
37. Amizuka N, Lee HS, Kwan MY, et al. Cell-specific expression of the parathyroid hormone (PTH)/PTH-related peptide receptor gene in kidney from kidney-specific and ubiquitous promoters. Endocrinology 1997;138:469–81.
38. Ba J, Brown D, Friedman PA. CaSR regulation of PTH-inhibitable proximal tubule phosphate transport. Am J Physiol Renal Physiol 2003;285:F1233–43.
39. Capuano P, Bacic D, Roos M, et al. Defective coupling of apical PTH receptors to phospholipase C prevents internalization of the Na+-phosphate cotransporter NaPi-IIa in Nherf1-deficient mice. Am J Physiol Cell Physiol 2007;292:C927–34.

40. Traebert M, Völkl H, Biber J, et al. Luminal and contraluminal action of 1–34 and 3–34 PTH peptides on renal type IIa Na-Pi cotransporter. Am J Physiol Ren Physiol 2000;278:F792–8.

41. Bacic D, Lehir M, Biber J, et al. The renal Na+/phosphate cotransporter NaPi-IIa is internalized via the receptor-mediated endocytic route in response to parathyroid hormone. Kidney Int 2006;69:495–503.

42. Segawa H, Yamanaka S, Onitsuka A, et al. Parathyroid hormone-dependent endocytosis of renal type IIc Na-Pi cotransporter. Am J Physiol Ren Physiol 2007;292:F395–403.

43. Kaminsky NI, Broadus AE, Hardman JG, et al. Effects of parathyroid hormone on plasma and urinary adenosine 3′,5′-monophosphate in man. J Clin Invest 1970;49:2387–95.

44. Ullrich KJ, Rumrich G, Kloss S. Active Ca2+ reabsorption in the proximal tubule of the rat kidney. Dependence on sodium- and buffer transport. Pflugers Arch 1976;364:223–8.

45. Hebert SC. Extracellular calcium-sensing receptor: implications for calcium and magnesium handling in the kidney. Kidney Int 1996;50:2129–39.

46. Toka HR, Al-Romaih K, Koshy JM, et al. Deficiency of the calcium-sensing receptor in the kidney causes parathyroid hormone-independent hypocalciuria. J Am Soc Nephrol 2012;23(11):1879–90.

47. Loupy A, Ramakrishnan SK, Wootla B, et al. PTH-independent regulation of blood calcium concentration by the calcium-sensing receptor. J Clin Invest 2012;122:3355–67.

48. van Abel M, Hoenderop JG, van der Kemp AW, et al. Coordinated control of renal Ca(2+) transport proteins by parathyroid hormone. Kidney Int 2005;68:1708–21.

49. Cha SK, Wu T, Huang CL. Protein kinase C inhibits caveolae-mediated endocytosis of TRPV5. Am J Physiol Ren Physiol 2008;294:F1212–21.

50. Topala CN, Schoeber JP, Searchfield LE, et al. Activation of the Ca(2+)-sensing receptor stimulates the activity of the epithelial Ca(2+) channel TRPV5. Cell Calcium 2009;45:331–9.

51. Wagner CA, Devuyst O, Bourgeois S, et al. Regulated acid-base transport in the collecting duct. Pflugers Arch 2009;458:137–56.

52. Rouleau MF, Mitchell J, Goltzman D. Characterization of the major parathyroid hormone target cell in the endosteal metaphysis of rat long bones. J Bone Miner Res 1990;5:1043–53.

53. Boyle WJ, Simonet WS, Lacey DL. Osteoclast differentiation and activation. Nature 2003;423:337–42.

54. Li X, Liu H, Qin L, et al. Determination of dual effects of parathyroid hormone on skeletal gene expression in vivo by microarray and network analysis. J Biol Chem 2007;282:33086–97.

55. Yang D, Singh R, Divieti P, et al. Contributions of parathyroid hormone (PTH)/PTH-related peptide receptor signaling pathways to the anabolic effect of PTH on bone. Bone 2007;40:1453–61.

56. Guo J, Liu M, Yang D, et al. Phospholipase C signaling via the parathyroid hormone (PTH)/PTH related peptide receptor is essential for normal bone responses to PTH. Endocrinology 2010;151:3502–13.

57. Miao D, He B, Karaplis AC, et al. Parathyroid hormone is essential for normal fetal bone formation. J Clin Invest 2002;109:1173–82.

58. Ren Y, Liu B, Feng Y, et al. Endogenous PTH deficiency impairs fracture healing and impedes the fracture-healing efficacy of exogenous PTH(1–34). PLoS One 2011;6:e23060.

59. Miao D, Li J, Xue Y, et al. Parathyroid hormone-related peptide is required for increased trabecular bone volume in parathyroid hormone-null mice. Endocrinology 2004;145:3554–62.

60. Zhu Q, Zhou X, Zhu M, et al. Endogenous parathyroid hormone-related protein compensates for the absence of parathyroid hormone in promoting bone accrual in vivo in a model of bone marrow ablation. J Bone Miner Res 2013;28:1898–911.

61. Miao D, Su H, He B, et al. Severe growth retardation and early lethality in mice lacking the nuclear localization sequence and C-terminus of PTH-related protein. Proc Natl Acad Sci U S A 2008;105:20309–14.

62. Toribio RE, Brown HA, Novince CM, et al. The midregion, nuclear localization sequence and C terminus of PTHrP regulate skeletal development, hematopoiesis, and survival in mice. FASEB J 2010;24:1947–57.

63. McCauley LK, Koh AJ, Beecher CA, et al. Proto-oncogene c-fos is transcriptionally regulated by parathyroid hormone (PTH) and PTH-related protein in a cyclic adenosine monophosphate-dependent manner in osteoblastic cells. Endocrinology 1997;138:5427–33.

64. Swarthout JT, Doggett TA, Lemker JL, et al. Stimulation of extracellular signal-regulated kinases and proliferation n rat osteoblastic cells by parathyroid hormone is protein kinaseC-dependent. J Biol Chem 2001;276:7586–92.

65. Miao D, Tong X, Chan G, et al. Parathyroid hormone-related peptide stimulates osteogenic cell proliferation through protein kinase C activation of the Ras/mitogen-activated protein kinase signaling pathway. J Biol Chem 2001;276:32204–12.

66. Krishnan V, Moore TL, Ma YL, et al. Parathyroid hormone bone anabolic action requires Cbfa1/Runx2-dependent signaling. Mol Endocrinol 2003;17:423–35.

67. Hisa I, Inoue Y, Hendy GN, et al. Parathyroid hormone-responsive Smad3-related factorTmem119, promotes osteoblast differentiation and interacts with the bone morphogenetic protein-Runx2 pathway. J Biol Chem 2011;286:9787–96.

68. Qin L, Li X, Ko JK, et al. Parathyroid hormone uses multiple mechanisms to arrest the cell cycle progression of osteoblastic cells from G1 to S phase. J Biol Chem 2005;280:3104–11.

69. Onishi T, Hruska K. Expression of p27Kip1 in osteoblast-like cells during differentiation with parathyroid hormone. Endocrinology 1997;138:1995–2004.

70. Datta NS, Kolailat R, Fite A, et al. Distinct roles for mitogen-activated protein kinase phosphatase-1 (MKP-1) and ERK-MAPK in PTH1R signaling during osteoblast proliferation and differentiation. Cell Signal 2010;22:457–66.

71. Jilka RL, Weinstein RS, Bellido T, et al. Increased bone formation by prevention of osteoblast apoptosis with parathyroid hormone. J Clin Invest 1999;104:439–46.

72. Schnoke M, Midura SB, Midura RJ. Parathyroid hormone suppresses osteoblast apoptosis by augmenting DNA repair. Bone 2009;45:590–602.

73. van Bezooijen RL, Roelen BA, Visser A, et al. Sclerostin is an osteocyte-expressed negative regulator of bone formation, but not a classical BMP antagonist. J Exp Med 2004;199:805–14.

74. Keller H, Kneissel M. SOST is a target gene for PTH in bone. Bone 2005;37(2):148–58.

75. Leupin O, Kramer I, Collette NM, et al. Control of the SOST bone enhancer by PTH using MEF2 transcription factors. J Bone Miner Res 2007;22:1957–67.

76. Sims NA. Building bone with a SOST–PTH partnership. J Bone Miner Res 2010;25:175–7.

77. Kramer I, Keller H, Leupin O, et al. Does osteocytic SOST suppression mediate PTH bone anabolism? Trends Endocrinol Metab 2010;21:237–44.

78. McCarthy TL, Centrella M, Canalis E. Parathyroid hormone enhances the transcript and polypeptide levels of insulin-like growth factor I in osteoblast-enriched cultures from fetal rat bone. Endocrinology 1989;124:1247–53.

79. Hurley MM, Okada Y, Xiao L, et al. Impaired bone anabolic response to parathyroid hormone in Fgf2−/− and Fgf2+/− mice. Biochem Biophys Res Commun 2006;341:989–94.

80. Dobnig H, Sipos A, Jiang Y, et al. Early changes in biochemical markers of bone formation correlate with improvements in bone structure during teriparatide therapy. J Clin Endocrinol Metab 2005;90:3970–7.

81. Lane NE, Sanchez S, Genant HK, et al. Short-term increases in bone turnover markers predict parathyroid hormone-induced spinal bone mineral density gains in post-menopausal women with glucocorticoid-induced osteoporosis. Osteoporos Int 2000;11:434–42.

82. Kurland ES, Cosman F, McMahon DJ, et al. Parathyroid hormone as a therapy for idiopathic osteoporosis in men: effects on bone mineral density and bone markers. J Clin Endocrinol Metab 2000;85:3069–76.

83. Rubin MR, Bilezikian JP. Parathyroid hormone as an anabolic skeletal therapy. Drugs 2005;65:2481–98.

84. Girotra M, Rubin MR, Bilezikian JP. The use of parathyroid hormone in the treatment of osteoporosis. Rev Endocr Metab Disord 2006;7:113–21.

85. Lindsay R, Cosman F, Zhou H, et al. A novel tetracycline labeling schedule for longitudinal evaluation of the short-term effects of anabolic therapy with a single iliac crest bone biopsy: early actions of teriparatide. J Bone Miner Res 2006;21:366–73.

86. Compston JE. Skeletal actions of intermittent parathyroid hormone: effects on bone remodelling and structure. Bone 2007;40:1447–52.

87. Lindsay R, Zhou H, Cosman F, et al. Effects of a one-month treatment with PTH(1–34) on bone formation on cancellous, endocortical, and periosteal surfaces of the human ilium. J Bone Miner Res 2007;22:495–502.

88. Zanchetta JR, Bogado CE, Cisari C, et al. Treatment of postmenopausal women with osteoporosis with PTH(1–84) for 36 months: treatment extension study. Curr Med Res Opin 2010;26:2627–33.

89. Boyce BF. Advances in the regulation of osteoclasts and osteoclast functions. J Dent Res 2013;92:860.

90. Lee S-K, Lorenzo J. Parathyroid hormone stimulates TRANCE and inhibits osteoprotegerin messenger ribonucleic acid expression in murine bone marrow cultures: correlation with osteoclast-like cell formation. Endocrinology 1999;140:3552–61.

91. Locklin RM, Khosla S, Turner RT, et al. Mediators of the biphasic responses of bone to intermittent and continuously administered parathyroid hormone. J Cell Biochem 2003;89:180–90.

92. Mundy GR. The effects of TGF-beta on bone. Ciba Found Symp 1991;157:137–43.

93. Tang Y, Wu X, Lei W, et al. TGF-beta1-induced migration of bone mesenchymal stem cells couples bone resorption with formation. Nat Med 2009;15:757–65.

94. Zhao C, Irie N, Takada Y, et al. Bidirectional ephrinB2-EphB4 signaling controls bone homeostasis. Cell Metab 2006;4:111–21.

95. Ryu J, Kim HJ, Chang EJ, et al. Sphingo-sine 1-phosphate as a regulator of osteoclast differentiation and osteoclast-osteoblast coupling. EMBO J 2006;25: 5840–51.

96. Pederson L, Ruan M, Westendorf JJ, et al. Regulation of bone formation by osteoclasts involves Wnt/BMP signaling and the chemokine sphingosine-1-phosphate. Proc Natl Acad Sci USA 2008;105:20764–9.

Signs and Symptoms of Hypoparathyroidism

Natalie E. Cusano, MD, MS[a],*, John P. Bilezikian, MD[b]

KEYWORDS

- Hypoparathyroidism • Complication • Renal failure • Basal ganglia calcification
- Cataract

KEY POINTS

- Hypoparathyroidism is associated with a large spectrum of clinical manifestations in the acute and chronic settings, from mild to debilitating.
- Although the acute symptoms of hypoparathyroidism are primarily due to neuromuscular irritability associated with hypocalcemia, the chronic manifestations may be due to the disease itself or to complications of therapy.
- The chronic complications of hypoparathyroidism can affect multiple organ systems, including the renal, neurologic, neuropsychiatric, skeletal, and immune systems.
- Further research is needed to determine the pathophysiology of complications in hypoparathyroidism and whether interventions can decrease the risk of these complications in the disease.

INTRODUCTION

Hypoparathyroidism is associated with a spectrum of clinical manifestations in the acute and chronic settings, from mild to debilitating. There are large interindividual differences in the threshold of calcium that may elicit symptoms. Some patients may be asymptomatic, even in the setting of severe hypocalcemia, whereas others may present with life-threatening manifestations. The presence of symptomatic hypocalcemia is a function not only of the degree of hypocalcemia but also of the rate at which the serum calcium has declined. Although the acute symptoms of hypocalcemia are primarily due to neuromuscular irritability, the chronic manifestations of

Disclosure Statement: Dr J.P. Bilezikian is a consultant for Amgen, Radius, Shire, and Ultragenyx. Dr N.E. Cusano is a consultant for Shire.
Funding Source: National Institutes of Health grant DK32333.
[a] Department of Medicine, Bone Metabolism Program, Lenox Hill Hospital, Zucker School of Medicine at Hofstra/Northwell, 110 East 59th Street, 8th Floor, Suite 8B, New York, NY 10022, USA; [b] Division of Endocrinology, Department of Medicine, Columbia University College of Physicians and Surgeons, 630 West 168th Street, PH 8W-864, New York, NY 10032, USA
* Corresponding author.
E-mail address: ncusano@northwell.edu

hypoparathyroidism may be due to the disease itself or to complications of therapy or to both. The chronic complications of hypoparathyroidism can affect multiple organ systems, including the renal, neurologic, neuropsychiatric, skeletal, and immune systems (**Table 1**). Further research is needed to determine the pathophysiology of complications in hypoparathyroidism and whether interventions can decrease the risk of these complications.

ACUTE MANIFESTATIONS OF HYPOPARATHYROIDISM

The maintenance of a normal extracellular ionized calcium concentration is critical for multiple tissues and organ systems, including the brain, heart, and skeletal muscles. Acute or severe hypocalcemia can cause well-recognized manifestations, some life-threatening, and potentially leading to respiratory or cardiac arrest.[1,2] The rate of development and severity of hypocalcemia may affect the presentation. Other factors, such as hypomagnesemia or concomitant alkalosis in which the partition between bound and free calcium favors bound calcium, can influence the variability of frequency and the severity of symptoms. There is also a large interindividual variation in description of symptoms. Patients with acute post-parathyroidectomy reductions in parathyroid hormone (PTH) concentrations may complain of severe tetany despite a serum calcium concentration that is close to the normal range. The symptoms are due primarily to the rapid reduction in the serum calcium and not the actual level per se. In contrast, patients with autoimmune hypoparathyroidism that develops over a long period may be asymptomatic despite severe biochemical disturbances and evidence for ectopic soft tissue calcifications.[3] Symptomatic patients or those with an electrocardiogram that shows a prolonged QTc interval should be considered for urgent treatment by infusion of intravenous calcium as detailed in Muriel Babey and colleagues' article, "Conventional Treatment of Hypoparathyroidism," in this issue.

Neuromuscular Irritability

Neuromuscular irritability is the hallmark of acute hypocalcemia, presenting clinically with both sensory nerve and muscle dysfunction. Hypocalcemia heightens the excitability of neurons, and on electromyographic testing, a single stimulus provokes repetitive, high-frequency discharges and muscle spasms (ie, tetany).[4] Symptoms can be mild, with perioral numbness, tingling of the hands or feet, myalgias, or muscle cramping. Severe tetany can lead to generalized muscle contractions. Bronchospasm or laryngospasm can occur with severe hypocalcemia and can lead to respiratory arrest.

The Chvostek and Trousseau signs are physical manifestations of neuromuscular irritability. The mechanism is thought to be a decreased threshold for transmission of the nerve impulse that is potentiated by mechanical stimulation or ischemia, respectively.[5] The Chvostek sign is a twitching of the ipsilateral facial muscles elicited by tapping over the facial nerve in front of the tragus. Depending on the degree of hypocalcemia, the response may vary from twitching of the lip to spasm of all facial muscles, and even bilateral spasm. The Chvostek sign is neither a sensitive nor specific test for hypocalcemia. Approximately 10% to 25% of healthy individuals will have a positive Chvostek sign,[6] and it can be negative in approximately 30% of hypocalcemic patients.[7] By contrast, the Trousseau sign has a sensitivity approaching 94% to 99% and is present in only 1% of normocalcemic individuals.[7,8] To elicit the Trousseau sign, a blood pressure cuff is placed on the upper arm and inflated above the systolic blood pressure for 3 minutes, occluding the brachial artery and vasa nervosum. In the presence of neuropathic ischemia, hypocalcemia will induce carpopedal spasm. There is flexion of the wrist and metacarpophalangeal joints, extension of the distal and

Table 1
Acute and chronic manifestations of hypocalcemia and hypoparathyroidism

Organ System	Acute and Chronic Manifestations
Cardiovascular	Hypotension Bradycardia Impaired cardiac contractility Prolonged QTc Torsade de pointes/arrhythmias Cardiomyopathy/congestive heart failure ST, QS, T-wave changes on electrocardiography suggestive of myocardial infarction Increased risk of ischemic heart disease and all cardiovascular outcomes in nonsurgical hypoparathyroidism
Dental	Dental aplasia or hypoplasia Failure of tooth eruption Enamel hypoplasia Defective root formation Severe dental caries
Dermatologic	Dry, rough, puffy, coarse skin Brittle hair with hair loss Brittle nails with transverse grooves
Immune	Increased risk of infection, particularly urinary tract infection
Neurologic and neuromotor	Seizures, most commonly tonic-clonic or focal motor, although atypical absence or akinetic seizures also described Spikes and bursts of high-voltage, paroxysmal slow waves on electroencephalogram Basal ganglia and other brain calcifications Extrapyramidal or cerebellar dysfunction
Neuromuscular	Fatigue Neuromuscular irritability Perioral/extremity numbness/tingling Muscle cramping with carpal/pedal spasms or generalized muscle contractions Bronchospasm and laryngospasm Chvostek sign Trousseau sign
Neuropsychiatric	Reduced quality of life Depression Bipolar disease Delirium Cognitive impairment Irritability Depression/anxiety Psychosis
Ophthalmologic	Papilledema Cataract (primarily posterior subcapsular)
Renal	Hypercalciuria Nephrocalcinosis Nephrolithiasis Renal insufficiency and renal failure
Skeletal	Elevated bone density compared with healthy, age-matched controls Markedly reduced bone remodeling

proximal interphalangeal joints, and adduction of the fingers.[5] The sign has also been described as main d'accoucheur in French ("hand of the obstetrician") due to a resemblance to the positioning of the obstetrician's hand during delivery.

Cardiovascular

The cardiovascular manifestations of acute hypocalcemia can include hypotension, bradycardia, impaired cardiac contractility, and arrhythmias. In the setting of an acute drop in serum calcium, there can be diminished vascular smooth muscle tone. This generalized state of vasodilatation can be refractory to fluid repletion and pressors until calcium is corrected.[1] In addition, the vital role of calcium in myocardial excitation-contraction coupling and myocardial relaxation has been well characterized. By prolonging the duration of phase 2 of the action potential of cardiac muscle, hypocalcemia subsequently increases the ST segment and the QT interval. A more rapid drop in serum calcium is associated with additional prolongation of the QT interval.[9] Torsades de pointes is a specific form of polymorphic ventricular tachycardia associated with a long QT interval. Although hypocalcemia can cause torsades de pointes, this unusual cardiac condition is more often reported in the presence of hypokalemia and hypopmagnesemia.[10,11] Hypocalcemia can also cause ST, QS, and T-wave changes suggestive of myocardial infarction.[12,13]

Seizures

Generalized tonic-clonic and focal motor seizures have been reported among the presenting symptoms of hypocalcemia, even in the absence of frank tetany. Atypical absence or akinetic seizures also have been reported, although much less frequently.[14-16] Patients with hypocalcemic seizures have both spikes and bursts of high-voltage, paroxysmal slow waves on electroencephalogram (EEG).[17,18] There is no correlation linking a specific serum calcium level to the seizure threshold or to EEG changes in hypocalcemia.

Papilledema

Papilledema can be a finding in severe hypocalcemia from any etiology. The pathophysiological mechanism remains poorly understood. Papilledema may be accompanied by elevated cerebrospinal fluid pressure (eg, benign intracranial hypertension), but pressure is normal in many cases, and the term "pseudopapilledema" has also been used. It has been postulated that hypocalcemia decreases axonal transport, leading to swelling of the axons and optic disc. Papilledema, if present, improves with resolution of hypocalcemia.[19]

Psychiatric Symptoms

Delirium and cognitive impairment have been the most frequently reported psychiatric symptoms associated with acute hypocalcemia; also, irritability, depression, and anxiety.[20] Psychosis is an uncommon presentation of acute hypocalcemia.[21]

CHRONIC MANIFESTATIONS OF HYPOPARATHYROIDISM

The chronic complications of hypoparathyroidism can affect multiple organ systems, including the renal, neurologic, neuropsychiatric, skeletal, and immune systems. These manifestations of hypoparathyroidism may be due to the disease itself or to complications of therapy. Low PTH concentrations, chronic hypocalcemia, relative hypercalcemia, hyperphosphatemia, an elevated calcium × phosphate product, and hypercalciuria have all been postulated to cause the chronic manifestations of hypoparathyroidism. Further research is needed to determine the pathophysiology of complications in hypoparathyroidism and whether interventions can decrease the risk of these complications.

Renal

Retrospective longitudinal analyses of cohorts of hypoparathyroid patients from the United States and Denmark have better characterized the renal complications of the disease. Mitchell and colleagues[22] retrospectively analyzed records from the Massachusetts General Hospital in Boston from 1988 to 2009. They found 120 patients with hypoparathyroidism with an average age of 52 ± 19 years; 73% were women and 66% had a postsurgical etiology with an average duration of 17 ± 16 years. In their cohort, 41% of patients had an estimated glomerular filtration rate less than 60 mL/min per 1.73 m^2, defining stage 3 to 5 chronic kidney disease. They demonstrated that stage 3 to 5 chronic kidney disease in patients with hypoparathyroidism was 2-fold to 35-fold greater than age-appropriate normal values from the National Health and Nutrition Examination Survey. Two patients (1.7%) had undergone renal transplantation for nephrocalcinosis and chronic kidney disease. Age, disease duration, and proportion of time with relative hypercalcemia (defined as serum calcium >9.5 mg/dL) were all significantly negatively associated with renal function. In this cohort, 54 patients had renal imaging during the study period with ultrasound, computed tomography, or both. Of these patients, 31% had evidence of renal calcification.

Underbjerg and colleagues[23,24] retrospectively analyzed medical records from Denmark over a 23-year period (1988–2011) for patients with postoperative hypoparathyroidism, and over a 34-year period (1977–2011) for patients with nonoperative hypoparathyroidism.[25] They identified 688 patients with hypoparathyroidism after neck surgery for nonmalignant disease. The average age was 49 years and 88% were women, with a median disease duration of 8 years. They found 180 patients with nonoperative hypoparathyroidism, and in this cohort the average age was 50 years with 53% female predominance. Most patients in the nonsurgical group presumably had hypoparathyroidism since birth. They matched both cohorts 3:1 with age-matched and sex-matched controls and searched hospital discharge codes for diagnoses. Their study noted that renal insufficiency was threefold higher in postsurgical (hazard ratio [HR] 3.10, 95% confidence interval [CI] 1.73–5.55) and sixfold higher in nonsurgical hypoparathyroidism (HR 6.01, 95% CI 2.45–14.75). Renal stones were fourfold higher in postsurgical hypoparathyroidism (HR 4.02, 95% CI 1.64–9.90) after adjustment for prior diabetes and renal disease.

Due to the very elevated risk of renal disease in patients with hypoparathyroidism, the European Society of Endocrinology guidelines recommend measurement of 24-hour urine calcium and creatinine at least annually and renal imaging if serum creatinine rises or if there are symptoms of nephrolithiasis.[26] The recommended target for urinary calcium excretion is the sex-specific reference range. The First International Workshop on the Management of Hypoparathyroidism also recommends measurement of 24-hour urine calcium and creatinine at least annually and renal imaging at baseline and every 5 years, or earlier if symptoms of stone disease arise.[27–30] Although not certain, ultrasound may be superior to computed tomography in the measurement of intrarenal calcification in patients with hypoparathyroidism.[31]

Neurologic and Neuromotor

As noted under acute manifestations, seizures can occur in the setting of hypocalcemia. In the studies from Underbjerg and colleagues,[23–25] the risk of seizure was more than 10-fold elevated in nonsurgical hypoparathyroidism (HR 10.05, 95% CI

5.39–18.72), and patients with postoperative hypoparathyroidism had a 3.8-fold risk of hospitalization due to seizures (HR, 3.82; 95% CI, 2.15–6.79). Although a matter of clinical judgment, therapy with antiepileptic drugs may not be necessary for patients with epileptic seizures in the setting of hypocalcemia in hypoparathyroidism, even those with subcortical calcification.[32,33]

Basal ganglia calcification was first noted in association with hypoparathyroidism in 1939.[34] The etiology for ectopic calcifications in hypoparathyroidism is thought to be due to an elevated calcium × phosphate product. Another mechanism for basal ganglia calcification specifically may be through the actions of elevated serum phosphorus to activate the inorganic phosphate transporter pit1 (SLC20A1) resulting in the expression of osteogenic molecules in the caudate nucleus and gray matter.[35] Basal ganglia calcification occurs in various infections and other diseases without metabolic disturbances, however, and the exact pathogenic mechanisms require further study.

In the cohort described by Mitchell and colleagues,[22] among 31 patients who had head imaging, 52% were noted to have basal ganglia calcification. Other studies systematically using head imaging have found a prevalence of 69% to 78%, primarily in cohorts of patients with nonsurgical hypoparathyroidism. A study from Goswami and colleagues[36] from India found that 107 (74%) of 145 patients with nonsurgical hypoparathyroidism had basal ganglia calcification and also noted calcifications in the cerebellum and thalamus. They found that the presence of intracerebral calcification was related to the duration of hypocalcemia, presence of cataracts, and the calcium × phosphate ratio. Forman and colleagues[37] from South Africa found that 7 (78%) of 9 patients had basal ganglia calcification, 5 of 7 with surgical and 2 of 2 with nonsurgical disease. They also noted that calcification was related to disease duration and the presence of cataracts.

Neuromotor abnormalities have been described in hypoparathyroidism, in particular symptoms of parkinsonism, including bradykinesia, shuffling gait, and resting tremor.[38] Other extrapyramidal symptoms (chorea, hemiballismus)[39] and cerebellar findings (truncal ataxia, disordered coordination) have also been described.[40] In the study of Mitchell and colleagues,[3,22] only 2 (1.7%) of the 120 patients were noted to have parkinsonism by chart review. The prevalence of extrapyramidal symptoms in smaller case series of patients with hypoparathyroidism has been 4.0% to 12.5%.[38] Whereas brain calcification may be responsible in part for the neuromotor symptoms described in hypoparathyroid patients, in various cases, neuromotor abnormalities were partially, if not completely, reversible with treatment for hypocalcemia.[38,39,41,42]

Aggarwal and colleagues[43] systemically studied 62 patients with idiopathic hypoparathyroidism (age 37 ± 15 years, 44% women, duration 12 ± 9 years) and found that neurologic signs were present in 35.5% of patients with hypoparathyroidism, with extrapyramidal findings in 16.1% and cerebellar findings in 20.9%. Of note, these patients on average were not at biochemical goal as recommended by recent guidelines, with mean serum calcium 5.4 ± 0.9 mg/dL (normal: 8.1–8.5) and serum phosphate 7.0 ± 1.5 mg/dL (normal: 2.5–4.5). They did not find associations between extrapyramidal or cerebellar dysfunction and volume of basal ganglia calcification or number of sites with intracranial calcification.

The First International Workshop on the Management of Hypoparathyroidism recommends central nervous system imaging as clinically indicated.[30]

Neuropsychiatric

In the studies from Underbjerg and colleagues,[23–25] the risk of depression and bipolar disorders was twofold higher in surgical hypoparathyroidism (HR 2.01, 95% CI 1.16–3.50) after adjustment for prior psychiatric diagnosis with a more than twofold risk of hospitalization for psychiatric disease in nonsurgical hypoparathyroidism (HR 2.45, 95% CI 1.78–3.35).

In the investigation referenced previously, Aggarwal and colleagues[43] studied 62 patients with idiopathic hypoparathyroidism compared with 70 controls using a battery of cognitive tests. Age, gender, and level of education between the 2 groups were similar. The investigators used the cognitive dysfunction score, compiling results from the battery of 9 standard tests used in the study and demonstrating increased scores for greater cognitive impairment. The cognitive dysfunction score increased by 2.1 for each 10-year increase in duration of illness and by 5.5 for each 1-unit increase in the calcium-phosphate product (P = .01). The score decreased by 0.27 for each mg/dL increase in serum calcium (P = .001).

Cataracts

The association between hypoparathyroidism and cataract, primarily of the posterior subcapsular type in patients with nonsurgical hypoparathyroidism, was first described in 1880.[44] Pohjola[45] found a 58% prevalence of cataract in 69 patients with nonsurgical hypoparathyroidism. Goswami and colleagues[36] found a 51% prevalence of cataract in nonsurgical disease, correlated to duration of disease and presence of basal ganglia calcification, as noted previously. Saha and colleagues[46] studied 27 patients with idiopathic hypoparathyroidism from the Pohjola cohort undergoing cataract surgery compared with controls. Patients with hypoparathyroidism underwent cataract surgery at a younger age than the control cohort (34 vs 58 years; P<.001) and had a higher incidence of posterior capsular opacification after surgery, requiring subsequent laser capsulotomy.

In the studies from Underbjerg and colleagues,[23–25] patients with nonsurgical hypoparathyroidism were more likely to develop cataracts than controls (HR 4.21, 95% CI 2.13–8.34), with a younger age of onset (53 vs 60 years). There was no difference between patients with postoperative hypoparathyroidism and controls in incidence (HR 1.17, 95% CI 0.66–2.09) or age of onset. As these data are based on hospital discharge codes and not direct clinical examination, the values may be an underrepresentation.

Cardiac

In the studies from Underbjerg and colleagues,[23–25] there were no excess adverse cardiovascular outcomes in patients with surgical hypoparathyroidism, including acute myocardial infarction, cardiac arrest, ischemic heart disease, stroke, or arrhythmia. In nonsurgical patients, there was an increased risk of ischemic heart disease (HR 2.01, 95% CI 1.31–3.09) and all cardiovascular outcomes (HR 1.91, 95% CI 1.29–2.81). As noted previously, the median disease duration in the postsurgical group was 8 years, with most patients in the nonsurgical group having hypoparathyroidism since birth. Chronic hypocalcemia can also cause cardiomyopathy and congestive heart failure that is reversible with treatment of hypocalcemia.[12,47,48]

Quality of Life

Studies using well-defined metrics have demonstrated that quality of life in patients with hypoparathyroidism is reduced. Quality of life is reduced even when patients are taking sufficient calcium and active vitamin D therapy to maintain serum calcium levels at goal.[49–53] PTH2 receptors are expressed in the brains of mammals,[54] and there is evidence that PTH may cross the blood-brain barrier,[55] demonstrating a potential role for PTH in the central nervous system. The effects of hypoparathyroidism on quality of life are underestimated by surgeons and healthy controls.[56] Most investigations in patients with hypoparathyroidism have used the 36-Item Short Form Health Survey (SF-36), a validated measure of health-related quality of life covering 8 domains of physical and mental health. Patients with hypoparathyroidism have reduced quality of life in both physical and mental health domains. In a cohort of 69 patients with hypoparathyroidism, patients with hypoparathyroidism scored below the normative reference range in all physical and mental health domains of the SF-36 survey, with T-scores ranging from -0.9 to -1.4 ($P<.0001$ for all).[51] Of note, the SF-36 quality-of-life instrument is generic and lacks specificity for any disease. At this time, there is no disease-specific questionnaire for hypoparathyroidism. Nevertheless, the fact that such dramatic reductions in quality of life are noted with a general health questionnaire is all-the-more noteworthy.

Skeletal Manifestations

Bone remodeling is markedly reduced in patients with hypoparathyroidism, and bone mineral density values are typically greater than healthy, age-matched controls. The skeletal effects of hypoparathyroidism have been further studied using iliac crest bone biopsies and other high-resolution techniques.[57] The skeletal manifestations of hypoparathyroidism are further covered in detail in Mishaela R. Rubin's article, "Skeletal Manifestations of Hypoparathyroidism," in this issue.

Infection

In the studies from Underbjerg and colleagues,[23–25] the risk of hospitalization due to infection was increased in postsurgical (HR 1.42, 95% CI 1.20–1.67) and nonsurgical disease (HR 1.94, 95% CI 1.55–2.44), particularly urinary tract infections in patients with nonsurgical disease. The excess risk of hospitalization for infection remained significant even after exclusion of urinary tract infections.

Malignancy

In the studies from Underbjerg and colleagues,[23–25] there were no differences in the overall risk of malignancy between patients with postoperative hypoparathyroidism and controls. Patients with postoperative hypoparathyroidism had a lower risk of gastrointestinal malignancy (HR 0.63, 95% CI 0.44–0.93). In nonsurgical disease, there was a lower overall risk of malignancy compared with controls (HR 0.44, 95% CI 0.24–0.82).

Dermatologic

Chronic hypocalcemia is associated with dermatologic manifestations, including dry, rough, puffy, coarse skin; coarse and brittle hair with hair loss; and brittle nails with transverse grooves. The etiology for the nail disorders and dermatologic findings is believed to be angiospasm. These findings are not specific to hypoparathyroidism and can be reversed with treatment of hypocalcemia.[58,59]

Dental

Enamel hypoplasia is the most common dental abnormality in patients with hypocalcemia. In the setting of hypocalcemia during early development before the teeth have entirely formed, dental aplasia or hypoplasia, failure of tooth eruption, defective root formation, and severe dental caries can occur.[60–62] These dental abnormalities are obviously much more common among those with autoimmune forms of hypoparathyroidism.

Manifestations Specific to the Etiology of Disease

Autoimmune polyendocrine syndrome type 1 is characterized by hypoparathyroidism, mucocutaneous candidiasis, and adrenal insufficiency and is associated with other clinical manifestations, including vitiligo and steatorrhea.[63] Genetic etiologies of the disease are associated with a number of other manifestations depending on the genetic defect. Manifestations specific to the etiology of disease are further detailed in Namrah Siraj and colleagues' article, "Medical Hypoparathyroidism," in this issue.

MORTALITY

There are very few data regarding mortality in patients with hypoparathyroidism compared with controls. In the studies from Underbjerg and colleagues,[23–25] mortality was not increased in surgical (HR 0.98, 95% CI 0.76–1.26) or nonsurgical hypoparathyroidism (HR 1.25, 95% CI 0.90–1.73). Of note, Underbjerg and colleagues[23–25] excluded patients with multiple endocrine neoplasia syndrome, individuals with hypoparathyroidism resulting from surgery for thyroid or parathyroid cancer or radiation-induced disease, and those with stage 3 to 5 chronic kidney disease before parathyroid surgery.

SUMMARY

The acute symptoms of hypoparathyroidism are primarily due to neuromuscular irritability associated with hypocalcemia, and can include tetany, seizures, papilledema, delirium, and cognitive impairment. The chronic manifestations may be due to the disease itself or to complications of therapy. In particular, there is concern for the renal system, with patients at increased risk of nephrocalcinosis, nephrolithiasis, and renal insufficiency. Basal ganglia calcification and decreased quality of life are also common. Further research is needed to determine the pathophysiology of complications in hypoparathyroidism and whether interventions can decrease the risk of these complications.

REFERENCES

1. Tohme JF, Bilezikian JP. Hypocalcemic emergencies. Endocrinol Metab Clin North Am 1993;22(2):363–75.
2. Cooper MS, Gittoes NJ. Diagnosis and management of hypocalcaemia. BMJ 2008;336(7656):1298–302.
3. Mannstadt M, Mitchell DM. Clinical manifestations of hypoparathyroidism. In: Bilezikian JP, Marcus R, Levine MA, et al, editors. The parathyroids: basic and clinical concepts. 3rd edition. Waltham (MA): Academic Press; 2015. p. 761–8.
4. Han P, Trinidad BJ, Shi J. Hypocalcemia-induced seizure: demystifying the calcium paradox. ASN Neuro 2015;7(2) [pii:1759091415578050].
5. Urbano FL. Signs of hypocalcemia: Chvostek's and Trousseau's signs. Hosp Physician 2000;36(3):43–5.
6. Hoffman E. The Chvostek sign: a clinical study. Am J Surg 1958;96(1):33 7.
7. Fonseca OA, Calverloy JN. Neurological manifestations of hypoparathyroidism. Arch Intern Med 1967;120(2):202–6.
8. Schaaf M, Payne CA. Effect of diphenylhydantoin and phenobarbital on overt and latent tetany. N Engl J Med 1966;274(22):1228–33.
9. Davis TM, Singh B, Choo KE, et al. Dynamic assessment of the electrocardiographic QT interval during citrate infusion in healthy volunteers. Br Heart J 1995;73(6):523–6.

10. Akiyama T, Batchelder J, Worsman J, et al. Hypocalcemic torsades de pointes. J Electrocardiol 1989;22(1):89–92.

11. Novick T, McMahon BA, Berliner A, et al. Cinacalcet-associated severe hypocalcemia resulting in torsades de pointes and cardiac arrest: a case for caution. Eur J Clin Pharmacol 2016;72(3):373–5.

12. Rallidis LS, Gregoropoulos PP, Papasteriadis EG. A case of severe hypocalcaemia mimicking myocardial infarction. Int J Cardiol 1997;61(1):89–91.

13. Lehmann G, Deisenhofer I, Ndrepepa G, et al. ECG changes in a 25-year-old woman with hypocalcemia due to hypoparathyroidism. Hypocalcemia mimicking acute myocardial infarction. Chest 2000;118(1):260–2.

14. Oki J, Takedatsu M, Itoh J, et al. Hypocalcemic focal seizures in a one-month-old infant of a mother with a low circulating level of vitamin D. Brain Dev 1991;13(2): 132–4.

15. Mrowka M, Knake S, Klinge H, et al. Hypocalcemic generalised seizures as a manifestation of iatrogenic hypoparathyroidism months to years after thyroid surgery. Epileptic Disord 2004;6(2):85–7.

16. Riggs JE. Neurologic manifestations of electrolyte disturbances. Neurol Clin 2002;20(1):227–39.

17. Basser LS, Neale FC, Ireland AW, et al. Epilepsy and electroencephalographic abnormalities in chronic surgical hypoparathyroidism. Ann Intern Med 1969; 71(3):507–15.

18. Swash M, Rowan AJ. Electroencephalographic criteria of hypocalcemia and hypercalcemia. Arch Neurol 1972;26(3):218–28.

19. McLean C, Lobo R, Brazier DJ. Optic disc involvement in hypocalcaemia with hypoparathyroidism: papilloedema or optic neuropathy? Neuroophthalmology 1998;20(3):117–24.

20. Velasco PJ, Manshadi M, Breen K, et al. Psychiatric aspects of parathyroid disease. Psychosomatics 1999;40(6):486–90.

21. Ang AW, Ko SM, Tan CH. Calcium, magnesium, and psychotic symptoms in a girl with idiopathic hypoparathyroidism. Psychosom Med 1995;57(3):299–302.

22. Mitchell DM, Regan S, Cooley MR, et al. Long-term follow-up of patients with hypoparathyroidism. J Clin Endocrinol Metab 2012;97(12):4507–14.

23. Underbjerg L, Sikjaer T, Mosekilde L, et al. Postsurgical hypoparathyroidism—risk of fractures, psychiatric diseases, cancer, cataract, and infections. J Bone Miner Res 2014;29(11):2504–10.

24. Underbjerg L, Sikjaer T, Mosekilde L, et al. Cardiovascular and renal complications to postsurgical hypoparathyroidism: a Danish nationwide controlled historic follow-up study. J Bone Miner Res 2013;28(11):2277–85.

25. Underbjerg L, Sikjaer T, Mosekilde L, et al. The epidemiology of nonsurgical hypoparathyroidism in Denmark: a nationwide case finding study. J Bone Miner Res 2015;30(9):1738–44.

26. Bollerslev J, Rejnmark L, Marcocci C, et al, European Society of Endocrinology. European Society of Endocrinology Clinical Guideline: Treatment of chronic hypoparathyroidism in adults. Eur J Endocrinol 2015;173(2):G1–20.

27. Brandi ML, Bilezikian JP, Shoback D, et al. Management of hypoparathyroidism: summary statement and guidelines. J Clin Endocrinol Metab 2016;101(6): 2273–83.

28. Clarke BL, Brown EM, Collins MT, et al. Epidemiology and diagnosis of hypoparathyroidism. J Clin Endocrinol Metab 2016;101(6):2284–99.

29. Shoback DM, Bilezikian JP, Costa AG, et al. Presentation of hypoparathyroidism: etiologies and clinical features. J Clin Endocrinol Metab 2016;101(6):2300–12.

30. Bilezikian JP, Brandi ML, Cusano NE, et al. Management of Hypoparathyroidism: Present and Future. J Clin Endocrinol Metab 2016;101(6):2313–24.
31. Boyce AM, Shawker TH, Hill SC, et al. Ultrasound is superior to computed tomography for assessment of medullary nephrocalcinosis in hypoparathyroidism. J Clin Endocrinol Metab 2013;98(3):989–94.
32. Modi S, Tripathi M, Saha S, et al. Seizures in patients with idiopathic hypoparathyroidism: effect of antiepileptic drug withdrawal on recurrence of seizures and serum calcium control. Eur J Endocrinol 2014;170(5):777–83.
33. Liu MJ, Li JW, Shi XY, et al. Epileptic seizure, as the first symptom of hypoparathyroidism in children, does not require antiepileptic drugs. Childs Nerv Syst 2017;33(2):297–305.
34. Eaton ML, Camp JD, Love JG. Symmetric cerebral calcification, particularly of the basal ganglia, demonstrable roentgenographically calcification of the finer cerebral blood vessels. Arch Neurol Psychiatry 1939;41(5):921–42.
35. Goswami R, Millo T, Mishra S, et al. Expression of osteogenic molecules in the caudate nucleus and gray matter and their potential relevance for basal ganglia calcification in hypoparathyroidism. J Clin Endocrinol Metab 2014;99(5):1741–8.
36. Goswami R, Sharma R, Sreenivas V, et al. Prevalence and progression of basal ganglia calcification and its pathogenic mechanism in patients with idiopathic hypoparathyroidism. Clin Endocrinol (Oxf) 2012;77(2):200–6.
37. Forman MB, Sandler MP, Danziger A, et al. Basal ganglia calcification in postoperative hypoparathyroidism. Clin Endocrinol (Oxf) 1980;12(4):385–90.
38. Abe S, Tojo K, Ichida K, et al. A rare case of idiopathic hypoparathyroidism with varied neurological manifestations. Intern Med 1996;35(2):129–34.
39. Baumert T, Kleber G, Schwarz J, et al. Reversible hyperkinesia in a patient with autoimmune polyglandular syndrome type I. Clin Investig 1993;71(11):924–7.
40. Gay JD, Grimes JD. Idiopathic hypoparathyroidism with impaired vitamin B 12 absorption and neuropathy. Can Med Assoc J 1972;107(1):54–6, passim.
41. Berger JR, Ross DB. Reversible Parkinson syndrome complicating postoperative hypoparathyroidism. Neurology 1981;31(7):881–2.
42. Tambyah PA, Ong BK, Lee KO. Reversible parkinsonism and asymptomatic hypocalcemia with basal ganglia calcification from hypoparathyroidism 26 years after thyroid surgery. Am J Med 1993;94(4):444–5.
43. Aggarwal S, Kailash S, Sagar R, et al. Neuropsychological dysfunction in idiopathic hypoparathyroidism and its relationship with intracranial calcification and serum total calcium. Eur J Endocrinol 2013;168(6):895–903.
44. Granström KO, Hed R. Idiopathic hypoparathyroidism with cataract and spontaneous hypocalcaemic hypercalciuria. Acta Med Scand 1965;178(4):417–21.
45. Pohjola S. Ocular manifestations of idiopathic hypoparathyroidism. Acta Ophthalmol (Copenh) 1962;40:255–65.
46. Saha S, Gantyala SP, Aggarwal S, et al. Long-term outcome of cataract surgery in patients with idiopathic hypoparathyroidism and its relationship with their calcemic status. J Bone Miner Metab 2017;35(4):405–11.
47. Bashour T, Basha HS, Cheng TO. Hypocalcemic cardiomyopathy. Chest 1980; 78(4):663–5.
48. Wong CK, Lau CP, Cheng CH, et al. Hypocalcemic myocardial dysfunction: short- and long-term improvement with calcium replacement. Am Heart J 1990; 120(2):381–6.
49. Arlt W, Fremerey C, Callies F, et al. Well-being, mood and calcium homeostasis in patients with hypoparathyroidism receiving standard treatment with calcium and vitamin D. Eur J Endocrinol 2002;146(2):215–22.

50. Cusano NE, Rubin MR, McMahon DJ, et al. The effect of PTH(1-84) on quality of life in hypoparathyroidism. J Clin Endocrinol Metab 2013;98(6):2356–61.
51. Cusano NE, Rubin MR, McMahon DJ, et al. PTH(1-84) is associated with improved quality of life in hypoparathyroidism through 5 years of therapy. J Clin Endocrinol Metab 2014;99(10):3694–9.
52. Sikjaer T, Rolighed L, Hess A, et al. Effects of PTH(1-84) therapy on muscle function and quality of life in hypoparathyroidism: results from a randomized controlled trial. Osteoporos Int 2014;25(6):1717–26.
53. Sikjaer T, Moser E, Rolighed L, et al. Concurrent hypoparathyroidism is associated with impaired physical function and quality of life in hypothyroidism. J Bone Miner Res 2016;31(7):1440–8.
54. Usdin TB, Gruber C, Bonner TI. Identification and functional expression of a receptor selectively recognizing parathyroid hormone, the PTH2 receptor. J Biol Chem 1995;270(26):15455–8.
55. Care AD, Bell NH. Evidence that parathyroid hormone crosses the blood-brain barrier. In: Cohn DV, Martin TJ, Meunier PJ, editors. Calcium regulation and bone metabolism: basic and clinical aspects: proceedings of the 9th International Conference on Calcium Regulating Hormones and Bone Metabolism, Nice, France. October 25-November 1, 1986. New York: Elsevier; 1987. p. 540.
56. Cho NL, Moalem J, Chen L, et al. Surgeons and patients disagree on the potential consequences from hypoparathyroidism. Endocr Pract 2014;20(5):427–46.
57. Silva BC, Rubin MR, Cusano NE, et al. Bone imaging in hypoparathyroidism. Osteoporos Int 2017;28(2):463–71.
58. Learner N, Brown CL. Ectodermal disorders in chronic hypoparathyroidism. J Clin Endocrinol Metab 1943;3(5):261–4.
59. Fuleihan Gel-H, Rubeiz N. Dermatologic manifestations of parathyroid-related disorders. Clin Dermatol 2006;24(4):281–8.
60. Albright F. The parathyroids—physiology and therapeutics. JAMA 1941;117(7):527–33.
61. Goepferd SJ, Flaitz CM. Enamel hypoplasia associated with congenital hypoparathyroidism. Pediatr Dent 1981;3(2):196–200.
62. Gallacher AA, Pemberton MN, Waring DT. The dental manifestations and orthodontic implications of hypoparathyroidism in childhood. J Orthod 2017;30:1–5.
63. Ahonen P, Myllärniemi S, Sipilä I, et al. Clinical variation of autoimmune polyendocrinopathy-candidiasis-ectodermal dystrophy (APECED) in a series of 68 patients. N Engl J Med 1990;322(26):1829–36.

Epidemiology and Complications of Hypoparathyroidism

Bart L. Clarke, MD

KEYWORDS

- Hypoparathyroidism • Hypocalcemia • Hyperphosphatemia • Parathyroid hormone
- Prevalence • Incidence • Epidemiology

KEY POINTS

- Hypoparathyroidism is a rare endocrine disorder.
- Recent studies have evaluated the prevalence of this disorder in a number of countries as ranging between 10.1 and 40.0 per 100,000.
- Two studies have provided incidence estimates for hypoparathyroidism of 0.8 and 2.6 per 100,000 person-years.
- The risk of complications of hypoparathyroidism are defined by studies from Denmark and Boston.
- Mortality from hypoparathyroidism is not thought to be increased.

INTRODUCTION

Anterior neck surgery is the most common cause of the rare endocrine disorder of hypoparathyroidism. Other than anterior neck surgery, causes may include autoimmunity, iron or copper overload, tumor infiltration of the parathyroid glands, radiation treatment, and inherited causes including isolated hypoparathyroidism and forms of hypoparathyroidism associated with other syndromic features.

Mild to moderate hypocalcemia resulting from hypoparathyroidism frequently manifests with symptoms including neuromuscular irritability leading to tingling paresthesias of the finger tips, toe tips, or lips, and muscle cramps or tetany. More severe hypocalcemia due to hypoparathyroidism may result in other symptoms or signs, including bronchospasm, laryngospasm, seizures, cardiac rhythm disturbances, or sudden death. Classic signs of hypocalcemia due to hypoparathyroidism include Chvostek and Trousseau signs, QTc interval prolongation, and brain and other soft tissue calcification.

Disclosure Statement: The author has nothing to disclose.
Division of Endocrinology, Diabetes, Metabolism, and Nutrition, Mayo Clinic, E18-A, 200 1st Street SW, Rochester, MN 55905, USA
E-mail address: clarke.bart@mayo.edu

Endocrinol Metab Clin N Am 47 (2018) 771–782
https://doi.org/10.1016/j.ecl.2018.07.004
0889-8529/18/© 2018 Elsevier Inc. All rights reserved.

endo.theclinics.com

Until recently, very few studies have described the epidemiology of this rare disorder. A number of large population-based studies have recently been published from different countries describing the prevalence and incidence of hypoparathyroidism. Some of these studies have included information regarding the epidemiology of both postsurgical and nonsurgical hypoparathyroidism. In addition, a number of studies have now been published describing the prevalence of complications of this disorder. This review summarizes the published medical literature regarding the prevalence and incidence of this disorder, and the risk of known complications of hypoparathyroidism.

EPIDEMIOLOGY

Surgical procedures on the anterior neck lead to the most common form of adult hypoparathyroidism. Postsurgical hypoparathyroidism is responsible for approximately 75% of all cases of hypoparathyroidism.[1,2] The next most common cause in adults is thought to be autoimmune disease, either affecting only the parathyroid glands, or multiple other endocrine glands.[3] Remaining cases are due to a variety of rare disorders in which the parathyroid glands are infiltrated by cancer or iron or copper overload, or radiation treatment, or rare genetic isolated or syndromic disorders.[4]

PREVALENCE

The best prevalence estimate of chronic hypoparathyroidism in the United States is based on analysis of a large health plan claims database, which identified a total of 77,000 cases.[5] This figure was derived by interpolation from a large US claims database with 77 million patients from 75 health plans during October 2007 to September 2008. The interpolation resulted in an estimated 58,793 US adult patients in these insurance plans that had been diagnosed with chronic hypoparathyroidism. This prevalence estimate was based on the number of new diagnoses of hypoparathyroidism in the database over the interval studied. A surgical incidence estimate was also performed, based on calculation of the proportion of total neck operations that resulted in transient (<6 months) or chronic (>6 months) hypoparathyroidism. A physician primary market research study was performed to assess disease severity in postsurgical hypoparathyroid patients, and to determine the percentage of new nonsurgical patients having this disorder. The surgical incidence data were entered into an epidemiologic model to derive a surgical prevalence estimate. The surgical prevalence approach estimated that 117,342 relevant neck surgeries had been performed during this interval, resulting in 8901 new cases of hypoparathyroidism over 12 months. It was estimated that 7.6% of surgeries resulted in hypoparathyroidism, with 75% of these cases being transient, and 25% chronic. The prevalence estimate of insured patients with chronic hypoparathyroidism in the surgical database was 58,625, similar to that obtained in the diagnostic estimate. Assuming that 15.4% of the US population did not have medical insurance at the time this study was done, these findings were extrapolated to give an estimate of 77,000 total insured and uninsured individuals in the United States with hypoparathyroidism.

The longitudinal population-based Rochester Epidemiology Project was used to derive a separate prevalence estimate of hypoparathyroidism. This system used medical records linkage resources to identify all persons residing in Olmsted County, Minnesota, in 2009 with any diagnosis of hypoparathyroidism assigned by a health care provider since 1945.[6] Detailed medical records were reviewed to confirm the diagnosis of hypoparathyroidism and to assign an etiology. All patients with hypoparathyroidism were assigned 2 age-matched and sex-matched controls. Fifty-four cases of hypoparathyroidism were confirmed, with mean age 58 ± 20 years, and 71% women, giving a prevalence estimate of 37 per 100,000 (**Table 1**). This prevalence estimate was used to estimate that approximately 115,000 patients in the United States have hypoparathyroidism of any cause. In this Olmsted County cohort, hypoparathyroidism was caused by neck surgery in 78% of cases, other secondary causes in 9%, familial disorders in 7%, and idiopathic in 6%.

In the nationwide Danish historic cohort study, the prevalence of hypoparathyroidism was estimated using data from the Danish National Patient Registry.[7–9] This study assessed mortality and comorbidities by comparing patients with hypoparathyroidism with age-matched and sex-matched population-based controls. Search of the Danish National Patient Registry revealed a total of 1849 patients with postsurgical hypoparathyroidism, and 180 patients with nonsurgical hypoparathyroidism. Among these, 1127 patients with postsurgical hypoparathyroidism and 123 patients with nonsurgical hypoparathyroidism, respectively, were alive at the time of follow-up. The estimated prevalence of postsurgical hypoparathyroidism was 22.0 per 100,000, and estimated prevalence of nonsurgical hypoparathyroidism was 2.3 per 100,000, respectively (see **Table 1**). Of the postsurgical cases, approximately 33% had acquired postsurgical hypoparathyroidism due to surgery for malignant diseases (mainly thyroid cancer), 33% due to surgery for nontoxic goiter, 25% due to surgery for toxic goiter, and 10% due to surgery for primary hyperparathyroidism.[7]

A population-based study was undertaken to describe the prevalence and incidence of hypoparathyroidism in Tayside, Scotland.[10] The investigators evaluated electronically linked data on biochemistry, hospital admissions, prescriptions, and death records in this city area from 1988 to 2015. Inclusion criteria required that patients have at least 3 serum albumin-corrected calcium concentrations below the reference range taken in an outpatient setting to be included in the study. Patients who had developed severe chronic kidney disease before low calcium levels were detected were excluded from the study. Patients with hypocalcemia were further screened for previous neck surgery or irradiation, low serum parathyroid hormone (PTH), or treatment with vitamin D. Patients were categorized as having either a postsurgical or nonsurgical cause, or having secondary hypoparathyroidism due to a recognized cause, for example, hypomagnesemia. Overall, 18,955 patients were identified with hypocalcemia. Of these, 222 patients were identified as having hypoparathyroidism, and 116 with postsurgical and 106 with nonsurgical chronic hypoparathyroidism. In 2015, the prevalence estimate for primary hypoparathyroidism was calculated to be 40 per 100,000, with a rate of 23 per 100,000 for postsurgical hypoparathyroidism, and rate of 17 per 100,000 for nonsurgical hypoparathyroidism (see

Table 1
Prevalence of hypoparathyroidism

Country	Hypoparathyroidism per 100,000	Postsurgical Hypoparathyroidism per 100,000	Nonsurgical Hypoparathyroidism per 100,000
Rochester, Minnesota[6]	37.0	29.0	8.0
Denmark[7–9]	24.3	22.0	2.3
Scotland[10]	40.0	23.0	17.0
Italy[11]	34.0	—	—
Italy[12]	27.0	—	—
Norway[13]	10.1	6.4	3.0

Table 1). Of the postsurgical hypoparathyroidism cohort, 80% were women, and 64% were women in the nonsurgical hypoparathyroidism group. Mean serum calcium at diagnosis for these patients was 7.28 ± 0.96 (SD) mg/dL (1.82 ± 0.24 mmol/L). The annual incidence rate over the 27-year interval studied was estimated to vary from 1 to 4 per 100,000. Overall, 71% of the patients were prescribed calcium and/or vitamin D, whereas activated vitamin D was prescribed for 48% of the postsurgical cases and 43% of the nonsurgical cases. Thyroxine and/or hydrocortisone were prescribed to more than 90% of the postsurgical cases and to 64% of the nonsurgical cases. This study concluded that the prevalence of surgical chronic hypoparathyroidism was similar to that reported in previous studies, but that nonsurgical chronic hypoparathyroidism in this population-based study was greater than previously reported. Many of the patients categorized as having chronic hypoparathyroidism had mild hypocalcemia and were not prescribed any treatment.

A retrospective register-based study investigated the prevalence of different forms of hypoparathyroidism among hospitalized patients in Italy over an 8-year period.[11] The investigators evaluated data from hospital discharge records maintained by the Italian Health Ministry from 2006 to 2013, and analyzed the codes corresponding to hypoparathyroidism-related diagnoses. The inpatient prevalence of the disease was calculated after excluding repeated hospitalizations for the same diagnosis. Overall, 27,692 hospitalization episodes for hypoparathyroidism were identified during this interval. Of these episodes, 72.2% occurred in women, and 27.8% in men, with mean age of 49.5 ± 22.9 years. The mean length of hospital stay was 7.4 ± 9.8 days, with 25.9% of the episodes requiring fewer than 3 days of hospital stay. The mean hospitalization rate for hypoparathyroidism was 5.9 per 100,000 inhabitants per year, and a significant decrease was observed to occur during the interval of 2006 to 2013 ($P<.0001$) (see Table 1). The mean hospitalization rate for postsurgical hypoparathyroidism was estimated to be 1.4 per 100,000 inhabitants per year, and this rate also showed a significant reduction over the same years ($P<.0001$). The mean prevalence of hypoparathyroidism among inpatients was 5.3 per 100,000 inhabitants, and a significant decrease also occurred in the prevalence over these same years ($P<.0001$). The study concluded that hypoparathyroidism, particularly the postsurgical form of this disorder, is not uncommon among hospitalized patients in Italy, and that there seemed to be a decrease in the frequency of hospitalization for this condition during the period 2006 to 2013.

Another study in Italy[12] assessed the prevalence of permanent hypoparathyroidism and incidence of surgical hypoparathyroidism by analysis of an electronic anonymous public health care database in the Region of Tuscany. Data corresponding to the 5-year period from 2009 to 2013 were analyzed, with the assumption that this sample was representative of the entire Mediterranean European population, with an estimated mean population of 3,750,000 inhabitants. Data were retrieved by analyzing a national pharmaceutical distribution dataset, containing data related to drugs reimbursed by the public health system, hospital discharge and procedure codes, and *International Classification of Diseases, Ninth Revision* (ICD-9) exemption codes for chronic diseases. A specific algorithm was applied to indirectly identify people with permanent hypoparathyroidism by requiring chronic therapy with active vitamin D metabolites. The number of people taking active vitamin D metabolites for a period equal to or longer than 6 months until the end of the study period, with ICD-9 exemption code for hypoparathyroidism, and with a disease-related discharge code were identified. Within this restricted group, patients with chronic kidney disease and osteoporosis were excluded. The indirect estimate of the prevalence of permanent hypoparathyroidism in this Mediterranean European population by means of the analysis of chronic therapy with active vitamin D metabolites was 27 per 100,000 in-habitants, with the female-to-male ratio 2.2:1.0, and mean age 63.5 ± 16.7 years (see **Table 1**). The risk of developing permanent hypoparathyroidism after neck sur-gery in this cohort was 1.5%. Although this epidemiologic approach based on disease codes and hospital discharge codes underestimates the prevalence of hypoparathy-roidism, the indirect estimate of this disease prevalence through the analysis of pre-scriptions of active vitamin D metabolites in a European region is in line with the results of studies performed in other regions of the world.

A group of investigators in Norway attempted to determine the prevalence, etiol-ogies, health-related quality of life (HRQoL), and treatment pattern for hospitalized pa-tients with hypoparathyroidism in this country.[13] Patients with hypoparathyroidism and patients with 22q11 deletion syndrome (DiGeorge syndrome) were identified by search of electronic hospital registries. All patients identified were invited to partici-pate in a survey. Among patients who responded, HRQoL was assessed using the Short Form-36 and Hospital Anxiety and Depression scale. Autoantibodies were measured, and candidate genes including calcium sensing receptor (CaSR), AIRE, GATA3, and 22q11-deletion were sequenced for mutations to classify the etiology of genetic forms of hypoparathyroidism. A total of 522 patients, 511 of whom were alive, were identified, with an estimated overall prevalence of 102 per million (10.2 per 100,000) (see **Table 1**). These cases were divided among postsurgical hypo-parathyroidism, with an estimated prevalence of 64 per million (6.4 per 100,000), nonsurgical hypoparathyroidism, with an estimated prevalence of 30 per million (3.0 per 100,000), and pseudohypoparathyroidism, with an estimated prevalence of 8 per million (0.8 per 100,000). The cohort with nonsurgical hypoparathyroidism included patients with autosomal dominant hypocalcemia (21%), autoimmune polyen-docrine syndrome type 1 (17%), DiGeorge/22q11 deletion syndrome (15%), idiopathic hypoparathyroidism (44%), and others (4%). Among the 283 survey respondents of median age 53 years (range, 9–89), 75% were female individuals, and 7 patients formerly classified as idiopathic were reclassified after genetic and immunologic ana-lyses were completed, whereas 26 cases (37% of the nonsurgical hypoparathyroidism cohort) remained idiopathic. Most patients were treated with vitamin D (94%) and cal-cium (70%), and 10 received PTH therapy. Patients with hypoparathyroidism scored significantly worse than the normative population on Short Form-36 and Hospital Anx-iety and Depression scales. Patients with postsurgical hypoparathyroidism scored worse than those with nonsurgical hypoparathyroidism and pseudohypoparathyroid-ism, especially with regard to physical health. The study concluded that the preva-lence of nonsurgical hypoparathyroidism in Norway was higher than reported elsewhere. Genetic testing and autoimmunity screening of patients with idiopathic hy-poparathyroidism identified a specific cause in 21%. Further research was felt to be necessary to identify the causes of idiopathic hypoparathyroidism, and to improve the reduced HRQoL reported by patients with hypoparathyroidism.

An estimate of the prevalence of hypoparathyroidism in Hungary was facilitated by a single state health insurance company that insures most residents, with information on the population of 10 million maintained in a single database. Evaluation of this data base by diagnosis of permanent hypoparathyroidism from 2004 to 2013 demonstrated a prevalence estimate of approximately 1000 patients with permanent hypoparathy-roidism in 2013. The yearly prevalence estimate of hypoparathyroidism increased by more than 60% over this period, whereas the ratio of females to males of 4:1 did not change. Regional differences and trends in the incidence of hypoparathyroidism over time were reported as relatively constant across the country, after adjusting for the population in each region. An annual average of 5000 thyroid-related operations are performed in Hungary. Transient postsurgical hypoparathyroidism was estimated to occur in 31% of these cases, whereas permanent postsurgical hypoparathyroidism was estimated to occur in 1.9%. Surgical centers with experienced endocrine surgeons reported lower rates of post-thyroid surgical permanent hypoparathyroidism of 0.1% to 5.8%. Several confounding factors were thought to influence these estimates. The incidence of hypoparathyroidism was reported to increase dramatically to approximately 15% after a second neck operation. The study concluded that postsurgical hypoparathyroidism is the most common cause of hypoparathyroidism in Hungary, as in other countries.[13]

Postsurgical hypoparathyroidism is thought to be the cause of 95% of cases of permanent hypoparathyroidism in Russia, which is significantly higher than in other countries.[14] In Russia, estimates of rates of postsurgical permanent hypoparathyroidism vary between 1% and 40%.[15]

INCIDENCE

Acquired hypoparathyroidism typically occurs due to irreversible damage to, or removal of parathyroid glands, or due to damage to the vascular supply of the parathyroid glands. The incidence of postsurgical hypoparathyroidism depends on the surgical center, type of surgical intervention, and expertise of the surgeons involved. Transient postsurgical hypoparathyroidism lasting for less than 6 months is estimated to occur in 25.4% to 83.0% of patients worldwide after neck surgery,[16] whereas permanent postsurgical hypoparathyroidism lasting for more than 6 months has been estimated to occur in 0.12% to 4.6% of cases.[17,18] Incidence estimates of nonsurgical causes of hypoparathyroidism are generally not available in the United States and most other countries due to the infrequency of the causes that lead to hypoparathyroidism.

In the Danish historic cohort study, the incidence of postsurgical hypoparathyroidism was reported to be 0.8 per 100,000 per year[7] (**Table 2**). No other European studies have reported the incidence of postsurgical hypoparathyroidism. Estimates of the incidence of nonsurgical causes of hypoparathyroidism are generally not available in most other European countries either, but the incidence of autoimmune hypoparathyroidism due to autoimmune polyendocrinopathy syndrome type 1 in Hungary was estimated at 1 per million.[19]

A group of investigators investigated the incidence of various parathyroid disorders in a cohort of health care personnel in India who were followed over a long interval.[20] This retrospective, descriptive epidemiologic study was performed using data from the electronic medical records of health care personnel enrolled between 1990 and 2015. Subjects in the study were recruited between the ages of 17 and 20 years and in good health. The study calculated the incidence rates of parathyroid disorders in person-years using appropriate statistical methods. The analysis included 51,217 participants of median age 33 years (range, 17–54 years), with mean follow-up of 12.5 years. Yearly evaluation of the data gave a cumulative follow-up duration of

Table 2 Incidence of hypoparathyroidism	
	Hypoparathyroidism per 100,000
Denmark[7]	0.8
India[20]	2.6

613,925 person-years. Hypoparathyroidism was diagnosed in 16 patients, giving an incidence rate of 2.6 per 100,000 person-years (see **Table 2**). One patient was diagnosed with pseudohypoparathyroidism, for an incidence rate of 0.16 per 100,000 person-years. Of 37 patients identified with primary hyperparathyroidism in the study, 16 (43%) developed postsurgical hypoparathyroidism. The study concluded that this cohort had a low incidence of hypoparathyroidism, similar to that reported in the Danish historic cohort study. Long-term epidemiologic studies were felt to be essential to identify the demographic trends of metabolic bone disorders in India.

COST AND HOSPITALIZATION

Leibson and colleagues[21] performed a population-based study to assess the overall cost of medical care for patients with hypoparathyroidism in Olmsted County, Minnesota. Yearly cost of medical care for patients with hypoparathyroidism in 2007 to 2009 was estimated to be approximately 3 times that for healthy patients. This study was unable to quantify expenditures related to, or the frequency of utilization of, outpatient clinics, hospitals, emergency departments, or pharmacies. No other studies have yet reported the frequency of hospitalization of patients with hypoparathyroidism relative to healthy controls, but it is probable that hospitalization for complications of hypoparathyroidism, such as tetany, bronchospasm, laryngospasm, seizures, or cardiac dysrhythmias, is higher than in the general population. If one were to factor in these cost estimates for care of patients with hypoparathyroidism, they are likely to be much higher than that reported in the Olmsted County experience.

MORBIDITIES

The morbidities reported to be associated with hypoparathyroidism are thought to be directly related to hypocalcemia and/or to hyperphosphatemia, or indirectly due to treatment effects from excessive or insufficient amounts of calcium and/or active vitamin D. Patients who are inadequately treated commonly experience symptoms and signs of neuromuscular excitability, including tetany, due mainly to hypocalcemia. Patients who are overtreated with excessive amounts of calcium and vitamin D frequently develop hypercalcemia and/or hypercalciuria. Changes in quality of life experienced by these patients, such as alteration in sense of well-being and mood, may be related to the disorder itself, or to its treatment. This is apparently also true for ectopic calcifications that can occur in the basal ganglia and gray-white matter interface in the brain, in the kidney, and rarely, in other tissues. Other complications of hypoparathyroidism include posterior subcapsular cataracts and reduced skeletal remodeling.

Clarke and colleagues[6] demonstrated that patients with hypoparathyroidism in Olmsted County, Minnesota, were significantly more likely than healthy age-matched and sex-matched controls to have at least 1 diagnosis within 7 of 17 major disease categories, and 16 of 113 subcategories of disease within the major categories, as defined by the ICD-9-CM (Clinical Modification) system. Mitchell and colleagues[22] evaluated the prevalence of various morbidities associated with permanent hypoparathyroidism in a large Boston health system from 1988 to 2009. A total of 120 patients aged 52 ± 19 years were identified, with 73% women. Of the 54 patients who had renal imaging during follow-up over this interval, 31% had renal calcifications. Of 31 patients with head imaging, 52% had basal ganglia calcifications. The study showed that stage 3 to 5 chronic kidney disease was 2-fold to 17-fold greater than age-appropriate renal function.

In a more detailed analysis, the Danish national cohort study[7] reported that renal disease of all types was more than threefold greater in patients with postsurgical (hazard ratio [HR] 3.67; 95% confidence interval [CI] 2.41–5.59) and nonsurgical hypoparathyroidism (HR 3.39; 95% CI 1.67–6.88) compared with the general population (**Table 3**). The risk of renal insufficiency was reported to be threefold higher in postsurgical (HR 3.10; 95% CI 1.73–5.55) and sixfold higher in nonsurgical hypoparathyroidism (HR 6.01; 95% CI 2.45–14.75) compared with the general population. Patients with postsurgical hypoparathyroidism had a fourfold increased risk of being hospitalized due to renal stone disease (HR 4.02; 95% CI 1.64–9.90), whereas an estimate was not reported for the nonsurgical cohort.

In the Danish national cohort study,[8] cardiovascular disease was not increased in postsurgical hypoparathyroidism, but patients with nonsurgical hypoparathyroidism had a significantly increased risk of ischemic heart disease (HR 2.01; 95% CI 1.31–3.09) and any cardiovascular disease (HR 1.91; 95% CI 1.29–2.81) compared with the general population (see **Table 3**). The study also reported that a higher proportion of patients with nonsurgical hypoparathyroidism had been hospitalized due to stroke (HR 1.84; 95% CI 0.95–3.94; $P = .03$) or arrhythmia (HR 1.78; 95% CI 0.96–3.30; $P = .03$), whereas risk of stroke and arrhythmia in the postsurgical hypoparathyroidism cohort was not different from in the general population.

Hospitalization for neuropsychiatric disease in the Danish national cohort study[8] was significantly increased by 2.45-fold in patients with postsurgical hypoparathyroidism, and by 1.78-fold in patients with nonsurgical hypoparathyroidism (HR 2.45, 95% CI 1.78–3.35), compared with the general population (see **Table 3**). Among patients with surgical hypoparathyroidism, risk of depression and bipolar disorders was significantly increased (HR 2.01; 95% CI 1.16–3.50), but not in patients with nonsurgical hypoparathyroidism.

Risk of being hospitalized due to an infection in the Danish national cohort study[8] was significantly increased among patients with postsurgical (HR 1.42; 95% CI 1.20–1.67) and nonsurgical hypoparathyroidism (HR 1.94; 95% CI 1.55–2.44), compared with the general population (see **Table 3**). Risk of urinary tract infections was borderline significantly increased in postsurgical (HR 1.36; 95% CI 0.97–1.91) and significantly increased in nonsurgical hypoparathyroidism (HR 3.84; 95% CI 2.24–6.60), compared with the general population. Risk of hospitalization due to infection remained significantly increased after exclusion of hospitalizations due to urinary

Table 3		
Risk of mortality and hospitalization for complications of hypoparathyroidism		
	Postsurgical Hypoparathyroidism	**Nonsurgical Hypoparathyroidism**
Mortality[7]	0.96 (0.76–1.26)	1.25 (0.90–1.73)
Renal insufficiency[7,9]	3.10 (1.73–5.55)	6.01 (2.45–14.75)
Renal stones[7,9]	4.02 (1.54–9.90)	—
Ischemic cardiovascular disease[7,9]	1.09 (0.83–1.45)	2.01 (1.31–3.09)
Neuropsychiatric disease[8,9]	1.26 (1.01–1.56)	2.45 (1.78–3.36)
Seizures[8,9]	3.82 (2.15–6.79)	10.05 (5.39–18.72)
Cataracts[8,9]	1.17 (0.66–2.09)	4.21 (2.13–8.34)
Upper extremity fractures[8,9]	0.69 (0.49–0.97)	1.93 (1.31–2.85)
Intracerebral calcifications, %[26–29]	56	69–74

Values are hazard ratio (95% confidence interval) unless otherwise indicated.

tract infections. Calcium is known to serve many physiologic functions, so it is not surprising that hypocalcemia might affect the immune response to infections. Calcium has been reported to act as a second messenger in infection-fighting neutrophils, which in part depends on extracellular calcium.[23]

Hospitalization for seizures in the Danish national cohort study[8] was significantly increased in postsurgical (HR 3.82; 95% CI 2.15–6.79) and in nonsurgical hypoparathyroidism (HR 10.05; 95% CI 5.39–18.72), compared with the general population (see **Table 3**). Cataracts were significantly increased in nonsurgical hypoparathyroidism (HR 4.21; 95% CI 2.13–8.34), but not in postsurgical hypoparathyroidism (HR 1.17; 95% CI 0.66–2.09). Risk of fractures, as well as risk of fractures at specific skeletal sites, did not differ between patients and controls. However, patients with postsurgical hypoparathyroidism had a decreased risk of upper extremity fracture (HR 0.69; 95% CI 0.49–0.97), whereas patients with nonsurgical hypoparathyroidism had an increased risk of upper extremity fracture (HR 1.93; 95% CI 1.31–2.85), compared with the general population, including risk of fractures at the forearm (HR 2.83; 95% CI 1.43–5.63) and proximal humerus (HR 2.81; 95% CI 1.34–5.85). Another study from India reported an increased risk of vertebral fractures in patients with idiopathic hypoparathyroidism.[24] In light of these conflicting reports, the effect of postsurgical and nonsurgical hypoparathyroidism on fracture risk remains uncertain.

Hypoparathyroidism is associated with increased risk of a variety of morbidities, with some risks seen in both postsurgical and nonsurgical hypoparathyroidism, but others seen mainly in one form of hypoparathyroidism or the other. Only a few data are available on risk factors for the various morbidities and complications, however. A Danish study used a case-control design to assess associations between biochemical findings and risk of different complications within a subpopulation of the previously identified Danish national cohort patients.[25] The investigators retrieved all biochemical data available on 431 (81% women) patients from the central region of Denmark, covering approximately 20% of the Danish population. Average age of patients was 41 years at time of diagnosis. Most patients (88%) had hypoparathyroidism due to surgery, mainly due to atoxic goiter, and more than 95% were on treatment with calcium supplements and activated vitamin D. On average, time-weighted (tw) plasma levels of ionized calcium (Ca^{2+} tw) was 1.17 mmol/L (4.68 mg/dL) (interquartile range, 1.14–1.21 mmol/L; 4.56–4.84 mg/dL), and the tw calcium-phosphate product ($Ca^{2+} \times$ P tw) was 2.80 (interquartile range, 2.51–3.03) $mmol^2/L^2$. High phosphate tw levels were associated with increased mortality and risk of any infections, including infections of the upper airways. A high $Ca^{2+} \times$ P tw product was associated with an increased mortality and risk of renal disease. Compared with levels around the lower part of the reference interval, lower Ca^{2+} tw levels were associated with an increased risk of cardiovascular diseases. Mortality and risk of infections, cardiovascular disease, and renal disease all increased with the number of episodes of hypercalcemia and with increased disease duration. Treatment with a relatively high dose of active vitamin D was associated with decreased mortality and risk of renal diseases and infections. The study concluded that risk of complications in hypoparathyroidism is closely associated with disturbances in calcium-phosphate homeostasis.

In a small case series from Denmark of 16 patients with nonsurgical hypoparathyroidism and 8 patients with pseudohypoparathyroidism,[26] the presence of intracranial calcifications was systematically investigated by computed tomography (CT) imaging. Calcifications were detected in 69% of the patients with nonsurgical hypoparathyroidism, and in all patients with pseudohypoparathyroidism. In all 19 patients identified to have intracerebral calcifications, the globus pallidus was affected. In 5 patients, calcifications were found only in the globus pallidus, whereas the remaining 14 patients also had calcifications in their caudate nucleus. The putamen was affected in 11 cases, the thalamus in 10, and the cerebral cortex in 9 patients. Calcifications in the cerebellum and brainstem were found in 4 cases and 3 cases, respectively. Similar findings were reported in a study from India,[27] including 145 patients with nonsurgical hypoparathyroidism, among whom 74% had intracranial calcifications. In this study, independent predictors of progression of calcification were a history of seizures at presentation (odds ratio [OR] 9.42; 95% CI 1.68–52.74), and the calcium/phosphorus ratio during follow-up. For every 1% increase in the calcium/phosphorus ratio during follow-up, the odds of progression decreased by 5% (OR 0.95; 95% CI 0.93–0.99). Intracranial calcifications have also been reported in longstanding postsurgical hypoparathyroidism, and may be associated with Parkinson-like symptoms,[28] but these symptoms resolved with control of blood calcium. In a small case series of 9 patients with postsurgical hypoparathyroidism, calcifications were detected by CT imaging in 5 patients.[29] These studies suggest that intracerebral calcifications are commonly associated with longer-standing hypoparathyroidism, but that the association between these intracerebral calcifications and Parkinson-like symptoms is not yet established.

In the Danish cohort study,[8] risk of gastrointestinal cancer was significantly decreased in postsurgical hypoparathyroidism (HR 0.63; 95% CI 0.44–0.93), with a tendency toward lower risk of any malignant disease (HR 0.83; 95% CI 0.61–1.13). Risk of malignant disease was also significantly decreased in nonsurgical hypoparathyroidism (HR 0.44; 95% CI 0.24–0.82).

Some of the comorbidities seen with hypoparathyroidism are related to extraskeletal calcifications, such as cataracts, intracerebral calcifications, and renal stones or nephrocalcinosis. Increased risk of cardiovascular disease in nonsurgical hypoparathyroidism may be related to a tendency to precipitate calcium salts in vascular tissues. In the Danish cohort study, patients with postsurgical hypoparathyroidism[7,8] had a median duration of disease of only 8 years. Patients in the Danish cohort study with nonsurgical hypoparathyroidism[9] were of mean age 49.7 years, and most had had nonsurgical hypoparathyroidism since birth. More studies are needed to assess whether longstanding postsurgical hypoparathyroidism increases the risk of cardiovascular disease similar to what is seen in nonsurgical hypoparathyroidism.

Conventional treatment of hypoparathyroidism with calcium and active vitamin D causes an increase in serum calcium and relief of the classic symptoms of hypocalcemia. However, although serum calcium levels improve to the low-normal range, they typically do not completely normalize, and calcium and phosphorus homeostasis does not normalize in a physiologic manner in response to conventional treatment.

MORTALITY

The effects of chronic hypocalcemia, intermittent hypercalcemia, significant hypercalciuria, and multiple comorbidities on mortality in patients with hypoparathyroidism are uncertain. No studies have yet quantified overall or cause-specific mortality due to hypoparathyroidism in the United States. Analyses of mortality and comorbidities among patients with postsurgical hypoparathyroidism in the Danish historic cohort study[7] was limited to patients who developed hypoparathyroidism after neck surgery for nonmalignant diseases (toxic or nontoxic goiter, or primary hyperparathyroidism), and also excluded patients with postsurgical hypoparathyroidism following parathyroidectomy due to severe renal insufficiency. Analyses were adjusted for history of the disease in question before the diagnosis of postsurgical hypoparathyroidism. Mortality was not increased among patients in the Danish national cohort study with postsurgical (HR 0.98; 95% CI 0.76–1.26) or nonsurgical hypoparathyroidism

(HR 1.25; 95% CI 0.90–1.73), but the more recent central region of Denmark study[25] noted increased mortality in patients with increased serum phosphate, increased calcium × phosphate product, increased frequency of hypercalcemia, and longer duration of hypoparathyroidism. In light of these conflicting findings, the association between mortality and hypoparathyroidism is not yet clear.

SUMMARY

Hypoparathyroidism is a rare disorder, with prevalence now reported from various countries as between 10.1 per 100,000 in Norway, and 40 per 100,000 in Tayside, Scotland. Most studies show the prevalence to be the 20 to 30 per 100,000 range. Studies evaluating the incidence of hypoparathyroidism are much fewer, with the incidence in Denmark estimated at 0.8 per 100,000 per year, and the incidence in India estimated at 2.6 per 100,000 per year. Medical costs associated with hypoparathyroidism were reported to be approximately 3 times the costs of caring for average patients in one study from Olmsted County, Minnesota, with no other studies available. Morbidities associated with hypoparathyroidism are reported from a number of studies, with the most detailed information coming from the Danish national cohort study. Patients with hypoparathyroidism in general are at increased risk of renal disease, neuropsychiatric disease, seizures, and intracerebral calcifications. Patients with postsurgical hypoparathyroidism are also at increased risk of kidney stones. Patients with nonsurgical hypoparathyroidism are also at increased risk of ischemic cardiovascular disease and cataracts, and may be at increased risk of upper extremity fractures. Patients with nonsurgical hypoparathyroidism appear to have greater risk of renal disease, neuropsychiatric disease, seizures, and intracerebral calcifications than patients with postsurgical disease. The best national studies from Denmark have shown no increased risk of overall or cause-specific mortality.

REFERENCES

1. Bilezikian JP, Khan A, Potts JT Jr, et al. Hypoparathyroidism in the adult: epidemiology, diagnosis, pathophysiology, target-organ involvement, treatment, and challenges for future research. J Bone Miner Res 2011;26:2317–37.
2. Shoback D. Clinical practice. Hypoparathyroidism. N Engl J Med 2008;359: 391–400.
3. Clarke BL, Brown EM, Collins MT, et al. Epidemiology and diagnosis of hypoparathyroidism. J Clin Endocrinol Metab 2016;101:2284–99.
4. Shoback DM, Bilezikian JP, Costa AG, et al. Presentation of hypoparathyroidism: etiologies and clinical features. J Clin Endocrinol Metab 2016;101:2300–12.
5. Powers J, Joy K, Ruscio A, et al. Prevalence and incidence of hypoparathyroidism in the USA using a large claims database. J Bone Miner Res 2013; 28:2570–6.
6. Clarke BL, Leibson C, Emerson J, et al. Co-morbid-medical conditions associated with prevalent hypoparathyroidism: a population-based study. J Bone Miner Res 2011;26:S182 [abstract: SA1070].
7. Underbjerg L, Sikjaer T, Mosekilde L, et al. Cardiovascular and renal complications to postsurgical hypoparathyroidism: a Danish nationwide controlled historic follow-up study. J Bone Miner Res 2013;28:2277–85.
8. Underbjerg L, Sikjaer T, Mosekilde L, et al. Post-surgical hypoparathyroidism—risk of fractures, psychiatric diseases, cancer, cataract, and infections. J Bone Miner Res 2014;29:2504–10.

9. Underbjerg L, Sikjaer T, Mosekilde L, et al. The epidemiology of non-surgical hypoparathyroidism in Denmark: a nationwide case finding study. J Bone Miner Res 2015;30:1738–44.
10. Vadiveloo T, Donnan PT, Leese GP. A population-based study of the epidemiology of chronic hypoparathyroidism. J Bone Miner Res 2018;33:478–85.
11. Cipriani C, Pepe J, Biamonte F, et al. The epidemiology of hypoparathyroidism in Italy: an 8-year register-based study. Calcif Tissue Int 2017;100:278–85.
12. Cianferotti L, Parri S, Gronchi G, et al. Prevalence of chronic hypoparathyroidism in a Mediterranean region as estimated by the analysis of anonymous healthcare database. Calcif Tissue Int 2018;103(2):144–50.
13. Astor MC, Løvås K, Debowska A, et al. Epidemiology and health-related quality of life in hypoparathyroidism in Norway. J Clin Endocrinol Metab 2016;101:3045–53.
14. Romanchishen AF. The use of chromothyrolymphography for selection of surgical volume in patients with thyroid cancer. Vopr Onkol 1989;35:1037–40 [in Russian].
15. Romanchishen AF. Surgery of thyroid and parathyroid glands. Saint Petersburg (Russia): Vesty; 2009. p. 675.
16. Page C, Strunski V. Parathyroid risk in total thyroidectomy for bilateral, benign, multinodular goitre: report of 351 surgical cases. J Laryngol Otol 2007;121:237–41.
17. Asari R, Passler C, Kaczirek K, et al. Hypoparathyroidism after total thyroidectomy: a prospective study. Arch Surg 2008;143:132–7.
18. Ito Y, Kihara M, Kobayashi K, et al. Permanent hypoparathyroidism after completion total thyroidectomy as a second surgery: how do we avoid it? Endocr J 2014; 61:403–8.
19. Betterle C, Garelli S, Presotto F. Diagnosis and classification of autoimmune parathyroid disease. Autoimmun Rev 2014;13:417–22.
20. Hari Kumar KVS, Patnaik SK. Incidence of parathyroid disorders in Indian adult male population: a 25-year follow-up study. Clin Endocrinol (Oxf) 2017;87:605–8.
21. Leibson C, Clarke BL, Ransom JE, et al. Medical care costs for persons with and without prevalent hypoparathyroidism: a population-based study. J Bone Miner Res 2011;26:S183 [abstract: SA1071].
22. Mitchell DM, Regan S, Cooley MR, et al. Long-term follow-up of patients with hypoparathyroidism. J Clin Endocrinol Metab 2012;97:4507–14.
23. Krause KH, Campbell KP, Welsh MJ, et al. The calcium signal and neutrophil activation. Clin Biochem 1990;23:159–66.
24. Chawla H, Saha S, Kandasamy D, et al. Vertebral fractures and bone mineral density in patients with idiopathic hypoparathyroidism on long-term follow-up. J Clin Endocrinol Metab 2017;102:251–8.
25. Underbjerg L, Sikjaer T, Rejnmark L. Long-term complications in patients with hypoparathyroidism evaluated by biochemical findings: a case-control study. J Bone Miner Res 2017;33(5):822–31.
26. Illum F, Dupont E. Prevalences of CT-detected calcification in the basal ganglia in idiopathic hypoparathyroidism and pseudohypoparathyroidism. Neuroradiology 1985;27:32–7.
27. Goswami R, Sharma R, Sreenivas V, et al. Prevalence and progression of basal ganglia calcification and its pathogenic mechanism in patients with idiopathic hypoparathyroidism. Clin Endocrinol 2012;77:200–6.
28. Tambyah PA, Ong BK, Lee KO. Reversible parkinsonism and asymptomatic hypocalcemia with basal ganglia calcification from hypoparathyroidism 26 years after thyroid surgery. Am J Med 1993;94:444–5.
29. Forman MB, Sandler MP, Danziger A, et al. Basal ganglia calcification in postoperative hypoparathyroidism. Clin Endocrinol (Oxf) 1980;12:385–90.

Surgical Hypoparathyroidism

Hadiza S. Kazaure, MD[a], Julie Ann Sosa, MD, MA[b],*

KEYWORDS

- Hypoparathyroidism • Parathyroid • Surgery • Hypocalcemia • Parathyroidectomy
- Thyroidectomy

KEY POINTS

- Surgical hypoparathyroidism is the most common cause of hypoparathyroidism and is responsible for approximately 75% of cases.
- There is no standard definition of surgical hypoparathyroidism.
- Surgeon expertise is crucial in preventing surgical hypoparathyroidism.
- Postoperative hypoparathyroidism is a potentially fatal medical emergency; prevention and early recognition of symptoms are essential.

HISTORICAL PERSPECTIVE

The original description of the parathyroid gland in humans is attributed to Ivor V. Sandström (1852–1889), a medical student at the University of Uppsala, who independently described the parathyroid gland in a variety of species, including the first description in humans. He drew exacting illustrations describing parathyroid gland anatomy, histology, and blood supply. Sandström's original and detailed manuscript, entitled "*On a new gland in man and fellow animals*," went unnoticed for years until the function of the parathyroid glands was described.

Recognition of surgical hypoparathyroidism and eventual understanding of its prevention and management is closely intertwined with the history of thyroid surgery. Indeed, the functional significance of parathyroid glands remained unrecognized until Eugene Gley, a French physiologist, showed that removal of parathyroid glands during thyroidectomy resulted in postoperative tetany. This was further corroborated by Giulio Versale and Francesco Generali, two Italian scientists who demonstrated that

Disclosure Statement: Dr J.A. Sosa is a member of the Data Monitoring Committee of the Medullary Thyroid Cancer Consortium Registry supported by Novo Nordisk, GlaxoSmithKline, AstraZeneca, and Eli Lilly. Dr H.S. Kazaure has nothing to disclose.
[a] Section of Endocrine Surgery, Department of Surgery, Duke Cancer Institute, Duke University Medical Center, Box 2945, Durham, NC 27710, USA; [b] Department of Surgery, University of California, San Francisco, 513 Parnassus Avenue, Suite S320, Box 0104, San Francisco, CA 94143, USA
* Corresponding author.
E-mail address: julie.sosa@ucsf.edu

removal of the parathyroid glands in experimental animals led to paralytic and convulsive symptoms. Years later, while working at Johns Hopkins Hospital, Carl Voegtlin and William McCallum described postoperative tetany in parathyroidectomized dogs.[1,2]

In 1892, Anton von Eiselberg, an assistant to Sir Theodore Billroth, began exploring the utility of parathyroid transplantation in animal species. In 1909, William Stewart Halsted showed that the transplantation of even a single parathyroid gland could be lifesaving. He also noted that postoperative tetany improved after administration of bovine parathyroid extract; McCallum and Voegtlin showed that tetany could be alleviated by intravenous calcium.[2,3] As the relationship between tetany and parathyroid glands became established, surgeons began advocating for the preservation of parathyroid glands during thyroid surgery, and the treatment of postoperative tetany using calcium or bovine parathyroid extract. Isolation of parathyroid hormone (PTH) in the 1920s and later identification of its polypeptide sequence in the 1960s spurred further research.[4,5] In the early 1990s, George Irvin demonstrated the use of the intraoperative PTH assay to assess surgical success of parathyroidectomy.[6]

DEFINITION

Hypoparathyroidism is a condition of impaired or inadequate PTH secretion leading to hypocalcemia and hyperphosphatemia. This may arise secondary to congenital anomalies; autoimmune destruction; metabolic derangements, such as hypomagnesemia; rare infiltrative disorders, such as Wilson disease; or peripheral tissue resistance to PTH stimulation as seen in pseudohypoparathyroidism syndromes. In line with the history of parathyroid surgery, operative misadventure remains the most common cause of hypoparathyroidism. Surgical hypoparathyroidism occurs after inadvertent trauma, devascularization, or removal of parathyroid glands during neck surgery. Indeed, anterior neck surgery is the most common cause of acquired hypoparathyroidism and is responsible for about 75% of cases.[7] Preservation of the parathyroid glands and their blood supply *in situ* is key to minimizing the risk of surgical hypoparathyroidism.

There is variability and lack of consensus on the definition and criteria of surgical hypoparathyroidism.[8] Some investigators use biochemical evidence of hypocalcemia as the criterion for defining hypoparathyroidism, whereas others use the presence of clinical symptoms of postoperative hypocalcemia requiring oral or intravenous calcium supplementation; others measure PTH values to provide definition around the diagnosis (**Box 1**).[8,9] Postoperative hypoparathyroidism may be transient or permanent. Permanent hypoparathyroidism is most commonly defined as failure of the parathyroid gland to regain normal function by 6 months after surgery. However, some

---

Box 1
Varied definitions of permanent surgical hypoparathyroidism in the literature

- Hypocalcemia lasting greater than 6 months
- Continuing need for vitamin D medication at 1-year postoperatively
- Intact parathyroid hormone level less than 13 pg/mL and need for calcium medication at 1 month after thyroidectomy
- Requirement of calcium supplementation 1 year after surgery
- Hypocalcemia persisting longer than 1 year

authors have suggested a period of time beyond 6 months after surgery before making this diagnosis (see **Box 1**).

INCIDENCE AND RISK FACTORS

Surgical hypoparathyroidism is the most common complication of thyroid surgery, reported in 0.33% to 68.0% of patients.[10–12] Wide variation in the incidence of surgical hypoparathyroidism in the surgical literature is in part caused by discrepancies in the determination of postoperative recovery of parathyroid gland function, and varying biochemical assays used at institutions. In addition, most data are derived from single institutions or surgeon series. One review of post-thyroidectomy outcomes showed that the incidence rate of surgical hypoparathyroidism ranges from 0% to 46% for the same cohort of patients, depending on the definition of surgical hypoparathyroidism used.[8] Using data from a large proprietary health plan claims database and projected to the US insured population, Powers and colleagues[13] modeled epidemiologic data involving more than 110,000 neck surgeries and determined that approximately 7.6% of surgeries resulted in hypoparathyroidism, with 75% of these cases described as transient ($\leq$6 months) and 25% as permanent (>6 months) hypoparathyroidism.

Type and extent of surgery, operative technique, surgeon expertise, and cause of disease contribute to the risk of surgical hypoparathyroidism (**Box 2**). A meta-analysis of outcomes following total thyroidectomy with central neck dissections compared with total thyroidectomy alone found a relative risk (RR) of temporary hypocalcemia of 2.52 (95% confidence interval [CI], 1.95–3.25); however, the increase in risk associated with the addition of prophylactic central lymph node dissection was not statistically significant for permanent hypocalcemia (RR, 1.82; 95% CI, 0.51–6.5).[14] Lateral neck dissections, especially when bilateral, are associated with a higher risk of surgical hypoparathyroidism. The study of McMullen and coworkers[15] of 62 patients who underwent bilateral lateral neck dissections reported a 37% risk of permanent hypoparathyroidism.

Improved technology has led to the introduction of minimally invasive techniques in thyroid surgery, including robotic, endoscopic, and transoral approaches. There are conflicting data on the rate of surgical hypoparathyroidism with these techniques as compared with conventional open thyroidectomy. One retrospective review of 700 robotic thyroid surgery cases using the transaxillary approach found that transient hypoparathyroidism was the most common complication (43.7%), and its incidence decreased steeply to a range of 9.1% to 25.0% after 300 consecutive cases. Permanent hypoparathyroidism was observed in 1.1% of patients.[16] A meta-analysis of patients who underwent robotic, endoscopic, and open thyroidectomy found that patients who underwent robotic thyroidectomy had a higher risk of developing

---

Box 2
Risk factors for surgical hypoparathyroidism

- Extensive neck dissection
- Bilateral neck exploration
- Reoperative thyroid or parathyroid surgery
- Pediatric patient
- Hyperthyroidism, especially Graves disease
- Malabsorptive conditions, such as a history of bariatric surgery

temporary hypocalcemia (RR, 1.25; 95% CI, 1.08–1.46; $P<.001$). They also found an RR of 0.46 (95% CI, 0.34–0.64; $P = .014$) between the robotic and endoscopic approaches. Comparing the incidence of permanent hypocalcemia showed an RR of 1.01 (95% CI, 0.48–2.01) between the open and robotic groups ($P = .658$), and an RR of 0.99 (95% CI, 0.35–2.77) between the endoscopic and robotic groups ($P = .519$).[17] Another meta-analysis reported rates of transient and permanent hypoparathyroidism in robotic thyroidectomy ranging from 0% to 53% and 0% to 3%, respectively. In 18 studies comparing robotic thyroidectomy with open thyroidectomy, all except three studies reported no significant difference between the two groups for the rates of transient hypoparathyroidism, and the rates of permanent hypoparathyroidism were comparable among all studies.[18]

In parathyroid surgery, patients undergoing a bilateral four-gland exploration are more likely to experience postoperative hypoparathyroidism than those undergoing a less extensive exploration. A meta-analysis of outcomes following minimally invasive parathyroidectomy versus bilateral neck explorations reported a hypocalcemia rate of 2.3% versus 13.6%, respectively ($P<.001$). In the study, minimally invasive parathyroidectomy included focused exploration and other approaches, such as video-assisted and radio-guided parathyroidectomy; postoperative hypocalcemia was not categorized into transient versus permanent.[19] Another meta-analysis specifically comparing focused parathyroidectomy with bilateral neck explorations reported a 1.6% versus 13.2% rate of transient hypocalcemia ($P = .03$); two patients (0.05%) versus eight patients (0.2%) experienced permanent hypoparathyroidism, respectively.[20]

A retrospective review of 621 patients who underwent thyroid or parathyroid surgery at a high-volume medical center reported an overall 17% rate of concomitant thyroid and parathyroid surgery. Approximately 11% of patients with thyroid disease had concomitant parathyroid disease, whereas 26% of patients with parathyroid disease had concomitant thyroid pathology.[21] Data suggest that concomitant thyroid and parathyroid surgery raises the risk of surgical hypoparathyroidism. Riss and colleagues[22] analyzed outcomes of patients undergoing parathyroidectomy only versus parathyroidectomy with thyroid resection; overall 17.9% of patients experienced transient hypoparathyroidism, with three patients (0.3%) experiencing permanent hypoparathyroidism. Compared with patients undergoing parathyroidectomy only, those undergoing parathyroidectomy with hemithyroidectomy were 2.3 times as likely to experience surgical hypoparathyroidism, whereas those undergoing concomitant total thyroidectomy were more than seven times as likely to experience this complication.

The risk of surgical hypoparathyroidism after a repeat thyroid, parathyroid, or anterior neck operation may be 30%.[23] In the reoperative setting, eutopic (and ectopic) parathyroid glands are more difficult to identify secondary to scarring, distorted neck anatomy, and obliteration of normal planes. During initial surgery, parathyroid glands left in situ may have been unknowingly devascularized or damaged. Therefore, review of the pathology report from the index operation can underestimate parathyroid reserve going into a remedial operation; a patient can be rendered hypoparathyroid without there being parathyroid glands in the surgical specimen. Subsequent removal or inadvertent injury of any remaining functional gland during reoperative neck surgery may result in permanent hypoparathyroidism. A recent study by Thompson and colleagues[24] reported a 13% rate of permanent hypocalcemia for patients undergoing reoperative parathyroidectomy; another study of 77 patients who underwent reoperative parathyroidectomy at a single institution reported an 8% rate of permanent hypocalcemia.[25]

Hyperthyroidism and specific patient characteristics, such as age and a prior history of bariatric surgery, increase the risk of surgical hypoparathyroidism. Among patients undergoing total thyroidectomy for benign pathology, those with hyperthyroidism, and particularly Graves disease, have been consistently shown to have a higher risk of surgical hypoparathyroidism.[26–28] In a meta-analysis evaluating Graves disease as a risk factor of hypocalcemia among 6681 patients pooled from four studies, patients with Graves disease had a significantly higher incidence of transient hypocalcemia compared with those without this condition (odds ratio [OR], 1.75 [1.34–2.28]).[26] Reasons for the increased risk of hypoparathyroidism among patients undergoing Graves disease surgery are thought to be related to increased bone turnover and difficult operations caused by increased vascularity of the thyroid gland.[26,28]

Bariatric surgery is associated with several vitamin and mineral deficiencies, with 15% to 48% of such patients experiencing low serum calcium levels after bariatric surgery; 30% to 60% experience vitamin D deficiency.[29–31] Existing data show that patients with a previous history of bariatric surgery undergoing thyroid or parathyroid surgery are at high risk of surgical hypoparathyroidism.[32–34] Chereau and colleagues[33] reported a 40% rate of surgical hypoparathyroidism among patients with a history of bariatric surgery undergoing thyroidectomy; the rate of transient and permanent surgical hypoparathyroidism was 29% and 10.4%, respectively. In particular, bypass surgery had a two-fold increased risk of hypocalcemia compared with other bariatric procedures (60% vs 30%; $P = .05$).

Pediatric patients are another high-risk group for endocrine complications after thyroid or parathyroid surgery because of smaller, more delicate, and subtle anatomic structures in a shorter neck, with considerable space constraints.[35,36] At the population level, Sosa and colleagues[36] found that pediatric patients had higher endocrine-specific complication rates than adults after parathyroidectomy (15.2% vs 6.2%, respectively; $P<.01$) and thyroidectomy (9.1% vs 6.3%; $P<.01$), and this was inversely related to patient age: children aged 0 to 6 years had higher complication rates (22% vs 15% for 7–12 years and 11% for 13–17 years; $P<.01$). The rate of surgical hypoparathyroidism was not specifically reported.

One of the largest single series of pediatric endocrine surgery outcomes examined 241 cases, including 177 thyroid procedures, 13 neck dissections, and 24 parathyroidectomies performed by high-volume surgeons at the Mayo Clinic.[37] Hypoparathyroidism was considered transient if it occurred for fewer than 6 months, and was noted in 32.7% of patients, whereas 2.3% of patients experienced permanent hypoparathyroidism. Of 26 patients younger than 10 years, nine had transient hypocalcemia (34%); there were no cases of permanent hypoparathyroidism among patients who underwent parathyroidectomy. Another study of pediatric thyroidectomies at a high-volume center found that 12.9% of patients experienced postoperative hypocalcemia, with 7.0% requiring intravenous calcium infusion. One patient (0.9%) experienced permanent hypoparathyroidism. Risk factors for postoperative hypocalcemia in the study included total thyroidectomy (OR, 7.39; $P<.01$), central and bilateral lateral neck dissection (OR, 22.26; $P = .01$), Graves disease (OR, 3.99; $P = .02$), and thyroid malignancy (OR, 2.96; $P = .03$).[38]

STRATEGIES TO REDUCE THE RISK OF SURGICAL HYPOPARATHYROIDISM

Surgical hypoparathyroidism has significant consequences for the health and quality of life of the patient, including expensive and potentially lifelong medication supplementation, frequent laboratory testing, the possibility of frequent hospital admissions, and an overall reduced quality of life. For patients with prolonged or permanent hypoparathyroidism, long-term systemic effects have been reported. These include premature cataract formation, cardiac dysfunction (including congestive heart failure), ectopic calcifications in the kidneys and basal ganglia, and neurocognitive derangement.

Regardless of disease cause or demographic characteristics, surgeon experience as measured by number of cases performed is associated with greatly reduced risk of postoperative hypoparathyroidism. Experienced endocrine surgeons and high-volume centers report rates of surgical hypoparathyroidism ranging from 0.9% to 1.8%, the lowest in the literature.[39–41] Meticulous preservation of the parathyroid glands and their vascular supply is critical during thyroid and parathyroid surgery. Tissue should be handled delicately to avoid damage to normal parathyroid glands. A parathyroid remnant on its native vascular pedicle is less likely to result in hypocalcemia than remnant implantation into muscles of the neck or nondominant forearm. The surgeon should use judgment about the extent of resection in multigland hyperplasia; typically, a remnant smaller than 50 mg is left in place after subtotal resection.

Inadvertent parathyroidectomy during thyroid surgery is a potentially remediable risk factor for surgical hypoparathyroidism that occurs in up to 20% of patients undergoing thyroidectomy,[42] and in up to 28% of patients undergoing total thyroidectomy with central neck dissection.[43] Therefore, after resection all thyroid specimens should be promptly examined in the operating room and before sending them to pathology to facilitate autotransplantation should a normal parathyroid gland have been inadvertently removed. Aspiration of suspected parathyroid tissue with immediate measurement of PTH using the intraoperative rapid PTH assay also is used to confirm parathyroid gland tissue. The authors recommend that parathyroid glands that have been inadvertently removed or those with questionable viability should be autotransplanted promptly into the ipsilateral sternocleidomastoid or strap muscle. A sample of the specimen intended for transplantation should be sent to pathology for frozen section or aspirated with the rapid PTH assay to confirm that it is, in fact, parathyroid tissue to avoid inadvertent transplantation of nonparathyroid tissue or a thyroid malignancy into a soft tissue location. The remaining gland is placed on sterile ice to slow down ischemic necrosis. Once histology is confirmed, the gland is then sliced into small pieces, each approximately 1 mm in size; a slurry also can be created. The sternocleidomastoid or strap muscle is exposed, and small pockets are created by bluntly separating the muscle fibers. Two or three pieces of the parathyroid specimen are placed into each pocket, and the pockets are then closed with a silk stitch or microclips to facilitate identification in case of future reoperation. This same technique is used in the autotransplantation of hyperplastic parathyroid tissue into the brachioradialis muscle of the nondominant forearm during subtotal or total parathyroidectomy. The brachioradialis muscle of the forearm is used most commonly, principally to aid future surgery under local anesthetic for recurrent disease. A clip on the transplant site is placed to facilitate identification of the remnant in the case of recurrent hyperparathyroidism.

Cryopreservation of parathyroid tissue provides another margin of safety against permanent surgical hypoparathyroidism. The decision to cryopreserve parathyroid tissue is made before surgery and may be considered for patients undergoing parathyroidectomy for multigland parathyroid disease, those undergoing near-total or total parathyroidectomy, or redo neck operations.[44,45] Cryopreservation is not immediately available at most surgical centers, however, and protocols may vary by institution. To be cryopreserved, a piece of the parathyroid gland is submitted to pathology for histologic confirmation. The remaining specimen for cryopreservation is sliced into small pieces, about 1 to 2 mm in size, and brought into suspension in sterile saline, which is then frozen based on the hospital's specific protocol and stored at subzero temperatures in the tissue bank.[44] The need to reimplant cryopreserved parathyroid tissue usually becomes evident within 6 months of surgery if the cervical remnants become nonfunctional. Pooled studies show that the success rate of delayed autotransplantation ranges from 17% to 83%.[46]

The utility of measuring serum PTH to identify patients at risk of postoperative hypocalcemia or surgical hypoparathyroidism is unsettled. Some studies have shown good reliability of PTH testing in the early postoperative period for predicting long-term hypocalcemia[47,48]; however, a nonrandomized prospective study by Lombardi and colleagues[49] including 523 patients who underwent total thyroidectomy showed that the serum level of PTH 4 hours after surgery did not predict the occurrence of hypocalcemia. Wang and colleagues[50] showed that postoperative PTH levels better predict long-term hypocalcemia requiring vitamin D supplementation than serum calcium levels. A study by Saba and colleagues[51] randomized 150 patients who underwent total thyroidectomy into an experimental group that had rapid PTH assay testing performed 6 hours after surgery and a control group that underwent daily monitoring of serum calcium and phosphate testing for 3 days postoperatively; this study demonstrated an early postoperative rate of hypocalcemia of 14.3% in both groups, presumably caused by hypoparathyroidism. When the sensitivities and specificities of calcium and phosphate levels in predicting hypocalcemia were analyzed using receiver operating characteristic curve analyses, PTH assay testing 6 hours after surgery (≤ 11 pg/mL) combined with serum calcium assay testing 24 hours after surgery (≤ 7.9 mg/dL) yielded the highest diagnostic accuracy for predicting early hypocalcemia, with 100% sensitivity and 100% specificity, and identifying those patients who would require the most intensive treatment with calcium and activated vitamin D. According to the authors, no patient was still suffering from hypocalcemia at the 6-month follow-up. Results of this single institution study have not been validated at a multi-institutional level or with a larger sample.

Strategies to decrease the risk of surgical hypoparathyroidism should be considered preoperatively and postoperatively (**Box 3**). Vitamin D deficiency or insufficiency should be corrected before elective thyroid or parathyroid surgery if possible. A randomized trial showed that perioperative vitamin D administration decreased the risk of transient hypocalcemia and related symptoms in patients undergoing total thyroidectomy.[52] Oltmann and colleagues[28] found that compared with patients with Graves disease pretreated with 1 g of calcium carbonate three times a day for 2 weeks before total thyroidectomy, those who did not receive this supplementation were more likely to experience numbness and tingling (symptoms of hypocalcemia) after surgery (26% vs 10% without preoperative supplementation; $P = .049$).

Box 3
Strategies to reduce risk of surgical hypoparathyroidism

- High-volume thyroid/parathyroid surgeon
- Preoperative localization of aberrant parathyroid glands to aid focused exploration
- Preoperative supplementation in select patients at high risk
- Prompt recognition and autotransplantation of devascularized or inadvertently removed normal glands
- Cryopreservation with delayed autotransplantation of parathyroid tissue
- Postoperative supplementation with oral calcium with or without vitamin D

In the postoperative setting, Carter and coworkers[53] showed that a postoperative protocol of calcium carbonate administration for patients with intact PTH levels greater than or equal to 10 pg/mL after surgery and calcium carbonate plus 0.25 µg calcitriol twice a day for intact PTH less than 10 pg/mL is associated with a decreased likelihood of hypocalcemia. Wang and colleagues[54] compared the incremental cost–utility of routine versus selective calcium and vitamin D supplementation in a hypothetical group of patients following completion or total thyroidectomy. Using a Markov decision model, the study showed that routine calcium supplementation after thyroidectomy was a cost-effective strategy associated with improved quality of life. Current American Thyroid Association guidelines for the management of hyperthyroidism recommend assessment of calcium and 25-hydroxy vitamin D preoperatively, repletion if necessary, or given prophylactically.[55] In addition, the 2015 American Thyroid Association guidelines for the management of hyperthyroidism and thyrotoxicosis, and also those for the management of differentiated thyroid cancer in pediatric patients, recommend that calcium and calcitriol should be considered preoperatively in patients at increased risk for transient or permanent hypoparathyroidism.[55,56] At this time, protocols for prophylactic and postoperative supplementation with calcium and calcitriol are not standardized.

CLINICAL MANIFESTATIONS AND TREATMENT

Clinically significant surgical hypoparathyroidism ultimately manifests with symptoms of hypocalcemia if biochemical abnormalities are not anticipated and/or corrected. The diagnosis is established based on laboratory tests that show a normal or inappropriately with low serum albumin–corrected total calcium or ionized calcium values with elevated serum phosphorus levels; concurrent low intact PTH levels are consistent with hypoparathyroidism, whereas elevated PTH levels with low phosphorus levels suggest the "hungry bones" phenomenon that can occur in patients with preoperative hyperthyroidism or hyperparathyroidism. Postoperative hypoparathyroidism may be asymptomatic. The severity and acuity of hypocalcemia determine the severity of symptoms. Severe hypocalcemia is life-threatening and should be considered an urgent or emergent situation. It may be evident acutely with tetany, seizures, bronchospasm, laryngeal spasms, or cardiac dysrhythmia, including prolongation of the QTc interval. Typical mild symptoms include tingling parasthesias in the perioral area and fingertips and muscle cramps secondary to neuromuscular irritability. Simple bedside maneuvers, such as testing for the presence of the Chvostek and Trousseau signs, are used to assess neuromuscular excitability caused by hypocalcemia.

The cornerstone for managing surgical hypoparathyroidism is correction of hypocalcemia with amelioration of symptoms. Treatment primarily involves calcium and vitamin D supplementation; oral calcium can help reduce elevated serum phosphorus levels (**Box 4**). In patients with severe hypocalcemia, intravenous calcium replacement is given in a continuous fashion with oral supplementation. Calcium gluconate is commonly used for intravenous treatment of hypocalcemia. Intravenous calcium chloride should be avoided because it is potentially sclerosing to veins.

In addition to boosting intake of dietary calcium and reducing dietary phosphate intake, oral calcium supplements are important. The amount of elemental calcium provided in an oral calcium supplement is an important consideration during treatment of hypoparathyroidism. The various calcium salts have different amounts of elemental calcium and varying bioavailability of elemental calcium. Calcium carbonate, which provides 40% elemental calcium, is a common choice, but it requires an acidic environment for optimal absorption if not given with meals; therefore, it may be less

---

Box 4
Treatment of surgical hypoparathyroidism

- Intravenous calcium gluconate for severe for symptomatic hypocalcemia

- Oral calcium salts

- Calcitriol, 0.25 to 2 μg

- Thiazide diuretics

- Increase dietary calcium intake

- Address alkalosis, hypomagnesemia, and hypokalemia, and monitor serum phosphate levels

- Discontinue proton pump inhibitors and H_2-blockers

- Trend electrolytes every 4 to 6 hours; titrate calcium and calcitriol supplementation accordingly

---

effective in patients taking proton pump inhibitors. Calcium citrate, an alternative calcium salt that provides 21% elemental calcium, may be useful in achlorhydric patients or those who have undergone bariatric surgery; diarrhea is a known complication. Other oral formulations include calcium lactate, calcium gluconate, and calcium glubionate, which contain 13%, 9%, and 6.6% elemental calcium, respectively. Calcium supplements are best given with meals to reduce absorption of dietary phosphate.

Calcitriol improves serum calcium, in part, by improving the efficiency of intestinal calcium absorption. The dosage of calcitriol administered ranges between 0.25 and 2.0 μg/d and usually is administered in two divided doses. Vitamin D therapy may result in hyperphosphatemia; therefore, phosphate levels should be monitored. Ectopic deposition of insoluble calcium phosphate complexes in soft tissues can occur because of hyperphosphatemia. Dietary intake of phosphate should be reduced. Specific phosphate binders may be needed in severe hyperphosphatemia.

Thiazide diuretics can complement efforts to improve renal tubular calcium reabsorption and retention. Because hypokalemia and hyponatremia may occur with these agents, serum electrolytes should be monitored. Loop diuretics should be avoided, because these medications promote urinary calcium loss. Alkalosis, hypokalemia, and hypomagnesemia exacerbate hypocalcemia; therefore, these conditions must be concurrently corrected.

Most patients with surgical hypoparathyroidism become eucalcemic without need for exogenous calcium supplementation within a few weeks to months after surgery.[57] For patients with permanent surgical hypoparathyroidism, the general goal of treatment is to preserve serum calcium in the low normal level with minimal or tolerable symptoms. These patients usually need life-long calcium and vitamin D supplementation. They are prone to fluctuations in calcium homeostasis necessitating long-term surveillance. Good communication between the surgeon and the patient about appropriate expectations and prognosis, and between the surgeon and the endocrinologist or primary care provider during transfer of care is important.

NEW AND EMERGING PROSPECTS FOR THE PREVENTION AND MANAGEMENT OF SURGICAL HYPOPARATHYROIDISM

There has been renewed interest in intraoperative parathyroid imaging to facilitate parathyroid identification and preservation. Because parathyroid glands autofluoresce in the near-infrared spectrum, near-infrared fluorescence imaging is a potential intraoperative adjunct.[58,59] A multi-institutional study of 210 patients undergoing thyroid resection found concordance in detecting parathyroid autofluorescence from 97% to 99% of parathyroid glands using near-infrared fluorescence imaging. However, there was variability (37%–67%) in rates of parathyroid gland identification by near-infrared imaging before conventional recognition by the surgeons in the study.[58]

Parathyroid autofluorescence may be enhanced by fluorophores, such as methylene blue and indocyanin green. Methylene blue is taken up readily by endocrine tissues and aids naked eye identification of enlarged parathyroid glands by staining culprit glands blue in the operating room. Disadvantages include discoloration of the surrounding surgical field and the possibility of hypersensitivity reactions.[60,61] In a Phase 1b interventional study involving 41 patients undergoing thyroid and/or parathyroid surgery, Hillary and colleagues[62] investigated the optimum dose of methylene blue and fluorescent patterns of thyroid and parathyroid glands. A protocol for the use of intravenous methylene blue emitted fluorescence was developed. The investigators found that the optimum dose of methylene blue to visualize thyroid and parathyroid glands was 0.4 mg/kg body weight and that parathyroid glands autofluoresce before methylene blue injection and fluoresce more intensely than thyroid glands after injection of methylene blue; these are findings that could aid in assessing parathyroid gland viability.

A recently published trial by Vidal Fortuny and colleagues[63] involving 196 patients who underwent indocyanin angiography during thyroid surgery demonstrated that a well-vascularized parathyroid gland could be identified in 146 (74.5%). Patients in the study were then randomized into a control group that had standard follow-up consisting of measurement of calcium and PTH levels on postoperative day (POD) 1 and POD 10 to 15. Oral supplementation with 1 g calcium and 800 units 25-hydroxy vitamin D twice daily until the first follow-up appointment was also used (POD 10–15). Patients in the experimental group had postoperative clinical follow-up assessment for symptoms of hypocalcemia, but no blood tests to determine calcium or PTH levels on POD 1, and no oral calcium and vitamin D supplementation. The authors found that the intervention group was statistically noninferior to the control group (95% CI, −0.053 to 0.053; $P = .012$). More studies are needed to confirm efficacy, safety, appropriate dosage, and intraoperative protocols to facilitate widespread use of intraoperative parathyroid imaging.

Recombinant PTH and PTH analogues are the latest addition to the treatment armamentarium for surgical hypoparathyroidism. Teriparatide ($PTH_{[1-34]}$, Forteo) and $PTH_{(1-84)}$ (Natpara) are the two clinical forms of recombinant PTH under investigation. Clinical trials of human $PTH_{(1-34)}$ and $PTH_{(1-84)}$ for chronic hypoparathyroidism have shown that recombinant PTH is safe and effective in studies lasting 3 to 4 years.[64–66] Both forms are administered by subcutaneous injection. The longer in duration of effect in vivo of $PTH_{(1-84)}$ makes once-daily dosing more feasible than $PTH_{(1-34)}$. In 2015, the Food and Drug Administration approved recombinant human $PTH_{(1-84)}$ for the management of hypoparathyroidism not adequately controlled with conventional therapy. Approval was granted with a "black box" warning because of evidence that exogenous PTH is associated with the development of osteosarcoma in rats; this has not been reported in humans. Cost is a major disincentive for the use of recombinant $PTH_{(1-84)}$ to treat surgical hypoparathyroidism. Longer term data on safety and efficacy also are needed.

REFERENCES

1. Medvei VC. A history of endocrinology. Lancaster (England): MTP Press Ltd; 1982.

2. Eknoyan G. A history of the parathyroid glands. Am J Kidney Dis 1995;26(5): 801–7.

3. Halsted WS. Auto- and iso transplantation, in dogs of the parathyroid glandules. J Exp Med 1909;11:175–9.

4. Collip JB. The extraction of a parathyroid hormone which will prevent or control parathyroid tetany and which regulates the level of blood calcium. J Biol Chem 1925;63:395–438.

5. Rasmussen H, Craig LC. The parathyroid polypeptides. Recent Prog Horm Res 1962;18:269–95.

6. Irvin GL, Deriso GT. A new practical intraoperative parathyroid hormone assay. Am J Surg 1994;168:466–8.

7. Clarke BL, Brown EM, Collins MT, et al. Epidemiology and diagnosis of hypoparathyroidism. J Clin Endocrinol Metab 2016;101:2282–99.

8. Mehanna HM, Jain A, Randeva H, et al. Postoperative hypocalcemia: the difference a definition makes. Head Neck 2010;32:279–83.

9. Stack BC Jr, Bimston DN, Bodenner DL, et al. American Association of Clinical Endocrinologists and American College of Endocrinology Disease State Clinical Review: postoperative hypoparathyroidism-definitions and management. Endocr Pract 2015;21:674–85.

10. Shaha A, Jaffe B. Parathyroid preservation during thyroid surgery. Am J Otolaryngol 1998;19:113–7.

11. Rosato L, Avenia N, Bernante P, et al. Complications of thyroid surgery: analysis of a multicentric study on 14,934 patients operated on in Italy over 5 years. World J Surg 2004;28:271–6.

12. Wilson RB, Erskine C, Crowe PJ. Hypomagnesemia and hypocalcemia after thyroidectomy: a prospective study. World J Surg 2000;24:722–6.

13. Powers J, Joy K, Ruscio A, et al. Prevalence and incidence of hypoparathyroidism in the United States using a large claims database. J Bone Miner Res 2013; 28:2570–6.

14. Wang TS, Cheung K, Farrokhyar F, et al. A meta-analysis of the effect of prophylactic central compartment neck dissection on locoregional recurrence rates in patients with papillary thyroid cancer. Ann Surg Oncol 2013;20(11):3477–83.

15. McMullen C, Rocke D, Freeman J. Complications of bilateral neck dissection in thyroid cancer from a single high-volume center. JAMA Otolaryngol Head Neck Surg 2017;143(4):376–81.

16. Kim EB, Cho JW, Lee YM, et al. Postsurgical outcomes and surgical completeness of robotic thyroid surgery: a single surgeon's experience on 700 cases. J Laparoendosc Adv Surg Tech A 2018;28(5):540–5.

17. Kandil E, Hammad AY, Walvekar RR, et al. Robotic thyroidectomy versus nonrobotic approaches: a meta-analysis examining surgical outcomes. Surg Innov 2016;23(3):317–25.

18. Liu SY, Ng EK. Robotic versus open thyroidectomy for differentiated thyroid cancer: an evidence-based review. Int J Endocrinol 2016;2016:4309087.

19. Singh Ospina NM, Rodriguez-Gutierrez R, Maraka S, et al. Outcomes of parathyroidectomy in patients with primary hyperparathyroidism: a systematic review and meta-analysis. World J Surg 2016;40:2359.

20. Jinih M, O'Connell E, O'Leary DP, et al. Focused versus bilateral parathyroid exploration for primary hyperparathyroidism: a systematic review and meta-analysis. Ann Surg Oncol 2017;24(7):1924–34.

21. Wright MC, Jensen K, Mohamed H, et al. Concomitant thyroid disease and primary hyperparathyroidism in patients undergoing parathyroidectomy or thyroidectomy. Gland Surg 2017;6(4):368–74.

22. Riss P, Kammer M, Selberherr A, et al. Morbidity associated with concomitant thyroid surgery in patients with primary hyperparathyroidism. Ann Surg Oncol 2015; 22(8):2707–13.

23. Jaskowiak N, Norton JA, Alexander HR, et al. A prospective trial evaluating a standard approach to reoperation for missed parathyroid adenoma. Ann Surg 1996;224(3):308–20 [discussion: 320–1].

24. Thompson GB, Grant CS, Perrier ND, et al. Reoperative parathyroid surgery in the era of sestamibi scanning and intraoperative parathyroid hormone monitoring. Arch Surg 1999;134:699–704.

25. Morris LF, Lee S, Warneke CL, et al. Fewer adverse events after reoperative parathyroidectomy associated with initial minimally invasive parathyroidectomy. Am J Surg 2014;208(5):850–5.

26. Edafe O, Antakia R, Laskar N, et al. Systematic review and meta-analysis of predictors of post-thyroidectomy hypocalcaemia. Br J Surg 2014;101(4):307–20.

27. Pesce CE, Shiue Z, Tsai HL, et al. Postoperative hypocalcemia after thyroidectomy for Graves' disease. Thyroid 2010;20:1279–83.

28. Oltmann SC, Brekke AV, Schneider DF, et al. Preventing postoperative hypocalcemia in patients with Graves disease: a prospective study. Ann Surg Oncol 2015; 22(3):952–8.

29. Slater GH, Ren CJ, Siegel N, et al. Serum fat-soluble vitamin deficiency and abnormal calcium metabolism after malabsorptive bariatric surgery. J Gastrointest Surg 2004;8(1):48–55.

30. Newbury L, Dolan K, Hatzifotis M, et al. Calcium and vitamin D depletion and elevated parathyroid hormone following biliopancreatic diversion. Obes Surg 2003;13(6):893–5.

31. Chakhtoura MT, Nakhoul NN, Shawwa K, et al. Hypovitaminosis D in bariatric surgery: a systematic review of observational studies. Metabolism 2016;65(4): 574–85.

32. Durr ML, Saunders JR, Califano JA, et al. Severe hypocalcemia complicating thyroid surgery after Roux-en-Y gastric bypass procedure. Arch Otolaryngol Head Neck Surg 2009;135(5):507–10.

33. Chereau N, Vuillermet C, Tilly C, et al. Hypocalcemia after thyroidectomy in patients with a history of bariatric surgery. Surg Obes Relat Dis 2017;13(3):484–90.

34. McKenzie TJ, Chen Y, Hodin RA, et al. Recalcitrant hypocalcemia after thyroidectomy in patients with previous Roux-en-Y gastric bypass. Surgery 2013;154(6): 1300–6.

35. Machens A, Elwerr M, Thanh PN, et al. Impact of central node dissection on postoperative morbidity in pediatric patients with suspected or proven thyroid cancer. Surgery 2016;160(2):484–92.

36. Sosa JA, Tuggle CT, Wang TS, et al. Clinical and economic outcomes of thyroid and parathyroid surgery in children. J Clin Endocrinol Metab 2008;93:3058–65.

37. Kundel A, Thompson GB, Richards ML, et al. Pediatric endocrine surgery: a 20-year experience at the Mayo Clinic. J Clin Endocrinol Metab 2014;99(2):399–406.

38. Chen Y, Masiakos PT, Gaz RD, et al. Pediatric thyroidectomy in a high volume thyroid surgery center: risk factors for postoperative hypocalcemia. J Pediatr Surg 2015;50(8):1316–9.

39. Udelsman R, Donovan PI, Sokoll LJ. One hundred consecutive minimally invasive parathyroid explorations. Ann Surg 2000;232:331–9.

40. Allendorf J, DiGorgi M, Spanknebel K, et al. 1112 consecutive bilateral neck explorations for primary hyperparathyroidism. World J Surg 2007;31(11):2075–80.

41. Adam MA, Thomas S, Youngwirth L, et al. Is there a minimum number of thyroidectomies a surgeon should perform to optimize patient outcomes? Ann Surg 2017;265(2):402–7.

42. Zhou HY, He JC, McHenry CR. Inadvertent parathyroidectomy: incidence, risk factors, and outcomes. J Surg Res 2016;205(1):70–5.

43. Sitges-Serra A, Gallego-Otaegui L, Suárez S, et al. Inadvertent parathyroidectomy during total thyroidectomy and central neck dissection for papillary thyroid carcinoma. Surgery 2017;161(3):712–9.

44. Guerrero MA. Cryopreservation of parathyroid glands. Int J Endocrinol 2010; 2010:829540.

45. Shepet K, Alhefdhi A, Usedom R, et al. Parathyroid cryopreservation after parathyroidectomy: a worthwhile practice? Ann Surg Oncol 2013;20(7):2256–60.

46. McHenry CR, Stenger DB, Calandro NK. The effect of cryopreservation on parathyroid cell viability and function. Am J Surg 1997;174(5):481–4.

47. Sabour S, Manders E, Steward DL. The role of rapid PACU parathyroid hormone in reducing post-thyroidectomy hypocalcemia. Otolaryngol Head Neck Surg 2009;141(6):727–9.

48. Sywak MS, Palazzo FF, Yeh M, et al. Parathyroid hormone assay predicts hypocalcaemia after total thyroidectomy. ANZ J Surg 2007;77:667–70.

49. Lombardi CP, Raffaelli M, Princi P, et al. Early prediction of post thyroidectomy hypocalcemia by one single iPTH measurement. Surgery 2004;136:1236–41.

50. Wang TS, Cayo AK, Wilson SD, et al. The value of postoperative parathyroid hormone levels in predicting the need for long-term vitamin D supplementation after total thyroidectomy. Ann Surg Oncol 2011;18(3):777–81.

51. Saba A, Podda M, Messina Campanella A, et al. Early prediction of hypocalcemia following thyroid surgery. A prospective randomized clinical trial. Langenbecks Arch Surg 2017;402:1119.

52. Genser L, Tresallet C, Godiris-Petit G, et al. Randomized controlled trial of alfacalcidol supplementation for the reduction of hypocalcemia after total thyroidectomy. Am J Surg 2014;207:39–45.

53. Carter Y, Chen H, Sippel RS. An intact parathyroid hormone-based protocol for the prevention and treatment of symptomatic hypocalcemia after thyroidectomy. J Surg Res 2014;186:23–8.

54. Wang TS, Cheung K, Roman SA, et al. To supplement or not to supplement: a cost-utility analysis of calcium and vitamin D repletion in patients after thyroidectomy. Ann Surg Oncol 2011;18(5):1293–9.

55. Ross DS, Burch HB, Cooper DS, et al. 2016 American thyroid association guidelines for diagnosis and management of hyperthyroidism and other causes of thyrotoxicosis. Thyroid 2016;26(10):1343–421.

56. Francis GL, Waguespack SG, Bauer AJ, et al. Management guidelines for children with thyroid nodules and differentiated thyroid cancer: the American Thyroid Association guidelines task force on pediatric thyroid cancer. Thyroid 2015;25(7): 716–759..

57. Shoback DM, Bilezikian JP, Costa AG, et al. Presentation of hypoparathyroidism: etiologies and clinical features. J Clin Endocrinol Metab 2016;101(6):2300–12.

58. Kahramangil B, Dip F, Benmiloud F, et al. Detection of parathyroid autofluorescence using near-infrared imaging: a multicenter analysis of concordance between different surgeons. Ann Surg Oncol 2018;25(4):957–62.

59. Falco J, Dip F, Quadri P, et al. Cutting edge in thyroid surgery: autofluorescence of parathyroid glands. J Am Coll Surg 2016;223(2):374–80.
60. Dudley NE. Methylene blue for rapid identification of the parathyroids. Br Med J 1971;3(5776):680–1.
61. Kahramangil B, Berber E. The use of near-infrared fluorescence imaging in endocrine surgical procedures. J Surg Oncol 2017;115(7):848–55.
62. Hillary SL, Guillermet S, Brown NJ, et al. Use of methylene blue and near-infrared fluorescence in thyroid and parathyroid surgery. Langenbecks Arch Surg 2018; 403(1):111–8.
63. Vidal Fortuny J, Sadowski SM, Belfontali V, et al. Randomized clinical trial of intraoperative parathyroid gland angiography with indocyanine green fluorescence predicting parathyroid function after thyroid surgery. Br J Surg 2018;105(4): 350–7.
64. Mannstadt M, Clarke BL, Vokes T, et al. Efficacy and safety of recombinant human parathyroid hormone (1-84) in hypoparathyroidism (REPLACE): a double-blind, placebo-controlled, randomised, phase 3 study. Lancet Diabetes Endocrinol 2013;1:275.
65. Winer KK, Yanovski JA, Cutler GB Jr. Synthetic human parathyroid hormone 1-34 vs calcitriol and calcium in the treatment of hypoparathyroidism. JAMA 1996;276: 631–6.
66. Cusano NE, Rubin MR, McMahon DJ, et al. Therapy of hypoparathyroidism with PTH(1-84): a prospective four-year investigation of efficacy and safety. J Clin Endocrinol Metab 2013;98:137–44.

Medical Hypoparathyroidism

Namrah Siraj, MBBS, Yasser Hakami, MD, FRCPC, Aliya Khan, MD, FRCPC*

KEYWORDS

- Medical hypoparathyroidism
- Autoimmune polyendocrine syndrome type 1 hypocalcemia
- Pseudohypoparathyroidism • Autosomal dominant hypocalcemia • Genetics
- Parathyroid hormone

KEY POINTS

- The causes of nonsurgical hypoparathyroidism are broadly classified as autoimmune (as part of the autoimmune polyendocrine syndrome type 1 or isolated) genetic variants, infiltrative, metastatic, radiation destruction, mineral deposition (copper or iron), functional (magnesium deficiency or excess), or idiopathic.
- Autoimmune polyendocrine syndrome1 is associated with circulating autoantibodies and infiltration of the involved organs with lymphocytes leading to organ failure and is characterized by 3 major clinical features (chronic mucocutaneous candidiasis, hypoparathyroidism, and adrenal insufficiency); in addition, patients may have greater than 20 minor clinical features.
- Autoantibodies to 21-hydroxylase correlate with the development of adrenal insufficiency, and antibodies to NALP5 correlate with the development of hypoparathyroidism. A molecular diagnosis can be confirmed with DNA studies of the AIRE gene.
- Magnesium plays a key role in calcium homeostasis and should always be normalized.

INTRODUCTION

Hypoparathyroidism is a metabolic disorder characterized by low serum calcium, increased serum phosphorus, and inadequate production of parathyroid hormone (PTH). Hypoparathyroidism can be broadly classified as postsurgical (75%) and nonsurgical (25%) in cause. When hypoparathyroidism is not the result of surgical removal of too much parathyroid tissue, inadequate circulating levels of PTH are usually the result of genetic, autoimmune, environmental, or other conditions that affect either parathyroid gland function or mass.[1]

The authors have nothing to disclose.
Calcium Disorders Clinic, McMaster University, 50 Charlton Ave East, Hamilton, Ontario L8N 4A6, Canada
* Corresponding author.
E-mail address: aliya@mcmaster.ca

The diagnosis of hypoparathyroidism is confirmed by the presence of a low concentration of serum or plasma calcium (total corrected for albumin or ionized) in the presence of a low or inappropriately normal level of PTH. The reduced PTH level leads to increased renal tubular phosphate reabsorption and, consequently, elevated serum phosphate levels. Hyperphosphatemia contributes to extraskeletal calcification with mineral deposition in the basal ganglia, cornea, renal parenchyma, as well as other tissues. Functional hypoparathyroidism develops in the presence of magnesium deficiency or excess. The evaluation and causes of nonsurgical hypoparathyroidism are reviewed in detail next.

Autoimmune Hypoparathyroidism

Autoimmune hypoparathyroidism is the most common cause of nonsurgical hypoparathyroidism. This condition can occur as an isolated feature or as a part of the autoimmune polyglandular syndrome type I (APS-I).

APS-I, also known as autoimmune poly endocrinopathy candidiasis ectodermal dystrophy (APECED), is caused by mutations in the autoimmune regulator gene (AIRE), which is expressed in the lymph nodes, thymus, pancreas, adrenal cortex, and fetal liver.[2,3] The inheritance is autosomal recessive; however, dominant transmission has been reported.[4,5]

Chronic mucocutaneous candidiasis, hypoparathyroidism, and Addison disease represent the clinical hallmark of the syndrome; the clinical diagnosis of APECED requires the presence of at least 2 of these 3 major components. APECED typically presents in childhood with candidiasis, followed by hypoparathyroidism, which usually develops between 5 and 9 years of age and adrenal insufficiency during adolescence.[2,3,5,6] More than 80% of patients with APS-1 exhibit hypoparathyroidism, which may be their sole endocrinopathy.

Minor components include greater than 20 organ-specific components.[7] Genetic and environmental factors modify the phenotype resulting in diverse clinical presentations in the same family.[7] A large range of autoantibodies may be present in APS-1, including organ-specific autoantibodies as well as antibodies to cytokines and interferons.[7–9] Autoantibodies to intracellular enzymes restricted to specific organs in which the autoantigen is expressed can be measured and are useful for diagnostic screening.[10] Assays for autoantibodies to 21-hydroxylase and to NACHT leucine-rich-repeat protein 5 (NALP5) can be helpful in predicting the development of adrenal insufficiency and hypoparathyroidism, respectively. Autoantibodies to cytokines may also be present[5] as well as autoantibodies to type 1 interferon.[8,11]

The molecular diagnosis of APS-1 can be confirmed by DNA analysis of the AIRE gene.[12] The presence of minor components of APS-1 can be helpful in considering the diagnosis of APS-1. The minor features include keratitis, autoimmune hepatitis, primary ovarian insufficiency, enamel hypoplasia, enteropathy with chronic diarrhea or constipation, photophobia, periodic fever with rash, pneumonitis, nephritis, pancreatitis, and functional asplenia.[3,5]

A diagnosis of APS-1 is strongly suggested by the presence of at least one of the major syndrome components and positive antibodies to type 1 interferon; sequencing of the AIRE gene can provide confirmation of the diagnosis.

The worldwide incidence of APS-1 is 1 per 100,000, but it is more commonly observed in 3 genetically isolated populations: Finns (incidence 1:25,000), Sardinians (incidence 1:14,000), and Iranian Jews (incidence 1:9000).[2,3]

The association of AIRE mutations with isolated hypoparathyroidism is quite unusual. A kindred of 10 children, 3 of whom were diagnosed with hypoparathyroidism in the first decade of their life, were recently reported to have a mutation in the AIRE gene.[13] Only 1 of the 3 siblings with mutations in the AIRE gene developed additional features of APS-1 with the onset of premature ovarian failure at 33 years of age. The other 2 siblings (brothers) failed to develop any other clinical features of APS-1 even after 50 years of medical surveillance.[13] Other investigators have confirmed that APS-1 can present with isolated hypoparathyroidism; however, follow-up has been of limited duration.[14,15] Additional features of APS-1 can develop as late as the fifth decade of life.[16,17] Another investigator described 2 children aged 4 years and 5 years with biallelic AIRE mutations and no other features of APS-1 apart from hypoparathyroidism.[18] Two siblings with AIRE mutations have been reported with 1 brother aged 15 years demonstrating isolated hypoparathyroidism.[19]

Antibodies to the calcium sensing receptor (CaSR) that activate signaling can suppress PTH secretion leading to hypoparathyroidism. Kifor and colleagues[20] reported on 2 patients with activating anti-CaSR antibodies with direct functional actions on CaSR. One patient with long-standing hypoparathyroidism and Graves disease was noted to have a normal parathyroid gland at the time of subtotal thyroidectomy. The second patient was diagnosed with Addison's disease and transient mild hypoparathyroidism. The hypocalcemia subsequently remitted indicating that there had not been irreversible destruction of the parathyroid glands.[21]

Antibodies against the extracellular domain of the CaSR are present in a subset of patients with isolated hypoparathyroidism. In one study, 14 of 25 patients with autoimmune hypoparathyroidism had circulating antibodies that were reactive to the extracellular domain of the CaSR.[22] Antibodies to the parathyroid cell surface were present in 8 of 23 cases of idiopathic hypoparathyroidism.[23] Other studies have shown varying rates of anti-CaSR antibody positivity. It is not yet clear whether the anti-CaSR antibodies play a causal role or serve as markers of tissue injury.[24]

The management of an individual with APS-1 requires a multidisciplinary team at a specialized tertiary care center. Immediate family members, including the siblings, require further evaluation, including measuring autoantibodies for 21-hydroxylase, in order to determine the risk of developing adrenal insufficiency. Also measuring autoantibodies for NALP5 enables assessment of the risk of developing hypoparathyroidism. The management of hypoparathyroidism in APS-1 can be challenging if malabsorption is also present, as this may impact the absorption of calcium, cholecalciferol, as well as activated vitamin D.

Infiltrative Causes

Destruction of the parathyroid glands can occur secondary to granulomatous infiltration (eg, sarcoidosis, amyloidosis, Riedel thyroiditis); however, clinical hypoparathyroidism rarely occurs in these cases. There are a few case reports of possible infiltration of parathyroid glands by sarcoid granulomas leading to hypoparathyroidism.[25–27] Autopsy studies have indicated a high frequency of amyloid deposits in the parathyroid glands..[28] Several cases of hypoparathyroidism with Riedel thyroiditis have also been reported.[29–31]

Metastatic Cancer

Pathologic involvement of the parathyroid glands resulting in hypoparathyroidism can rarely occur due to infiltrating metastatic cancer.[32–34] However, metastases to the parathyroid glands are extremely rare with very few reported cases in the literature.[35] In an autopsy study evaluating sites of metastases in 1000 patients with malignancy, no patient was found to have parathyroid metastasis, even though several unusual locations for metastatic deposits were identified..[36] A prospective study of 160 consecutive necropsies in patients with various malignancies demonstrated metastatic involvement of at least one parathyroid gland in only 19 cases.[33] However, the same investigators in a retrospective study of 750 necropsies identified secondary malignant involvement of the parathyroid in 40 cases.[33] The most common primary sites of malignancy with parathyroid metastases in decreasing order of frequency were breast, blood (leukemia), skin (malignant melanoma), lung, soft tissue (spindle cell sarcomas), and lymphomas.[33]

Radiation Destruction

Another rare cause of hypoparathyroidism is exposure of the parathyroid glands to ionizing radiation. Radioactive iodine administered for the treatment of thyroid disease, particularly when high doses are given in the context of thyroid carcinoma, has been associated with hypoparathyroidism in reported cases.[37,38] A transient decline in PTH was observed 6 months after radioactive iodine therapy in 19 patients undergoing thyroid remnant ablation.[39] None of these patients were symptomatic despite low PTH and low serum calcium.[39] External beam radiotherapy used for the treatment of thyroid cancer has not been documented to impact parathyroid gland function.

Mineral Deposition

Hypoparathyroidism may occur because of accumulation or deposition of minerals in the parathyroid gland. Wilson's disease is among the rarest causes of hypoparathyroidism and results from destruction of parathyroid glands due to deposition of copper. This condition has been reported by a few investigators. Carpenter and colleagues[40] described a 11-year-old girl with hypoparathyroidism secondary to Wilson's disease. Fatima and colleagues[41] described an affected 16-year-old boy. Okada and colleagues[42] reported a case of Wilson's disease associated with hypoparathyroidism and amenorrhea.

Hemochromatosis with iron overload, either primary or secondary, due to chronic transfusions (eg, in thalassemia) has also been associated with hypoparathyroidism. The mainstay of treatment of severe beta thalassemia is regular blood transfusions. Hypoparathyroidism secondary to iron overload has been reported to occur in 13.5% to 20.0% of the patients.[43,44] There has been a decrease in the reported cases of hypoparathyroidism secondary to iron overload following introduction of improved chelation therapy regimen's suggesting chelation may prevent the development of hypoparathyroidism.[45]

Toxic Agents

Parathyroid tissue is highly resistant to chemotherapeutic and cytotoxic medications with the exceptions of L asparaginase, which has been associated with parathyroid necrosis[46] and ethiofos a radio and chemo-protective agent that causes reversible inhibition of PTH secretion.[47,48]

Transient Hypoparathyroidism

A transient form of hypoparathyroidism can occur in the context of severe burn injury as well as acute illness.

Children and adults who have sustained severe burn injuries can develop magnesium depletion (secondary to loss through the burn wound, abnormal intestinal secretion, and increased metabolic rate) hypocalcemia, and hypoparathyroidism. As discussed later, magnesium is an important cofactor in the production of cyclic adenosine monophosphate (cAMP) and inadequate magnesium levels block intracellular cyclic AMP generation in parathyroid cells impacting the secretion of parathyroid hormone.[49,50] Another possible mechanism for the development of hypoparathyroidism in burn injury is cytokine-mediated upregulation of the calcium-sensing receptor in the parathyroid glands resulting in hypoparathyroidism as well as urinary calcium wasting.[51]

Functional (Magnesium Deficiency or Excess)

Magnesium has a significant impact on parathyroid function and on the serum calcium level. Hypomagnesemia and hypermagnesemia can result in hypocalcemia and impair parathyroid function.

Both the magnesium ion (Mg^{2+}) and calcium ion (Ca^{2+}) activate the CaSR and affect PTH synthesis and secretion.[52] Intracellular Mg^{2+} is also involved in the activation of adenylate cyclase and in intracellular signaling of cyclic AMP.[53] Activation of the CaSR by Mg^{2+} results in stimulation of phospholipase C and A2 and inhibition of intracellular cyclic AMP formation with inhibition of PTH release.[54] Activation of the CaSR in the kidney decreases paracellular sodium, calcium, and magnesium transport and results in a loss of these cations through the kidneys. Heterozygous activating mutations of the CaSR result in autosomal-dominant hypocalcemia (ADH). Activation of the CaSR in the parathyroid glands leads to inappropriately low PTH levels. These patients may present with symptoms of hypocalcemia including seizures or muscle spasms. The hypocalcemia in ADH is associated with hypomagnesemia in many affected patients.[55] Salt and water loss due to inhibition of active transcellular sodium chloride reabsorption and a picture similar to Bartter's syndrome can also be seen in ADH.[56]

Approximately 70% of filtered Mg^{2+} is reabsorbed in the thick ascending limb of Henle loop (TAL) and is passively reabsorbed with calcium in a paracellular manner via specialized tight junctions. These tight junctions are composed of a specific set of proteins of the claudin family that allow selective passage of ions and seal the paracellular space for water and electrolytes. Claudin proteins claudin-16 and claudin-19 play a key role in regulating paracellular Ca^{2+} and Mg^{2+} transport.[57] Mutations affecting these two proteins result in impaired paracellular reabsorption of both Ca^{2+} and Mg^{2+} causing familial hypomagnesemia with hypercalciuria and nephrocalcinosis (FHHNC).[58] Patients with these mutations have hypomagnesemia and develop nephrocalcinosis in childhood due to the presence of hypercalciuria and often chronic renal failure by the second decade of life.[59,60]

Paracellular Ca^{2+} and Mg^{2+} transport in the TAL is regulated by the action of the basolaterally located CaSR. The CaSR senses extracellular Ca^{2+} as well as Mg^{2+} concentrations in the distal nephron as well as in other tissues and thereby plays an essential role in Ca^{2+} and Mg^{2+} homeostasis.[61] PTH increases Mg^{2+} reabsorption in the cortical TAL by enhancing paracellular permeability and also increases transcellular Mg^{2+} reabsorption in the distal convoluted tubule (DCT).[52,62] In the DCT only 5% to 10% of filtered Mg^{2+} is reabsorbed, and this is via active transcellular Mg^{2+} transport.[58,63]

Loss-of-function mutations in TRPM6 affect active transcellular Mg^{2+} transport in both the kidney and the intestine[64,65] and result in hypomagnesemia with secondary hypocalcemia (HSH). Familial HSH caused by mutations in transient receptor potential cation channel subfamily M member 6 (TRPM6) is an inherited disorder impairing intestinal magnesium absorption. The TRPM6 gene is involved in the formation of apical magnesium permeable ion channels in the intestine and kidney. Recessive mutations result in defective active transcellular magnesium uptake in the intestine and also impair renal magnesium conservation.[64,65] Children with this mutation have severe hypomagnesemia and seizures during infancy. In addition to hypomagnesemia, patients also have suppressed PTH levels with hypocalcemia. The severe hypomagnesemia leads to the suppression of PTH thought to be secondary to a block in PTH synthesis and secretion in the presence of profound hypomagnesemia.[66] This paradoxic inhibition of the parathyroid involves intracellular signaling pathways of the CaSR with an increase in the inhibitory G alpha subunit activity.[67] A resistance to PTH at the skeletal level is also seen in hypomagnesemia.[68–70] Intracellular Mg^{2+} is a cofactor of adenylate cyclase, and decreases in intracellular Mg^{2+} contributes to the resistance to PTH.[71–73]

The hypocalcemia in association with hypomagnesemia is resistant to treatment with Ca^{2+} or vitamin D and requires Mg^{2+} supplementation.

Deficiencies in intracellular Mg^{2+} may develop in the presence of a normal serum Mg^{2+}.[74,75] Intracellular Mg^{2+} may be a key regulator of serum PTH.[76]

Hypomagnesemia may be due to decreased intake, decreased intestinal absorption, increased losses, or redistribution of Mg^{2+}.[77] Mg^{2+} is widely present in all food groups.[77] Common causes of hypomagnesemia are decreased absorption due to malabsorption, short bowel syndrome, severe vomiting, diarrhea, or steatorrhea.[78]

Long-term proton pump inhibitor use contributes to enhanced gastrointestinal losses[79,80] most probably due to inhibition of TRPM6-mediated active transportation of Mg^{2+} secondary to altered intestinal pH. However, the exact mechanism leading to hypomagnesemia still needs to be clarified.[81]

The fractional excretion of magnesium (FEMg) enables us to determine if the magnesium deficiency is due to intestinal losses or due to renal wasting.

The formula for FEMg is as follows: urine Mg $\times$ plasma creatinine/plasma Mg $\times$ urine creatinine $\times$ 100%, where Mg is magnesium.

An FEMg greater than 4% in the presence of hypomagnesemia is consistent with renal magnesium wasting.

An intestinal or nonrenal cause is likely to be present if FEMg is less than 2%.[82] Low estimated glomerular filtration rate and severe hypomagnesemia can also lead to a reduced FEMg. A urinary magnesium excretion of more than 1 mmol/d in the presence of hypomagnesemia is consistent with renal magnesium wasting.[83]

Drugs can cause hypomagnesemia by promoting renal magnesium wasting as listed below:

Diuretics (thiazide and furosemide), antibiotics and antimycotics (foscarnet, amphotericin B, aminoglycosides, pentamidine, and rapamycin), anticancer agents (ie, platinum derivatives such as cisplatin, carboplatin), immunosuppressants (calcineurin inhibitors, such as tacrolimus and cyclosporine A), and also epidermal growth factor–receptor inhibitors (cetuximab).

Hypermagnesemia may also cause hypocalcemia due to the inhibition of PTH release.[68] Renal impairment decreases renal magnesium excretion and serum magnesium levels increase.[56] Hypermagnesemia is also associated with an increased fractional excretion of Mg^{2+} in order to maintain a normal serum Mg^{2+}. In familial hypocalciuric hypercalcemia, as well as with use of lithium, renal clearance of Mg^{2+} is mildly impaired; hence, serum magnesium levels are higher than in other forms of primary hyperparathyroidism.[84] Excess intake also results in high levels of serum magnesium (antacids, cathartics, laxatives, parenteral administrations of Mg^{2+}). Another important cause of clinically significant hypermagnesemia is the use of magnesium sulfate as a tocolytic therapy for eclampsia, which has been associated with hypocalcemia due to magnesium-induced suppression of PTH secretion.[85,86]

Mitochondrial Disorders Associated with Hypoparathyroidism

Several mitochondrial disorders have been associated with hypoparathyroidism.[87,88] These syndromes are caused by mutations and deletions in mitochondrial DNA and include the following:

Kearns-Sayer syndrome is a mitochondrial cytopathy that is characterized by encephalopathy, progressive external ophthalmoplegia, ptosis, retinitis pigmentosa, cardiomyopathy, cardiac conduction blocks, and ataxia.

Mitochondrial myopathy, encephalopathy, lactic acidosis, and strokelike episodes syndrome is a maternally inherited disorder caused by point mutations in mitochondrial transfer RNA. This syndrome usually manifests in childhood after a normal early development and affects the nervous system and muscles.

Mitochondrial trifunctional protein deficiency is a fatty acid oxidation disorder that manifests as nonketotic hypoglycemia, cardiomyopathy, hepatic dysfunction, skeletal myopathy, and developmental delays. In some cases, mothers of an affected fetus have acute liver degeneration during pregnancy.

Maternal Hyperparathyroidism/Hypercalcemia

The prevalence of primary hyperparathyroidism in the general population is 0.15%. It is more common in women, and 25% of cases of PHPT occur in women during the childbearing years. The true incidence during pregnancy, however, is not known; however, it is estimated that up to 80% of pregnant patients with primary hyperparathyroidism are asymptomatic, making the diagnosis of PHPT in pregnancy difficult. Complications associated with primary hyperparathyroidism in pregnancy have been reported to occur in up to 67% of mothers and 80% of fetuses. For the mother, hyperparathyroidism can present as hyperemesis, nephrolithiasis, and acute pancreatitis; in severe cases it may present as a hypercalcemic crisis. An infant who is exposed in utero to maternal primary hyperparathyroidism or hypercalcemia is at risk of having suppressed parathyroid function and hypocalcemia, which may lead to intrauterine growth retardation, preterm delivery, intrauterine fetal demise, or postpartum neonatal tetany if the mother remains untreated.[89–91]

Idiopathic

The hypoparathyroidism can be confirmed as idiopathic in cause following a careful review of all the possible causes of hypoparathyroidism. Such individuals should continue to be closely followed and monitored to ensure that target organ damage is prevented.

SUMMARY

Nonsurgical hypoparathyroidism remains an important cause of hypoparathyroidism. It is essential to diagnose this condition early and determine the underlying cause. In young individuals or in the presence of a positive family history of consanguinity it is advised that the patient and the family be referred for genetic counseling. Appropriate DNA studies can also be completed enabling a molecular diagnosis. Treatment is advised to ensure that serum calcium is maintained in the low-normal reference range with close monitoring of calcium, phosphate, magnesium, as well as renal function. Patients require monitoring for the development of extraskeletal calcification as well as other complications of hypoparathyroidism.

REFERENCES

1. Maedal SS, Fortes EM, Oliveira UM, et al. Hypoparathyroidism and pseudohypo-parathyroidism. Arq Bras Endocrinol Metabol 2006;50(4):664–73.
2. Lankisch TO, Jaeckel E, Strassburg CP. The autoimmune polyendocrinopathy-candidiasis-ectodermal dystrophy or autoimmune polyglandular syndrome type 1. Semin Liver Dis 2009;29(3):307–14.
3. Husebye E, Perheentupa J, Rautemaa R, et al. Clinical manifestations and management of patients with autoimmune polyendocrine syndrome type I. J Intern Med 2009;265(5):514–29.
4. Finnish-German APECED Consortium. An autoimmune disease, APECED, caused by mutations in a novel gene featuring two PHD-type zinc-finger domains. Nat Genet 1997;17(4):399–403.
5. Husebye E, Anderson M, Kämpe O. Autoimmune polyendocrine syndromes. N Engl J Med 2018;378(12):1132–41.
6. Blizzard RM, Chee D, Davis W. The incidence of parathyroid and other antibodies in the sera of patients with idiopathic hypoparathyroidism. Clin Exp Immunol 1966;1(2):119–28.
7. Orlova E, Sozaeva L, Kareva M, et al. Expanding the phenotypic and genotypic landscape of autoimmune polyendocrine syndrome type 1. J Clin Endocrinol Metab 2017;102(9):3546–56.
8. Meager A, Visvalingam K, Peterson P, et al. Anti-interferon autoantibodies in autoimmune polyendocrinopathy syndrome type 1. PLoS Med 2006;3(7):e289.
9. Meloni A, Furcas M, Cetani F, et al. Autoantibodies against type I interferons as an additional diagnostic criterion for autoimmune polyendocrine syndrome type I. J Clin Endocrinol Metab 2008;93(11):4389–97.
10. Söderbergh A, Myhre A, Ekwall O, et al. Prevalence and clinical associations of 10 defined autoantibodies in autoimmune polyendocrine syndrome type I. J Clin Endocrinol Metab 2004;89(2):557–62.
11. Dalin F, Nordling Eriksson G, Dahlqvist P, et al. Clinical and Immunological characteristics of autoimmune addison disease: a nationwide swedish multicenter study. J Clin Endocrinol Metab 2017;102(2):379–89.
12. Zhang J, Liu H, Liu Z, et al. A functional alternative splicing mutation in AIRE gene causes autoimmune polyendocrine syndrome type 1. PLoS One 2013;8(1): e53981.
13. Li D, Streeten EA, Chan A, et al. Exome sequencing reveals mutations in AIRE as a cause of isolated hypoparathyroidism. J Clin Endocrinol Metab 2017;102(5): 1726–33.
14. Sahoo S, Zaidi G, Srivastava R, et al. Identification of autoimmune polyendocrine syndrome type 1 in patients with isolated hypoparathyroidism. Clin Endocrinol (Oxf) 2016;85(4):544–50.
15. Oftedal B, Hellesen A, Erichsen M, et al. Dominant mutations in the autoimmune regulator AIRE are associated with common organ-specific autoimmune diseases. Immunity 2015;42(6):1185–96.
16. Perheentupa J. Autoimmune polyendocrinopathy-candidiasis-ectodermal dystrophy. J Clin Endocrinol Metab 2006;91(8):2843–50.
17. Ahonen P, Myllärniemi S, Sipilä I, et al. Clinical variation of autoimmune polyendocrinopathy-candidiasis-ectodermal dystrophy (APECED) in a series of 68 patients. N Engl J Med 1990;322(26):1829–36.

18. Cervato S, Morlin L, Albergoni M, et al. AIRE gene mutations and autoantibodies to interferon omega in patients with chronic hypoparathyroidism without APECED. Clin Endocrinol 2010;73(5):630–6.
19. Eyal O, Oren A, Jüppner H, et al. Hypoparathyroidism and central diabetes insipidus: in search of the link. Eur J Pediatr 2014;173(12):1731–4.
20. Kifor O, McElduff A, LeBoff MS, et al. Activating antibodies to the calcium-sensing receptor in two patients with autoimmune hypoparathyroidism. J Clin Endocrinol Metab 2004;89(2):548–56.
21. Bilezikian J, Khan A, Potts J Jr, et al. Hypoparathyroidism in the adult: epidemiology, diagnosis, pathophysiology, target organ involvement, treatment, and challenges for future research. J Bone Miner Res 2011;26(10):2317–37.
22. Li Y, Song YH, Rais N, et al. Autoantibodies to the extracellular domain of the calcium sensing receptor in patients with acquired hypoparathyroidism. J Clin Invest 1996;97(4):910–4.
23. Posillico J, Wortsman J, Srikanta S, et al. Parathyroid cell surface autoantibodies that inhibit parathyroid hormone secretion from dispersed human parathyroid cells. J Bone Mineral Res 1986;1(5):475–83.
24. Brown EM. Anti-parathyroid and anti-calcium sensing receptor antibodies in autoimmune hypoparathyroidism. Endocrinol Metab Clin North Am 2009;38(2): 437–45, x.
25. Brinkane A, Peschard S, Leroy-Terquem E, et al. Rare association of hypoparathyroidism and mediastinal-pulmonary sarcoidosis. Ann Med Interne (Paris) 2001;152(1):63–4.
26. Saeed A, Khan M, Irwin S, et al. Sarcoidosis presenting with severe hypocalcaemia. Ir J Med Sci 2011;180(2):575–7.
27. Badell A, Servitje O, Graells J, et al. Hypoparathyroidism and sarcoidosis. Br J Dermatol 1998;138(5):915–7.
28. Anderson TJ, Ewen SWB. Amyloid in normal and pathological parathyroid glands. J Clin Pathol 1974;27(8):656–63.
29. Yasmeen T, Khan S, Patel SG, et al. Riedel's thyroiditis: report of a case complicated by spontaneous hypoparathyroidism, recurrent laryngeal nerve injury, and horner's syndrome. J Clin Endocrinol Metab 2002;87(8):3543–7.
30. Casoli P, Tumiati B. Hypoparathyroidism secondary to Riedel's thyroiditis. A case report and a review of the literature. Ann Ital Med Int 1991;14(1):54–7.
31. McRorie ER, Chalmers J, Campbell JW. Riedel's thyroiditis complicated by hypoparathyroidism and hypothyroidism. Scott Med J 1993;38(1):27–8.
32. Goddard C, Mbewu A, Evanson J. Symptomatic hypocalcaemia associated with metastatic invasion of the parathyroid glands. Br J Hosp Med 1990;43(1):72.
33. Horwitz CA, Myers WL, Foote FW Jr. Secondary malignant tumors of the parathyroid glands: Report of two cases with associated hypoparathyroidism. Am J Med 1972;52(6):797–808.
34. Watanabe T, Adachi I, Satoshi K, et al. A case of advanced breast cancer associated with hypocalcemia. Jpn J Clin Oncol 1983;13(2):441–8.
35. Gattuso P, Khan N, Jablokow V, et al. Neoplasms metastatic to parathyroid glands. South Med J 1988;81(11):1467.
36. Abrams H, Spiro R, Goldstein N. Metastases in carcinoma; analysis of 1000 autopsied cases. Cancer 1950;3(1):74–85.
37. Glazebrook GA. Effect of decicurie doses of radioactive iodine 131 on parathyroid function. Am J Surg 1987;154(4):368–73.
38. Winslow CP, Meyers AD. Hypocalcemia as a complication of radioiodine therapy. Am J Otolaryngol 1998;19(6):401–3.

39. Guven A, Salman S, Boztepe H, et al. Parathyroid changes after high dose radio-active iodine in patients with thyroid cancer. Ann Nucl Med 2009;23(5):437–41.

40. Carpenter T, Carnes DJ, Anast C. Hypoparathyroidism in Wilson's disease. N Engl J Med 1983;309(15):873–7.

41. Fatima J, Karoli R, Jain V. Hypoparathyroidism in a case of Wilson's disease: rare association of a rare disorder. Indian J Endocrinol Metab 2013;17(2):361–2.

42. Okada M, Higashi K, Enomoto S, et al. A case of Wilson's disease associated with hypoparathyroidism and amenorrhea. Nihon Shokakibyo Gakkai Zasshi 1998; 95(5):445–9.

43. Angelopoulos N, Goula A, Rombopoulos G, et al. Hypoparathyroidism in transfusion-dependent patients with beta-thalassemia. J Bone Miner Metab 2006;24(2):138–45.

44. Aleem A, Al-Momen A, Al-Harakati M, et al. Hypocalcemia due to hypoparathy-roidism in beta-thalassemia major patients. Ann Saudi Med 2000;20(5–6):364–6.

45. De Satictis V, Vullo C, Bagni B, et al. Hypoparathyroidism in beta-thalassemia major: clinical and laboratory observations in 24 patients. Acta Haematol 1992; 88(2–3):105–8.

46. O'Regan S, Carson S, Chesney R, et al. Electrolyte and acid-base disturbances in the management of leukemia. Blood 1977;49(3):345–53.

47. Wadler S, Haynes H, Beitler J, et al. Management of hypocalcemic effects of WR2721 administered on a daily times five schedule with cisplatin and radiation therapy. The New York Gynecologic Oncology Group. J Clin Oncol 1993;11(8): 1517–22.

48. Attie MF, Fallon MD, Spar B, et al. Bone and parathyroid inhibitory effects of S-2(3-aminopropylamino)ethylphosphorothioic acid. Studies in experimental ani-mals and cultured bone cells. J Clin Invest 1985;75(4):1191–7.

49. Klein G, Herndon D. Magnesium deficit in major burns: role in hypoparathyroid-ism and end-organ parathyroid hormone resistance. Magnes Res 1998;11(2): 103–9.

50. Klein G, Nicolai M, Langman C, et al. Dysregulation of calcium homeostasis after severe burn injury in children: possible role of magnesium depletion. J Pediatr 1997;131(2):246–51.

51. Klein GL. Burns: where has all the calcium (and Vitamin D) gone? Adv Nutr 2011; 2(6):457–62.

52. Vetter T, Lohse M. Magnesium and the parathyroid. Curr Opin Nephrol Hypertens 2002;11(4):403–10.

53. Grubbs R, Maguire M. Magnesium as a regulatory cation: criteria and evaluation. Magnesium 1987;6(3):113–27.

54. Chang W, Pratt S, Chen T, et al. Coupling of calcium receptors to inositol phos-phate and cyclic AMP generation in mammalian cells and Xenopus laevis oo-cytes and immunodetection of receptor protein by region-specific antipeptide antisera. J Bone Mineral Res 1998;13(4):570–80.

55. Pearce S, Williamson C, Kifor O, et al. A familial syndrome of hypocalcemia with hypercalciuria due to mutations in the calcium-sensing receptor. N Engl J Med 1996;335:1115–22.

56. Watanabe S, Fukumoto S, Chang H, et al. Association between activating muta-tions of calcium-sensing receptor and Bartter's syndrome. Lancet 2002; 360(9934):692–4.

57. Hou J, Goodenough D. Claudin-16 and claudin-19 function in the thick ascending limb. Curr Opin Nephrol Hypertens 2010;19(5):483–8.

58. Ferrè S, Hoenderop JJ, Bindel RJ. Role of the distal convoluted tubule in renal Mg 2+ handling: molecular lessons from inherited hypomagnesemia. Magnes Res 2011;24(3). John Lippey Euro Text.

59. Weber S, Schneider L, Peters M, et al. Novel paracellin-1 mutations in 25 families with familial hypomagnesemia with hypercalciuria and nephrocalcinosis. J Am Soc Nephrol 2001;12(9):1872–81.

60. Konrad M, Hou J, Weber S, et al. CLDN16 genotype predicts renal decline in familial hypomagnesemia with hypercalciuria and nephrocalcinosis. J Am Soc Nephrol 2008;19(1):171–81.

61. Alfadda T, Saleh A, Houillier P, et al. Calcium-sensing receptor 20 years later. Am J Physiol Cell Physiol 2014;307(3):C221–31.

62. Wittner M, Mandon B, Roinel N, et al. Hormonal stimulation of Ca2+ and Mg2+ transport in the cortical thick ascending limb of Henle's loop of the mouse: evidence for a change in the paracellular pathway permeability. Pflugers Arch 1993;423(5–6):387–96.

63. Bindels R. 2009 Homer W. Smith award: minerals in motion: from new ion transporters to new concepts. J Am Soc Nephrol 2010;21(8):1263–9.

64. Schlingmann K, Weber S, Peters M, et al. Hypomagnesemia with secondary hypocalcemia is caused by mutations in TRPM6, a new member of the TRPM gene family. Nat Genet 2002;31(2):166–70.

65. Walder R, Landau D, Meyer P, et al. Mutation of TRPM6 causes familial hypomagnesemia with secondary hypocalcemia. Nat Genet 2002;31(2):171–4.

66. Anast C, Mohs J, Kaplan S, et al. Evidence for parathyroid failure in magnesium deficiency. Science 1972;177(4049):606–8.

67. Quitterer U, Hoffmann M, Friechel M, et al. Paradoxical block of parathormone secretion is mediated by increased activity of G alpha subunits. J Biol Chem 2001;276(9):6763–9.

68. Nijenhuis T, Vallon V, Van der kemp A, et al. Enhanced passive Ca2+ reabsorption and reduced Mg2+ channel abundance explains thiazide-induced hypocalciuria and hypomagnesemia. J Clin Invest 2005;115(6):1651–8.

69. Groenestege W, Thebault S, Van der Wijst J, et al. Impaired basolateral sorting of pro-EGF causes isolated recessive renal hypomagnesemia. J Clin Invest 2007;117(8):2260–7.

70. Hoorn E, Walsh S, McCormick J, et al. The calcineurin inhibitor tacrolimus activates the renal sodium chloride cotransporter to cause hypertension. Nat Med 2011;17(10):1304–9.

71. Mune T, Yasuda K, Ishii M, et al. Tetany due to hypomagnesemia induced by cisplatin and doxorubicin treatment for synovial sarcoma. Intern Med 1993;32(5):434–7.

72. Mori S, Harada S, Okazaki R, et al. Hypomagnesemia with increased metabolism of parathyroid hormone and reduced responsiveness to calcitropic hormones. Intern Med 1992;31(6):820–4.

73. Mihara M, Kamikubo K, Hiramatsu K, et al. Renal refractoriness to phosphaturic action of parathyroid hormone in a patient with hypomagnesemia. Intern Med 1995;34(7):666–9.

74. Dyckner T, Wester P. The relation between extra- and intracellular electrolytes in patients with hypokalemia and/or diuretic treatment. Acta Med Scand 1978;204(4):269–82.

75. Rob P, Bley N, Dick K, et al. Magnesium deficiency after renal transplantation and cyclosporine treatment despite normal serum-magnesium detected by a modified magnesium-loading-test. Transplant Proc 1995;27(6):3442–3.

76. Pironi L, Malucelli E, Guidetti M, et al. The complex relationship between magnesium and serum parathyroid hormone: a study in patients with chronic intestinal failure. Magnes Res 2009;22(1):37–43.

77. Steen O, Khan AA. Role of magnesium in parathyroid physiology," in hypoparathyroidism. Milano: Springer; 2015. p. 61–7.

78. Hoorn E, Zietse R. Disorders of calcium and magnesium balance: a physiology-based approach. Pediatr Nephrol 2013;28(8):1195–206.

79. Hess MW, Hoenderop JGJ, Bindels RJM, et al. Systematic review: hypomagnesaemia induced by proton pump inhibition. Aliment Pharmacol Ther 2012; 36(5):405–13.

80. Hoorn EJ, Van der Hoek J, de Man RA, et al. A case series of proton pump inhibitor–induced hypomagnesemia. Am J Kidney Dis 2010;56(1):112–6.

81. Cundy T, Dissanayake A. Severe hypomagnesaemia in long-term users of proton-pump inhibitors. Clin Endocrinol (Oxf) 2008;69(2):338–41.

82. Elisaf M, Panteli K, Theodorou J, et al. Fractional excretion of magnesium in normal subjects and in patients with hypomagnesemia. Magnes Res 1997; 10(4):315–20.

83. Sutton R, Domrongkitchaiporn S. Abnormal renal magnesium handling. Miner Electrolyte Metab 1993;19(4–5):232–40.

84. Marx S, Attie M, Levine M, et al. The hypocalciuric or benign variant of familial hypercalcemia: clinical and biochemical features in fifteen kindreds. Medicine 1981;60(6):397–412.

85. Mayan H, Hourvitz A, Schiff E, et al. Symptomatic hypocalcaemia in hypermagnesaemia-induced hypoparathyroidism, during magnesium tocolytic therapy–possible involvement of the calcium-sensing receptor. Nephrol Dial Transplant 1999;14(7):1764–6.

86. Cholst I, Steinberg S, Tropper P, et al. The influence of hypermagnesemia on serum calcium and parathyroid hormone levels in human subjects. N Engl J Med 1984;310(19):1221–5.

87. Zupanc M, Moraes C, Shanske S, et al. Deletion of mitochondrial DNA in patients with combined features of Kearns-Sayre and MELAS syndromes. Ann Neurol 1991;29(6):680–3.

88. Dionisi-Vici C, Garavaglia B, Burlina AB, et al. Hypoparathyroidism in mitochondrial trifunctional protein deficiency. J Pediatr 1996;129(1):159–62.

89. Ya H, Ming C, Zhengyi S, et al. Clinical presentation, management, and outcomes of primary hyperparathyroidism during pregnancy. Int J Endocrinol 2017;2017:7. Article ID 3947423.

90. Truong MT, Lalakea ML, Robbins P, et al. Primary hyperparathyroidism in pregnancy: a case series and review. Laryngoscope 2008;118(11):1966–9.

91. Schnatz P, Curry S. Primary hyperparathyroidism in pregnancy: evidence-based management. Obstet Gynecol Surv 2002;57(6):365–76.

Genetic Disorders of Parathyroid Development and Function

Rebecca J. Gordon, MD[a],*, Michael A. Levine, MD[b]

KEYWORDS

- Hypoparathyroidism • Parathyroid hormone • Genetics • Etiologies

KEY POINTS

- Hypoparathyroidism can be an isolated endocrine disorder or part of a complex syndrome.
- Genetic defects account for disorders of parathyroid gland formation, dysregulation of parathyroid hormone synthesis or secretion, and autoimmune destruction of the parathyroid glands.
- Genetic hypoparathyroidism may be sporadic or exhibit autosomal dominant, autosomal recessive, or X-linked recessive inheritance.

INTRODUCTION

Hypoparathyroidism may occur as an isolated endocrine disorder or as a component of a complex developmental, metabolic, or endocrinologic syndrome. Molecular genetics analyses over the past 20 years have identified mutations in a growing number of genes that have provided novel insights into embryologic development of the parathyroid glands, regulation of parathyroid hormone (PTH) synthesis and secretion, and maintenance of parathyroid gland homeostasis (**Table 1**). In the interest of taxonomy, pseudohypoparathyroidism, in which the biochemical manifestations of hypoparathyroidism are due to resistance to

Disclosures: The authors have received NIH grants (M.A. Levine: R01DK079970; R.J. Gordon: K12DK094723) in the preparation of this article. Dr M.A. Levine is an investigator and a member of an Advisory Board for Shire/NPS.
[a] Division of Endocrinology and Diabetes, The Center for Bone Health, The Children's Hospital of Philadelphia, Department of Pediatrics, University of Pennsylvania Perelman School of Medicine, 11 Northwest Tower, Suite 30, 3401 Civic Center Boulevard, Philadelphia, PA 19104, USA; [b] Division of Endocrinology and Diabetes, The Center for Bone Health, The Children's Hospital of Philadelphia, Department of Pediatrics, University of Pennsylvania Perelman School of Medicine, 3615 Civic Center Boulevard, Abramson Research Building, Room 510A, Philadelphia, PA 19104, USA
* Corresponding author.
E-mail address: gordonr4@email.chop.edu

Table 1
Genetic disorders associated with hypoparathyroidism

Disease	Inheritance	Gene	Locus	OMIM	Prevalence (if Known)	Associated Comorbidities
		Disorders of parathyroid gland formation				
Isolated parathyroid aplasia	AR or AD XR	GCM2 SOX3	6p23–24 Xq26–27	*603716 *307700	— —	
DiGeorge sequence	—	—	—	—	1:4000–1:7692	Thymic hypoplasia with immune deficiency, conotruncal cardiac defects, cleft palate, dysmorphic facies
DiGeorge type 1	Sporadic or AD	TBX1	22q11.21-q11.23	#188400	—	
DiGeorge type 2	Sporadic or AD	NEBL	10p13	%601362	—	
Charge syndrome	Sporadic or AD	CHD7 SEMA3E	8q12.2 7q21.11	#214800 #214800	1:8500	Cardiac anomalies, cleft palate, renal anomalies, ear abnormalities/deafness, and developmental delay
Hypoparathyroidism, deafness, and renal dysplasia	AD	GATA3	10p14–15	#146255	—	Deafness and renal dysplasia
Hypoparathyroidism, retardation, and dysmorphism	AR	TBCE	1q42–43	#241410	—	growth retardation, developmental delay, dysmorphic facies
Kenny-Caffey syndrome type 1	AR	TBCE	1q42–43	#244460	1:40,000–1:100,000 in Saudi Arabia	Short stature, medullary stenosis, dysmorphic facies, developmental delay
Kenny-Caffey syndrome type 2	AD	FAM111A	11q12.1	#127000	—	Similar to type 1, but clinically distinguished by the absence of mental retardation

Disease	Inheritance	Gene	Locus	OMIM	Frequency	Clinical features
Mitochondrial diseases						
Kearns-Sayre syndrome	Maternal	—	mtDNA	#530000	—	Encephalomyopathy, ophthalmoplegia, retinitis pigmentosa, and heart block
Pearson Marrow-Pancreas syndrome		—	mtDNA	#557000	—	Pancreatic dysfunction, sideroblastic anemia, neutropenia, and thrombocytopenia
MELAS		—	mt tRNA	#540000	—	Mitochondrial myopathy, encephalopathy, lactic acidosis, and strokelike episodes
LCHAD		MTP	2p23.3	#609016	—	
MCADD		ACADM	1p31.1	#201450	1:17,000	
Disorders of parathyroid hormone synthesis or secretion						
PTH gene mutations	AD or AR	PTH	11p15.3-p15.1	*168450	—	
AD hypocalcemia type 1	AD or sporadic	CASR	3q13.3-q21.1	#601198	—	Hypercalciuria
AD hypocalcemia type 2	AD or sporadic	GNA11	19p13.3	#615361	—	
Disorders of parathyroid gland destruction						
Autoimmune polyendocrinopathy candidiasis ectodermal dystrophy	AR, AD, or sporadic	AIRE	21q22.3	#240300	1:90,000–1:200,000	Mucocutaneous candidiasis and adrenal insufficiency

Abbreviations: AD, autosomal dominant; AR, autosomal recessive; mt tRNA, mitochondrial tRNA; mtDNA, mitochondrial DNA; OMIM, online Mendelian inheritance in man; XR, X-lir ked recessive.

PTH rather than to deficiency of PTH, is separately addressed (please see Agnès Linglart and colleagues' article, "Pseudohypoparathyroidism," in this issue).

DISORDERS OF PARATHYROID GLAND FORMATION
Isolated Parathyroid Aplasia: GCM2, SOX3

Some genetic defects will affect embryologic development of only the parathyroid glands and thereby lead to isolated hypoparathyroidism. The most common cause of isolated hypoparathyroidism is loss of function mutation in the GCM2 (previously GCMB) gene at 6p23-24.[1] GCM2 is a member of a small family of transcription factors that were first identified in Drosophila melanogaster. Family members show protein conservation that is limited to the N-terminal region which contains a unique GCM DNA binding domain. GCM2 is related to the Drosophila glial cells missing gene, which likely acts as a binary switch that determines cell fate between neuronal and glial cells. There are 2 mammalian homologs: GCM1, which is primarily expressed in the thymus and placenta, and regulates placental branching and vasculogenesis; and GCM2, which is principally if not exclusively expressed in the developing and mature parathyroid gland.[2] GCM2 is a master regulator of parathyroid gland development. Most cases of isolated hypoparathyroidism are due to autosomal recessive mutations that inactivate GCM2,[1,3] but in some cases GCM2 mutations produce an abnormal GCM2 protein with dominant-negative effects.[4,5]

In mice, Gcm2 is specifically expressed in the developing second and third pharyngeal pouches beginning at E9.5 days,[6] and studies with Gcm2 null mutant mice suggest that Gcm2 is not required for organogenesis, but is necessary for subsequent differentiation and survival of parathyroid cells with null mutant mice undergoing apoptosis by E12.5.[2] GCM2 is part of a network of transcription factors that are required for normal development of the parathyroid glands. The transcription factor GATA binding protein-3 (GATA3) is also necessary for development and survival of parathyroid glands and is highly expressed in parathyroid cell precursors in the pharyngeal pouch as well as in other tissues (see later discussion). GATA3 contains a carboxy-terminal zinc finger that is essential for DNA binding, and it induces GCM2 transcription by binding to specific GATA3 sites that are present in the promoter of the human GCM2 gene.[7] Remarkably, gain-of-function mutations of GCM2 are a cause of parathyroid hyperplasia[8] and familial isolated hyperparathyroidism.[9]

Another cause of isolated hypoparathyroidism shows X-linked recessive inheritance. Affected patients present with infantile hypocalcemic seizures, whereas heterozygous female patients are unaffected. The cause of hypoparathyroidism is complete agenesis of the parathyroid glands. Linkage analysis has localized the underlying mutation to a 1.5-Mb region on Xq26-27, in which there is a deletion-insertion involving chromosomes 2p25.3 and Xq27.1, near Sry-box 3 (SOX3), presumed to impact embryonic development of the parathyroid glands.[10]

DiGeorge Sequence: 22q11, TBX1, 10p13

DiGeorge sequence (DGS) refers to a well-characterized and yet highly variable constellation of developmental anomalies that can include parathyroid dysplasia. Typical features of DGS include thymic aplasia with impaired T-cell–mediated immunity, conotruncal cardiac defects, cleft palate, and dysmorphic facies with midface hypoplasia, hypertelorism, and external ear anomalies (**Fig. 1**). In addition, patients with DGS may have feeding difficulties, poor growth, and cognitive impairment. Notably, there is a range of DGS disease presentation, and various developmental syndromes with limited features of DGS have been described (eg, Shprintzen syndrome,

Patient 1

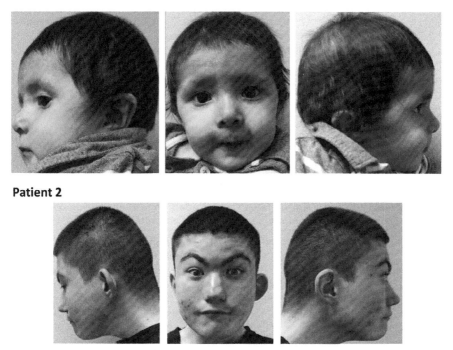

Patient 2

Fig. 1. DGS. Patient 1: Relatively nondysmorphic 1-year-old boy with DGS. Note, bitemporal narrowing, malar flatness, squared helices with a prominent antitragus, attached lobes, a prominent blue-tinged vessel over the nasal root, bulbous nasal tip with hypoplastic alae nasi, small mouth, and mild micrognathia. Patient 2: 19-year-old man with DGS. Note, malar flatness, mild upslanting palpebral fissures, unilateral helical protuberance, attached lobes, a broad nasal root, and bulbous tip with hypoplastic alae nasi.

velocardiofacial syndrome, and conotruncal anomaly face syndrome) that represent different manifestations of the same molecular defect, typically a large deletion at 22q11.[11–13] Not all patients with DGS have clinical hypoparathyroidism,[11] and several series have shown that hypoparathyroidism is present in only about 20% of older patients with DGS.[13] By contrast, up to 50% of patients in infancy can have hypoparathyroidism, which can vary from severe and symptomatic early-onset hypocalcemia associated with neonatal seizures, to mild and asymptomatic hypocalcemia that may only be discovered later in adulthood. Hypocalcemia can wax and wane during infancy and childhood, with some DGS patients even demonstrating complete resolution of hypocalcemia after 1 year of age. Nevertheless, the tendency for hypocalcemia to recur during times of stress (eg, surgery or severe illness) suggests that parathyroid hypoplasia is more common in DGS than is widely appreciated.[14–16] Under this proposition, it is likely that many subjects are able to produce sufficient PTH to maintain normal mineral homeostasis during ordinary conditions.

Most patients with DGS have hemizygous microdeletions within chromosome 22q11.21-23[17]; these microdeletions usually arise de novo but can also be inherited from a parent (5%–10%). 22q11 deletions are common, occur with an incidence of approximately 1 in 2000 to 5000 live births, and are the most common human contiguous gene deletion.[18] The relatively high frequency of spontaneous deletions is related to the presence of 4 distinct highly homologous blocks of low copy number repeats (LCRs) that flank the deletion region, which can lead to mispairing of the LCRs during meiosis and unequal meiotic exchange, leading to the microdeletion. Most affected individuals have a 3-Mb deletion of the chromosome 22q11.2 region (about 90% of cases), whereas a smaller 1.5-Mb deletion is present in about 7%. The 3-Mb deletion encompasses approximately 40 genes, but it is likely that loss of the *TBX1* gene, which encodes the T-box transcription factor gene 1, is responsible for most of the clinical findings in DGS. Patients with point mutations in *TBX1* will manifest several of the phenotypic findings of 22q11 syndrome, including hypocalcemia, cardiac defects, cleft palate, and facial anomalies, but notably not learning disabilities.[19]

A less common cause of DGS is a deletion at chromosome 10p13, termed the DiGeorge locus type II (DGS2).[20–22] The critical region for DGS2 has been mapped within a 1-cM interval in 10p13. DGS2 is likely caused by mutations in the nebulette (*NEBL*) gene, which is abundantly expressed in cardiac muscle.[23,24]

Coloboma, Heart Defects, Atresia Choanae, Retarded Growth and Development, Genital Hypoplasia, and Ear Anomalies/Deafness Syndrome: CHD7, SEMA3E

Hypoparathyroidism can be a component of the CHARGE (Coloboma, Heart defects, Atresia choanae, Retarded growth and development, Genital hypoplasia, and Ear anomalies/deafness) syndrome. CHARGE syndrome occurs with an incidence of 1 in 8500 to 10,000 live births, and in more than 75% of cases is due to a heterozygous loss-of-function mutation within the coding region of the *CHD7* gene at chromosome 8q12.2.[25,26] *CHD7* is a member of the chromodomain helicase DNA binding protein (CHD) family of adenosine triphosphate–dependent chromatin remodelers, which catalyzes nucleosome movement on DNA. Mutations are usually de novo mutations, but the syndrome can also be inherited in an autosomal dominant manner. A less common cause is due to abnormalities involving semaphorin 3E (*SEMA3E*), which controls cell positioning during embryonic development on chromosome 7q21.11.[27]

There is significant clinical overlap between DGS and CHARGE syndrome, with both having hypoparathyroidism, cardiac anomalies, cleft palate, renal anomalies, ear abnormalities/deafness, and developmental delay. Hypocalcemia, attributed to hypoparathyroidism, is more common in CHARGE syndrome newborns (72%) compared with DGS newborns (26%).[28]

Hypoparathyroidism, Deafness, and Renal Dysplasia/Barakat Syndrome: GATA3

Hypoparathyroidism, sensorineural deafness, and renal dysplasia syndrome (HDR), also known as Barakat syndrome, is an autosomal dominant inherited disorder[29] caused by haploinsufficiency of the GATA binding protein-3 (*GATA3*) gene, on chromosome 10p14-15, distal to the DGS2.[30–32] The GATA3 protein is a transcription factor with a carboxyterminal zinc finger that is essential for DNA binding and is expressed in the developing parathyroid gland, thymus, kidney, inner ear, and central nervous system. *GATA3* interacts with *GCM2* (see earlier discussion, isolated parathyroid aplasia) and *MafB*, two known transcriptional regulators of parathyroid development, and synergistically stimulates the PTH promoter, activating PTH gene transcription and serving as a critical regulator of PTH gene expression.[33]

There is wide phenotypic variability, and hypoparathyroidism ranges from asymptomatic and transient neonatal hypocalcemia that resolves in infancy to severe, symptomatic hypocalcemia with seizures and tetany from infancy that persists through adulthood. The sensorineural hearing loss is usually bilateral and is the most penetrant of the 3 HDR features. Deafness is present in more than 95% of HDR patients and is typically discovered during infancy or childhood.[34] Renal abnormalities are the least penetrant feature, present in 60% of patients, and are extremely variable, with only a minority (9%) of patients progressing to end-stage renal disease.[35] Notably, there are no cardiac, immunologic, or palatal abnormalities.

Hypoparathyroidism, Retardation, and Dysmorphism: TBCE, FAM111A

Hypoparathyroidism, retardation, and dysmorphism syndrome (HRD), also known as Sanjad-Sakati syndrome, consists of permanent hypoparathyroidism, severe prenatal and postnatal growth retardation, reduced T-cell subsets, and developmental delay.[36] Dysmorphic features include microcephaly, microphthalmia, micrognathia, ear abnormalities, depressed nasal bridge, thin upper lip, hooked small nose, and small hands and feet.[36] It is an autosomal recessive inherited disorder and usually due to mutations in the TBCE gene located on chromosome 1q42-43 that primarily affects patients of Arabic descent.[37]

Kenny-Caffey syndrome (KCS) is a clinically similar allelic syndrome, which includes hypocalcemia due to hypoparathyroidism, short stature, thickening of the long bones, thin marrow cavities (medullary stenosis), developmental delay, and facial abnormalities, including small eyes with hypermetropia and frontal bossing with triangular facies.[38] It may be inherited as an autosomal recessive[39] or autosomal dominant disorder. The autosomal recessive form has been mapped to the same locus (1q42-q43) as the HRD syndrome, and both are caused by mutations in the tubulin folding cofactor E (TBCE) gene and thus are allelic disorders due to a common founder mutation.[38] Mutations in the TBCE gene affect the synthesis of chaperone proteins that are involved in the normal folding of beta-tubulin, with abnormal tubulin formation affecting the Golgi apparatus and endosomes, suggesting a possible connection between tubulin physiology and development of the parathyroid gland. The autosomal dominant form of KCS, which is clinically distinguished from the autosomal recessive form of KCS by the absence of mental retardation, is due to a heterozygous mutation of the FAM111A gene (family with sequence similarity 111 member A), which is a chromatin-associated protein involved in DNA replication.[40]

Mitochondrial Disease: Kearns-Sayre Syndrome; Pearson Marrow-Pancreas Syndrome; Myopathy, Encephalopathy, Lactic Acidosis, and Strokelike Episodes; Long-Chain 3-Hydroxyacyl-CoA Dehydrogenase; Medium-Chain Acyl-CoA Dehydrogenase Deficiency

Several mitochondrial syndromes are associated with hypoparathyroidism. Kearns-Sayre syndrome is characterized by encephalomyopathy, ophthalmoplegia, retinitis pigmentosa, and heart block.[41] Pearson marrow-pancreas syndrome is characterized by pancreatic dysfunction, sideroblastic anemia, neutropenia, and thrombocytopenia.[42] The mitochondrial DNA deletion is identical in Kearns-Sayre syndrome and Pearson marrow-pancreas syndrome. They have different ages of disease onset, with Pearson marrow-pancreas syndrome presenting in infancy, whereas Kearns-Sayre syndrome presents later. Pearson marrow-pancreas syndrome frequently evolves into Kearns-Sayre syndrome. It is not uncommon to have hypoparathyroidism, with variable age of onset.

Other mitochondrial disorders associated with hypoparathyroidism include mitochondrial myopathy, encephalopathy, lactic acidosis, and strokelike episodes (MELAS) due to point mutations in mitochondrial tRNA[43]; LCAHD or combined mitochondrial trifunctional protein (MTP) deficiency due to mutations in MTP[44–46]; and medium-chain acyl-CoA dehydrogenase deficiency (MCADD) due to mutations in the ACADM gene.[47] The mechanism by which these mitochondrial defects affect parathyroid gland development or function is unknown.

DISORDERS OF PARATHYROID HORMONE SYNTHESIS OR SECRETION
PTH Gene Mutation

Isolated hypoparathyroidism can result from mutations in the PTH gene located on chromosome 11p15.3-p15.1 that impair synthesis of PTH. The PTH gene contains 3 exons that encode the 115-amino-acid preproPTH protein. Two proteolytic cleavages are required to produce the biologically active 84-amino-acid PTH molecule. The first cleavage occurs cotranslationally in the endoplasmic reticulum (ER) by the signalase enzyme, which removes the amino-terminal 25-amino-acid signal or prepeptide that directs the nascent preproPTH protein into the ER. The 6-amino-acid propeptide is subsequently removed by proprotein convertases, after trafficking to the Golgi apparatus, to generate the mature 84-amino-acid PTH polypeptide. In a few instances, autosomal dominant isolated hypoparathyroidism has been associated with heterozygous mutations in the PTH gene. In 2 families, PTH gene missense mutations were identified in exon 2, either p.C18R[48,49] or p.M14K,[50] that replace key amino acids in the hydrophobic core of the leader sequence. The mutations prevent normal removal of the leader sequence and impair translocation of the abnormal protein across the ER. The dominant negative mechanism is thought to be induction of an ER stress response that leads to apoptosis of the parathyroid cells.[50,51] In another hypoparathyroid patient, a heterozygous initiator codon mutation (M1T) was identified, predicting abnormal initiation of translation of the preproPTH mRNA at the +7 Met codon, thereby producing an N-terminally truncated protein with an abnormal leader sequence.[52]

Autosomal recessive forms of familial isolated hypoparathyroidism due to PTH gene mutations have also been described. Remarkably, in most cases these mutations also affect the leader sequence of the preproPTH molecule. In 2 instances, different mutations at codon 23 (p.S23P and p.S23X)[53,54] predict generation of a nonsecreted PTH molecule due to a defective or truncated leader sequence. In a third case, a donor splice site mutation at the exon 2–intron 2 junction of the PTH gene leads to exon skipping, with loss of the initiator methionine and the signal sequence encoded by exon 2.[53,55] In a most exceptional case, a bioinactive form of PTH was produced by an arginine-to-cysteine substitution at position 25 of the mature PTH(1–84) polypeptide that impairs recognition of the PTH molecule in some assays for intact PTH.[56]

Autosomal Dominant Hypocalcemia Type 1 and Type 2: Mutations in CASR and GNA11

Gain-of-function mutations in the genes encoding the calcium-sensing receptor (CASR)[57,58] or the alpha subunit of the G protein, Gα11 (GNA11),[59–61] that couples the CASR to activation of intracellular signaling pathways in the parathyroid cell, result in autosomal dominant hypocalcemic types 1 (ADH1) and 2 (ADH2), respectively.[62]

In ADH1, heterozygous mutations in the CASR increase the sensitivity of the calcium sensing receptor to extracellular ionized calcium. Consequently, PTH synthesis and secretion are suppressed at normal ionized calcium concentrations. Patients present with hypocalcemia, hyperphosphatemia, low magnesium levels, and low or low-normal levels of PTH. There is a wide range of clinical presentation, ranging from seizures in infancy to asymptomatic mild hypocalcemia in adulthood. Urinary calcium is usually elevated, because renal excretion of calcium is increased due to both the decrease in circulating PTH concentrations and the activation of calcium-sensing receptor in the distal renal tubule. Most activating mutations in the CASR gene on chromosome 3q13.3-q21.1 are familial,[57,58,63–66] but there have been a few sporadic cases due to de novo mutations.[63,67]

Increased sensitivity of the parathyroid cell to extracellular ionized calcium has also been proposed as the mechanism for hypoparathyroidism in patients with ADH2, but in this disorder the enhanced sensitivity to calcium is due to a gain of function in Gα11, which couples the calcium-sensing receptor to intracellular signal generators such as phospholipase C.[68] Patients with ADH2 do not appear to have increased fractional excretion of calcium by the kidney,[60] presumably because Gα11 is not the key transmembrane coupling protein for the calcium-sensing receptor in the distal renal tubule. By contrast, patients with ADH2 have short stature,[60] which may be a consequence of activated Gα11 signaling in the growth plates of long bones. Somatic missense mutations in GNA11 are considered proto-oncogenic and have been identified in some blue nevi, primary uveal melanomas, and uveal melanoma metastases.[69] However, GNA11 mutations in ADH2 are less activating than oncogenic GNA11 mutations.[60] These familial activating mutations in the GNA11 gene occur at chromosome 19p13.

As opposed to these gain-of-function mutations, mutations that inactivate the CASR and GNA11 genes reduce sensitivity of parathyroid cells to extracellular ionized calcium and are associated with the contrasting endocrine disorder familial hypocalciuric hypercalcemia.[59,70] All CASR mutations, as well as polymorphisms, are cataloged in a calcium-sensing receptor online database,[71] which is regularly updated and provides a highly useful resource.

Knowledge of the shared pathophysiology of hypoparathyroidism (ie, increased sensitivity to extracellular ionized calcium) in these 2 disorders, ADH1 and ADH2, has led to the development of calciolytic agents that reduce calcium sensitivity of the calcium-sensing receptor and which can reduce PTH secretion in animal models. To date, there has been one phase 2 study in adults with ADH treated with a calcium-sensing receptor antagonist (ClinicalTrials.gov Identifier: NCT02204579). Novel treatment therapies will be covered in greater detail in Gaia Tabacco and John P. Bilezikian's article, "New Directions in Treatment of Hypoparathyroidism," in this issue.

DISORDERS OF PARATHYROID GLAND DESTRUCTION
Autoimmune Polyendocrinopathy Candidiasis Ectodermal Dystrophy: AIRE

Autoimmune destruction of the parathyroids occurs most commonly in association with autoimmune polyendocrinopathy candidiasis ectodermal dystrophy (APECED), also known as autoimmune polyglandular syndrome type 1. The classic triad consists of mucocutaneous candidiasis, hypoparathyroidism, and adrenal insufficiency, and these features typically manifest in a corresponding chronologic order. There are many additional autoimmune features that may develop, including additional endocrinopathies such as ovarian failure, hypothyroidism, insulin-dependent diabetes, and hypophysitis. Nonendocrine manifestations include hepatitis, malabsorption, pernicious anemia, vitiligo, alopecia, nail and dental dystrophy.[72] There is wide variability in the clinical expression, with no significant correlation between genotype and phenotype.[73] This variability is exemplified by significant intrafamilial differences between siblings carrying the same mutation.

More than 100 different mutations of the autoimmune regulator (AIRE) gene[74] have been identified in patients with APECED.[75] AIRE encodes a transcription factor that functions as an important regulator in thymic epithelial cells. AIRE induces expression of important "self" identity proteins and T cells that respond to those proteins are eliminated in the thymus through apoptosis, thereby avoiding autoimmune disorders.[76,77] It is typically an autosomal recessive disorder caused by various different mutations in the AIRE gene, on chromosome 21q22.3.[78,79] It is most prevalent in Finns (prevalence 1/25,000),[78,80] Sardinians (1/14,400),[80] and Iranian Jews (1/6500–1/9000),[81] suggesting significant founder effects.[82] It is less commonly caused by autosomal dominant inheritance[83] and sporadic de novo mutations.[84] Interestingly, biallelic mutations in *AIRE* can cause isolated hypoparathyroidism, without additional clinical features of APECED.[85]

SUMMARY

Hypoparathyroidism consists of a heterogeneous group of disorders, with a broad phenotypic spectrum, that presents across the lifespan. Although genetic disorders are not a common cause of hypoparathyroidism, accurate diagnosis of the underlying genetic cause is essential, affecting treatment goals, screening for comorbidities, and family planning. Research has brought us closer to understanding the molecular mechanisms underlying the development of the parathyroid glands, disordered synthesis and secretion of PTH, and postnatal destruction of the parathyroid glands. However, further research is needed to elucidate the exact function of several genes that are known to result in hypoparathyroidism.

ACKNOWLEDGMENTS

The authors wish to thank Donna M. McDonald-McGinn, MS, CGC for the pictures of patients with DiGeorge sequence.

REFERENCES

1. Ding C, Buckingham B, Levine MA. Familial isolated hypoparathyroidism caused by a mutation in the gene for the transcription factor GCMB. J Clin Invest 2001; 108(8):1215–20.
2. Liu Z, Yu S, Manley NR. Gcm2 is required for the differentiation and survival of parathyroid precursor cells in the parathyroid/thymus primordia. Dev Biol 2007; 305(1):333–46.
3. Bowl MR, Mirczuk SM, Grigorieva IV, et al. Identification and characterization of novel parathyroid-specific transcription factor Glial Cells Missing Homolog B (GCMB) mutations in eight families with autosomal recessive hypoparathyroidism. Hum Mol Genet 2010;19(10):2028–38.
4. Canaff L, Zhou X, Mosesova I, et al. Glial cells missing-2 (GCM2) transactivates the calcium-sensing receptor gene: effect of a dominant-negative GCM2 mutant associated with autosomal dominant hypoparathyroidism. Hum Mutat 2009;30(1):85–92.
5. Mirczuk SM, Bowl MR, Nesbit MA, et al. A missense glial cells missing homolog B (GCMB) mutation, Asn502His, causes autosomal dominant hypoparathyroidism. J Clin Endocrinol Metab 2010;95(7):3512–6.
6. Gordon J, Bennett AR, Blackburn CC, et al. Gcm2 and Foxn1 mark early parathyroid- and thymus-specific domains in the developing third pharyngeal pouch. Mech Dev 2001;103(1):141–3.
7. Grigorieva IV, Mirczuk S, Gaynor KU, et al. Gata3-deficient mice develop parathyroid abnormalities due to dysregulation of the parathyroid-specific transcription factor Gcm2. J Clin Invest 2010;120(6):2144–55.
8. Maret A, Bourdeau I, Ding C, et al. Expression of GCMB by intrathymic parathyroid hormone-secreting adenomas indicates their parathyroid cell origin. J Clin Endocrinol Metab 2004;89(1):8–12.
9. Guan B, Welch JM, Sapp JC, et al. GCM2-Activating Mutations in Familial Isolated Hyperparathyroidism. Am J Hum Genet 2016;99(5):1034–44.
10. Bowl MR, Nesbit MA, Harding B, et al. An interstitial deletion-insertion involving chromosomes 2p25.3 and Xq27.1, near SOX3, causes X-linked recessive hypoparathyroidism. J Clin Invest 2005;115(10):2822–31.

11. Motzkin B, Marion R, Goldberg R, et al. Variable phenotypes in velocardiofacial syndrome with chromosomal deletion. J Pediatr 1993;123(3):406–10.

12. Goldberg R, Motzkin B, Marion R, et al. Velo-cardio-facial syndrome: a review of 120 patients. Am J Med Genet 1993;45(3):313–9.

13. Greig F, Paul E, DiMartino-Nardi J, et al. Transient congenital hypoparathyroidism: resolution and recurrence in chromosome 22q11 deletion. J Pediatr 1996;128(4): 563–7.

14. Cuneo BF, Langman CB, Ilbawi MN, et al. Latent hypoparathyroidism in children with conotruncal cardiac defects. Circulation 1996;93(9):1702–8.

15. Kapadia CR, Kim YE, McDonald-McGinn DM, et al. Parathyroid hormone reserve in 22q11.2 deletion syndrome. Genet Med 2008;10(3):224–8.

16. Fujii S, Nakanishi T. Clinical manifestations and frequency of hypocalcemia in 22q11.2 deletion syndrome. Pediatr Int 2015;57(6):1086–9.

17. Scambler PJ. The 22q11 deletion syndromes. Hum Mol Genet 2000;9(16): 2421–6.

18. Shprintzen RJ, Higgins AM, Antshel K, et al. Velo-cardio-facial syndrome. Curr Opin Pediatr 2005;17(6):725–30.

19. Yagi H, Furutani Y, Hamada H, et al. Role of TBX1 in human del22q11.2 syndrome. Lancet 2003;362(9393):1366–73.

20. Greenberg F, Elder FF, Haffner P, et al. Cytogenetic findings in a prospective series of patients with DiGeorge anomaly. Am J Hum Genet 1988;43(5): 605–11.

21. Monaco G, Pignata C, Rossi E, et al. DiGeorge anomaly associated with 10p deletion. Am J Med Genet 1991;39(2):215–6.

22. Lai MM, Scriven PN, Ball C, et al. Simultaneous partial monosomy 10p and trisomy 5q in a case of hypoparathyroidism. J Med Genet 1992;29(8):586–8.

23. Villanueva MP, Aiyer AR, Muller S, et al. Genetic and comparative mapping of genes dysregulated in mouse hearts lacking the Hand2 transcription factor gene. Genomics 2002;80(6):593–600.

24. Yatsenko SA, Yatsenko AN, Szigeti K, et al. Interstitial deletion of 10p and atrial septal defect in DiGeorge 2 syndrome. Clin Genet 2004;66(2):128–36.

25. Vissers LE, van Ravenswaaij CM, Admiraal R, et al. Mutations in a new member of the chromodomain gene family cause CHARGE syndrome. Nat Genet 2004; 36(9):955–7.

26. Aramaki M, Udaka T, Kosaki R, et al. Phenotypic spectrum of CHARGE syndrome with CHD7 mutations. J Pediatr 2006;148(3):410–4.

27. Lalani SR, Safiullah AM, Molinari LM, et al. SEMA3E mutation in a patient with CHARGE syndrome. J Med Genet 2004;41(7):e94.

28. Jyonouchi S, McDonald-McGinn DM, Bale S, et al. CHARGE (coloboma, heart defect, atresia choanae, retarded growth and development, genital hypoplasia, ear anomalies/deafness) syndrome and chromosome 22q11.2 deletion syndrome: a comparison of immunologic and nonimmunologic phenotypic features. Pediatrics 2009;123(5):e871–7.

29. Bilous RW, Murty G, Parkinson DB, et al. Brief report: autosomal dominant familial hypoparathyroidism, sensorineural deafness, and renal dysplasia. N Engl J Med 1992;327(15):1069–74.

30. Hasegawa T, Hasegawa Y, Aso T, et al. HDR syndrome (hypoparathyroidism, sensorineural deafness, renal dysplasia) associated with del(10)(p13). Am J Med Genet 1997;73(4):416–8.

31. Van Esch H, Groenen P, Nesbit MA, et al. GATA3 haplo-insufficiency causes human HDR syndrome. Nature 2000;406(6794):419–22.

32. Muroya K, Hasegawa T, Ito Y, et al. GATA3 abnormalities and the phenotypic spectrum of HDR syndrome. J Med Genet 2001;38(6):374–80.

33. Han SI, Tsunekage Y, Kataoka K. Gata3 cooperates with Gcm2 and MafB to activate parathyroid hormone gene expression by interacting with SP1. Mol Cell Endocrinol 2015;411:113–20.

34. Chien WW, Leiding JW, Hsu AP, et al. Auditory and vestibular phenotypes associated with GATA3 mutation. Otol Neurotol 2014;35(4):577–81.

35. Belge H, Dahan K, Cambier JF, et al. Clinical and mutational spectrum of hypoparathyroidism, deafness and renal dysplasia syndrome. Nephrol Dial Transplant 2017;32(5):830–7.

36. Sanjad SA, Sakati NA, Abu-Osba YK, et al. A new syndrome of congenital hypoparathyroidism, severe growth failure, and dysmorphic features. Arch Dis Child 1991;66(2):193–6.

37. Parvari R, Hershkovitz E, Kanis A, et al. Homozygosity and linkage-disequilibrium mapping of the syndrome of congenital hypoparathyroidism, growth and mental retardation, and dysmorphism to a 1-cM interval on chromosome 1q42-43. Am J Hum Genet 1998;63(1):163–9.

38. Diaz GA, Gelb BD, Ali F, et al. Sanjad-Sakati and autosomal recessive Kenny-Caffey syndromes are allelic: evidence for an ancestral founder mutation and locus refinement. Am J Med Genet 1999;85(1):48–52.

39. Franceschini P, Testa A, Bogetti G, et al. Kenny-Caffey syndrome in two sibs born to consanguineous parents: evidence for an autosomal recessive variant. Am J Med Genet 1992;42(1):112–6.

40. Unger S, Gorna MW, Le Bechec A, et al. FAM111A mutations result in hypoparathyroidism and impaired skeletal development. Am J Hum Genet 2013;92(6):990–5.

41. Tengan CH, Kiyomoto BH, Rocha MS, et al. Mitochondrial encephalomyopathy and hypoparathyroidism associated with a duplication and a deletion of mitochondrial deoxyribonucleic acid. J Clin Endocrinol Metab 1998;83(1):125–9.

42. Seneca S, De Meirleir L, De Schepper J, et al. Pearson marrow pancreas syndrome: a molecular study and clinical management. Clin Genet 1997;51(5):338–42.

43. Morten KJ, Cooper JM, Brown GK, et al. A new point mutation associated with mitochondrial encephalomyopathy. Hum Mol Genet 1993;2(12):2081–7.

44. Tyni T, Rapola J, Palotie A, et al. Hypoparathyroidism in a patient with long-chain 3-hydroxyacyl-coenzyme A dehydrogenase deficiency caused by the G1528C mutation. J Pediatr 1997;131(5):766–8.

45. Dionisi-Vici C, Garavaglia B, Burlina AB, et al. Hypoparathyroidism in mitochondrial trifunctional protein deficiency. J Pediatr 1996;129(1):159–62.

46. Naiki M, Ochi N, Kato YS, et al. Mutations in HADHB, which encodes the beta-subunit of mitochondrial trifunctional protein, cause infantile onset hypoparathyroidism and peripheral polyneuropathy. Am J Med Genet A 2014;164a(5):1180–7.

47. Baruteau J, Levade T, Redonnet-Vernhet I, et al. Hypoketotic hypoglycemia with myolysis and hypoparathyroidism: an unusual association in medium chain acyl-CoA desydrogenase deficiency (MCADD). J Pediatr Endocrinol Metab 2009;22(12):1175–7.

48. Arnold A, Horst SA, Gardella TJ, et al. Mutation of the signal peptide-encoding region of the preproparathyroid hormone gene in familial isolated hypoparathyroidism. J Clin Invest 1990;86(4):1084–7.

49. Karaplis AC, Lim SK, Baba H, et al. Inefficient membrane targeting, translocation, and proteolytic processing by signal peptidase of a mutant preproparathyroid hormone protein. J Biol Chem 1995;270(4):1629–35.

50. Cinque L, Sparaneo A, Penta L, et al. Autosomal Dominant PTH Gene Signal Sequence Mutation in a Family With Familial Isolated Hypoparathyroidism. J Clin Endocrinol Metab 2017;102(11):3961–9.

51. Datta R, Waheed A, Shah GN, et al. Signal sequence mutation in autosomal dominant form of hypoparathyroidism induces apoptosis that is corrected by a chemical chaperone. Proc Natl Acad Sci U S A 2007;104(50):19989–94.

52. Tomar N, Gupta N, Goswami R. Calcium-sensing receptor autoantibodies and idiopathic hypoparathyroidism. J Clin Endocrinol Metab 2013;98(9):3884–91.

53. Sunthornthepvarakul T, Churesigaew S, Ngowngarmratana S. A novel mutation of the signal peptide of the preproparathyroid hormone gene associated with autosomal recessive familial isolated hypoparathyroidism. J Clin Endocrinol Metab 1999;84(10):3792–6.

54. Ertl DA, Stary S, Streubel B, et al. A novel homozygous mutation in the parathyroid hormone gene (PTH) in a girl with isolated hypoparathyroidism. Bone 2012; 51(3):629–32.

55. Parkinson DB, Thakker RV. A donor splice site mutation in the parathyroid hormone gene is associated with autosomal recessive hypoparathyroidism. Nat Genet 1992;1(2):149–52.

56. Lee S, Mannstadt M, Guo J, et al. A Homozygous [Cys25]PTH(1-84) Mutation That Impairs PTH/PTHrP Receptor Activation Defines a Novel Form of Hypoparathyroidism. J Bone Miner Res 2015;30(10):1803–13.

57. Pollak MR, Brown EM, Estep HL, et al. Autosomal dominant hypocalcaemia caused by a Ca(2+)-sensing receptor gene mutation. Nat Genet 1994;8(3):303–7.

58. Pearce SH, Williamson C, Kifor O, et al. A familial syndrome of hypocalcemia with hypercalciuria due to mutations in the calcium-sensing receptor. N Engl J Med 1996;335(15):1115–22.

59. Nesbit MA, Hannan FM, Howles SA, et al. Mutations affecting G-protein subunit alpha11 in hypercalcemia and hypocalcemia. N Engl J Med 2013;368(26):2476–86.

60. Li D, Opas EE, Tuluc F, et al. Autosomal dominant hypoparathyroidism caused by germline mutation in GNA11: phenotypic and molecular characterization. J Clin Endocrinol Metab 2014;99(9):E1774–83.

61. Piret SE, Gorvin CM, Pagnamenta AT, et al. Identification of a G-Protein Subunit-alpha11 Gain-of-Function Mutation, Val340Met, in a Family With Autosomal Dominant Hypocalcemia Type 2 (ADH2). J Bone Miner Res 2016;31(6):1207–14.

62. Roszko KL, Bi RD, Mannstadt M. Autosomal dominant hypocalcemia (hypoparathyroidism) types 1 and 2. Front Physiol 2016;7:458.

63. Baron J, Winer KK, Yanovski JA, et al. Mutations in the Ca(2+)-sensing receptor gene cause autosomal dominant and sporadic hypoparathyroidism. Hum Mol Genet 1996;5(5):601–6.

64. Hirai H, Nakajima S, Miyauchi A, et al. A novel activating mutation (C129S) in the calcium-sensing receptor gene in a Japanese family with autosomal dominant hypocalcemia. J Hum Genet 2001;46(1):41–4.

65. Watanabe T, Bai M, Lane CR, et al. Familial hypoparathyroidism: identification of a novel gain of function mutation in transmembrane domain 5 of the calcium-sensing receptor. J Clin Endocrinol Metab 1998;83(7):2497–502.

66. D'Souza-Li L, Yang B, Canaff L, et al. Identification and functional characterization of novel calcium-sensing receptor mutations in familial hypocalciuric

hypercalcemia and autosomal dominant hypocalcemia. J Clin Endocrinol Metab 2002;87(3):1309–18.

67. De Luca F, Ray K, Mancilla EE, et al. Sporadic hypoparathyroidism caused by de Novo gain-of-function mutations of the Ca(2+)-sensing receptor. J Clin Endocrinol Metab 1997;82(8):2710–5.

68. Hannan FM, Babinsky VN, Thakker RV. Disorders of the calcium-sensing receptor and partner proteins: insights into the molecular basis of calcium homeostasis. J Mol Endocrinol 2016;57(3):R127–42.

69. Van Raamsdonk CD, Griewank KG, Crosby MB, et al. Mutations in GNA11 in uveal melanoma. N Engl J Med 2010;363(23):2191–9.

70. Brown EM, Pollak M, Chou YH, et al. The cloning of extracellular Ca(2+)-sensing receptors from parathyroid and kidney: molecular mechanisms of extracellular Ca(2+)-sensing. J Nutr 1995;125(7 Suppl):1965s–70s.

71. Pidasheva S, D'Souza-Li L, Canaff L, et al. CASRdb: calcium-sensing receptor locus-specific database for mutations causing familial (benign) hypocalciuric hypercalcemia, neonatal severe hyperparathyroidism, and autosomal dominant hypocalcemia. Hum Mutat 2004;24(2):107–11.

72. Betterle C, Greggio NA, Volpato M. Clinical review 93: Autoimmune polyglandular syndrome type 1. J Clin Endocrinol Metab 1998;83(4):1049–55.

73. Capalbo D, Mazza C, Giordano R, et al. Molecular background and genotype-phenotype correlation in autoimmune-polyendocrinopathy-candidiasis-ectodermal-distrophy patients from Campania and in their relatives. J Endocrinol Invest 2012; 35(2):169–73.

74. Scott HS, Heino M, Peterson P, et al. Common mutations in autoimmune polyendocrinopathy-candidiasis-ectodermal dystrophy patients of different origins. Mol Endocrinol 1998;12(8):1112–9.

75. De Martino L, Capalbo D, Improda N, et al. Novel findings into AIRE genetics and functioning: clinical implications. Front Pediatr 2016;4(86).

76. Bjorses P, Halonen M, Palvimo JJ, et al. Mutations in the AIRE gene: effects on subcellular location and transactivation function of the autoimmune polyendocrinopathy-candidiasis-ectodermal dystrophy protein. Am J Hum Genet 2000;66(2):378–92.

77. Abramson J, Giraud M, Benoist C, et al. Aire's partners in the molecular control of immunological tolerance. Cell 2010;140(1):123–35.

78. Aaltonen J, Bjorses P, Sandkuijl L, et al. An autosomal locus causing autoimmune disease: autoimmune polyglandular disease type I assigned to chromosome 21. Nat Genet 1994;8(1):83–7.

79. Aaltonen J, Horelli-Kuitunen N, Fan JB, et al. High-resolution physical and transcriptional mapping of the autoimmune polyendocrinopathy-candidiasis-ectodermal dystrophy locus on chromosome 21q22.3 by FISH. Genome Res 1997;7(8):820–9.

80. Rosatelli MC, Meloni A, Meloni A, et al. A common mutation in Sardinian autoimmune polyendocrinopathy-candidiasis-ectodermal dystrophy patients. Hum Genet 1998;103(4):428–34.

81. Zlotogora J, Shapiro MS. Polyglandular autoimmune syndrome type I among Iranian Jews. J Med Genet 1992;29(11):824–6.

82. Bjorses P, Aaltonen J, Vikman A, et al. Genetic homogeneity of autoimmune polyglandular disease type I. Am J Hum Genet 1996;59(4):879–86.

83. Cetani F, Barbesino G, Borsari S, et al. A novel mutation of the autoimmune regulator gene in an Italian kindred with autoimmune polyendocrinopathy-candidiasis-ectodermal dystrophy, acting in a dominant fashion and strongly cosegregating with hypothyroid autoimmune thyroiditis. J Clin Endocrinol Metab 2001;86(10): 4747–52.

84. Pearce SH, Cheetham T, Imrie H, et al. A common and recurrent 13-bp deletion in the autoimmune regulator gene in British kindreds with autoimmune polyendocrinopathy type 1. Am J Hum Genet 1998;63(6):1675–84.

85. Li D, Streeten EA, Chan A, et al. Exome Sequencing Reveals Mutations in AIRE as a Cause of Isolated Hypoparathyroidism. J Clin Endocrinol Metab 2017;102(5): 1726–33.

Skeletal Manifestations of Hypoparathyroidism

Mishaela R. Rubin, MD, MS

KEYWORDS

- Hypoparathyroidism • Bone • rhPTH(1-84) • Imaging • Histomorphometry

KEY POINTS

- Bone properties are altered in hypoparathyroidism; these include increased bone mineral density by dual-energy x-ray absorptiometry and decreased bone remodeling by biochemical and histomorphometric assessment.
- Fracture risk in hypoparathyroidism is uncertain.
- Parathyroid hormone treatment in hypoparathyroidism is associated with partial restoration of histomorphometric skeletal parameters.

INTRODUCTION

Chronic parathyroid hormone (PTH) deficiency has a marked effect on the skeleton. In healthy adults, bone mass is regulated by a specific balance between bone resorption and formation in the closely regulated process of bone remodeling. PTH is a key regulator of the rate of bone remodeling, and a reduction or absence of circulating PTH leads to characteristic decreases in bone remodeling[1–5] and increases in bone mass.[6–11] Numerous lines of evidence using biochemical, imaging, and histomorphometric methodologies have demonstrated that the skeleton is altered when PTH is absent[1,10] and that these abnormalities might be reversed with PTH treatment.[2,3,12]

SKELETAL MANIFESTATIONS OF HYPOPARATHYROIDISM
Biochemical Markers of Bone Turnover in Hypoparathyroidism

Low biochemical markers of bone turnover are a recognized feature of hypoparathyroidism.[13,14] Rubin and colleagues[2] measured biochemical markers of bone turnover in 64 subjects with hypoparathyroidism (48 women and 16 men) who were treated with calcitriol and/or vitamin D. The causes of the hypoparathyroid state were post–thyroid surgery (n = 32), autoimmune (n = 30), and DiGeorge syndrome (n = 2); the mean

Disclosure Statement: The author has received research support from Shire Pharmaceuticals (SHP634-402).
Metabolic Bone Disease Unit, Columbia University College of P&S, PH8W-864, 630 West 168th Street, New York, NY 10032, USA
E-mail address: mrr6@columbia.edu

duration of the disease was 15 ±13 (SD) years. Vitamin D intake ranged from 50 to 75,000 IU/d, and calcium supplementation varied between 0 and 9 g/d. Circulating markers of bone formation (procollagen type I amino-terminal propeptide, bone specific alkaline phosphatase, and osteocalcin) and of bone resorption (Tartrate-resistant acid phosphatase 5b and serum C-telopeptide [s-CTx]) were in the lower half of the normal reference range.[2] Other studies have shown similarly low biochemical markers of bone turnover.[3–5] Preliminary data suggest that the low biochemical markers of bone turnover might be associated with decreased circulating osteogenic precursor cells[15] and increased circulating sclerostin levels.[16]

Bone Mineral Density in Hypoparathyroidism

Chronically low bone turnover in hypoparathyroidism leads to bone mass that is relatively higher than age- and sex-matched controls.[6–9] For example, bone mass was 21% to 28% higher in 13 women, 10 to 13 years after thyroidectomies complicated by hypoparathyroidism as compared with 13 women whose thyroidectomies were not complicated by hypoparathyroidism.[6] The T- and Z-score differences in hypoparathyroidism typically exceed 1 at most sites that include trabecular and cortical bone, with the lumbar spine having the highest scores.[10] Bone mineral density (BMD) measured by dual-energy x-ray absorptiometry (DXA) in postmenopausal women with post-thyroidectomy hypoparathyroidism was found to be higher when compared with the age-predicted mean at the lumbar spine and proximal femur, although not at the distal radius.[17] Hypoparathyroidism was also found to delay the expected rate of postmenopausal bone loss as measured by DXA.[7] When a small number of subjects with hypoparathyroid were compared with those with primary hyperparathyroidism (PHPT), the subjects with hypoparathyroid did not show the catabolic effects of PTH to reduce bone density at the femoral neck.[17]

Greater insight into the architectural basis of the increase in bone mass has been obtained by peripheral quantitative computed tomography (pQCT). Using this technique, Chen and colleagues[11] compared volumetric BMD (vBMD) and geometry of the distal radius and midradius among postmenopausal women with postsurgical or idiopathic hypoparathyroidism, PHPT, and healthy control individuals. At the 4% distal radius site, which is enriched in cancellous bone, trabecular vBMD was higher in the rank order hypoparathyroidism > control > PHPT. At the 20% midradius site, cortical vBMD also was greater in the same rank order. The BMD differences among the 3 groups could be attributed to differences in bone geometry. At both radial sites, total bone area and both periosteal and endosteal surfaces were greater in PHPT than in patients with hypoparathyroidism and controls, and cortical thickness and area were higher in the rank order hypoparathyroidism > control > PHPT. High-resolution pQCT of the radius and tibia has further demonstrated an increase in cortical vBMD in men and women with hypoparathyroidism.[18] Decreased cortical porosity was also present at the radius and tibia in women and at the tibia in men. However, there was no difference between subjects with hypoparathyroidism and control subjects in estimated bone strength.[18]

Histomorphometry in Hypoparathyroidism

The most comprehensive information on the effects of hypoparathyroidism on the skeleton has come from histomorphometric analysis of iliac crest bone biopsies. The first histomorphometric study of bone in hypoparathyroidism, involving 12 patients with hypoparathyroid, suggested that PTH deficiency is associated with markedly abnormal bone turnover.[1] The study subjects, who had either postoperative or idiopathic hypoparathyroidism, were all treated with varying doses of vitamin D. As compared with euparathyroid age- and sex-matched controls, patients with hypoparathyroidism had a vastly protracted quiescent period (7.6 vs 1.7 years, $P<.001$), along with a reduced resorption rate (0.9 vs 3.8 $\mu m/d$, $P<.001$), formation rate (0.016 vs 0.081, $P<.001$), and reduced activation frequency (0.13 vs 0.6 year $^{-1}$, $P<.001$).[1] Despite the striking reduction in bone remodeling activity, variables reflecting the amount and microarchitecture of cancellous bone, such as cancellous bone volume, trabecular thickness, and marrow space star volume, were normal. A similarly profound suppression of bone turnover was reported in an earlier study on hypoparathyroid dogs, in which treatment with vitamin D was not able to restore normal bone turnover.[19]

The larger histomorphometric study of Rubin and colleagues[2,10] involved 64 subjects with hypoparathyroidism treated with calcitriol and/or vitamin D and 45 age- and sex-matched control subjects. In contrast to the earlier smaller study,[1] cancellous bone volume was elevated in the subjects with hypoparathyroid (**Figs. 1** and **2**). The structural basis for the higher cancellous bone volume in hypoparathyroidism was an increase in trabecular width; trabecular number and trabecular spacing were both similar to those in control subjects. Cortical width also tended to be greater in the subjects with hypoparathyroid, and cortical porosity was lower than in control subjects, but this difference was not statistically significant. Remodeling activity was assessed separately on cancellous, endocortical, and intracortical skeletal envelopes. Osteoid surface and width were reduced in the subjects with hypoparathyroidism on all 3 envelopes. The tetracycline-based bone formation rate (BFR) was significantly lower on all 3 envelopes in the subjects with hypoparathyroidism, with the greatest reduction observed on the cancellous envelope (**Fig. 3**). The reduction in BFR was a result of significant decreases in both mineralized surface and mineral apposition rate on all 3 envelopes. The eroded surface did not differ between the subjects with hypoparathyroidism and healthy subjects, but the bone-resorption rate was significantly lower in the subjects with hypoparathyroidism on all 3 envelopes. As in the earlier study,[1] these findings are all suggestive of a profound reduction in the bone turnover rate in hypoparathyroidism accompanied by an increase in bone mass in both cancellous and cortical compartments.

The effects of PTH deficiency on cancellous and cortical bone mass, which were observed initially by noninvasive imaging and by 2-dimensional histomorphometry, were confirmed by the 3-dimensional (3D) analytical capability of micro–computed tomography (μCT).[20] Results from this study corroborated the increase in cancellous

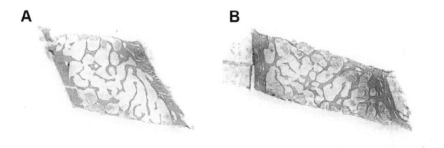

A   **B**

Fig. 1. Low-power view of iliac crest bone biopsies from a control subject (*A*) and a subject with hypoparathyroidism (*B*). Note the increase in cancellous bone volume and cortical thickness in the subject with hypoparathyroid (Goldner trichrome stain). (*From* Rubin MR, Dempster DW, Zhou H, et al. Dynamic and structural properties of the skeleton in hypoparathyroidism. J Bone Miner Res 2008;23:2021; with permission.)

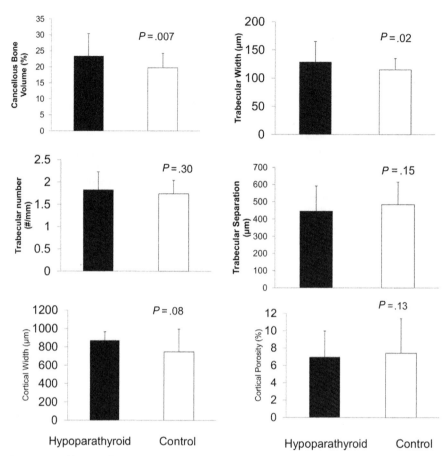

Fig. 2. Cancellous and cortical bone parameters obtained by histomorphometry in subjects with hypoparathyroidism (*black bars*) and controls (*white bars*). (*Adapted from* Rubin MR, Manavalan JS, Dempster DW, et al. Parathyroid hormone stimulates circulating osteogenic cells in hypoparathyroidism. J Clin Endocrinol Metab 2011;96:176–86; with permission.)

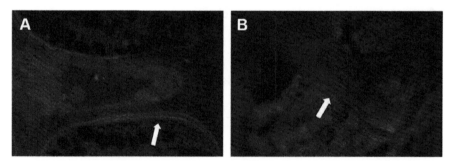

Fig. 3. Tetracycline labels (indicated by arrows) in a subject with hypoparathyroidism (*A*) and control (*B*). Tetracycline uptake was markedly reduced in the subject with hypoparathyroidism, reflecting the low bone turnover rate. (*From* Rubin MR, Dempster DW, Zhou H, et al. Dynamic and structural properties of the skeleton in hypoparathyroidism. J Bone Miner Res 2008;23:2022; with permission.)

bone volume and trabecular thickness in subjects with hypoparathyroidism and demonstrated a higher trabecular number and trabecular connectivity in comparison with matched control subjects. In addition, the structural model index was lower in hypoparathyroidism, indicating that the trabecular structure was more platelike than rodlike (**Fig. 4**).

The material composition of the bone matrix in hypoparathyroidism has also been studied. Using backscatter electron imaging, it was found that the mean mineralization density in iliac bone from subjects with hypoparathyroidism was similar to that of control subjects, although there was greater interindividual variation in mineralization parameters in the subjects with hypoparathyroidism than in the control subjects.[21] This result is surprising because one might have expected that mineralization density would be enhanced in hypoparathyroidism owing to the low turnover and attendant increase in mineralization as the bone ages. It suggests that mineralization density is controlled by other factors, in addition to the degree of secondary mineralization, and indicates that the higher BMD by densitometry in hypoparathyroidism is due in large part to the increase in bone tissue volume rather than an increase in the amount of mineral within the tissue.

Fracture Risk in Hypoparathyroidism

Prospective data on fracture risk in hypoparathyroidism are not available. Case-control studies show no differences in overall fracture rate as compared with the general population.[22,23] Analyses of specific fracture types showed that patients with nonsurgical hypoparathyroidism have an increased hazard ratio for upper extremity fractures (1.94; 95% confidence interval [CI]: 1.31–2.85) compared with controls and that patients with postsurgical hypoparathyroidism have a lower hazard ratio for the same fracture (0.69; CI: 0.49–0.97).[24] In a retrospective cohort, 21 of 120 patients (18%) had fractures over 7 years of follow-up.[25] A cohort of subjects with nonsurgical hypoparathyroidism had an increase in morphometric vertebral fractures, but a high rate of anticonvulsant use might have been a confounder.[26] A simulated strength study with stress loading of images by finite element analysis suggested

A   **B**

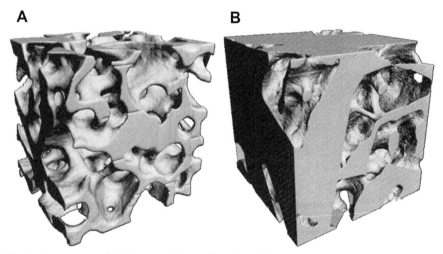

Fig. 4. Reconstructed μCT images of cancellous bone from a control (*A*) and a subject with hypoparathyroidism (*B*). Note the dense trabecular structure in hypoparathyroidism. (*From* Rubin MR, Dempster DW, Kohler T, et al. Three dimensional cancellous bone structure in hypoparathyroidism. Bone 2010;46:192; with permission.)

normal mechanical strength in hypoparathyroidism (**Fig. 5**).[27] Given the skeletal abnormalities that have been described, there is reason to be concerned about the fragility of bone in hypoparathyroidism[10]; but further data are necessary to address this point.

SKELETAL EFFECTS OF PARATHYROID HORMONE TREATMENT IN HYPOPARATHYROIDISM

Until recently, hypoparathyroidism was the only classic hormone deficiency state for which there was not an approved hormone replacement treatment. The skeletal

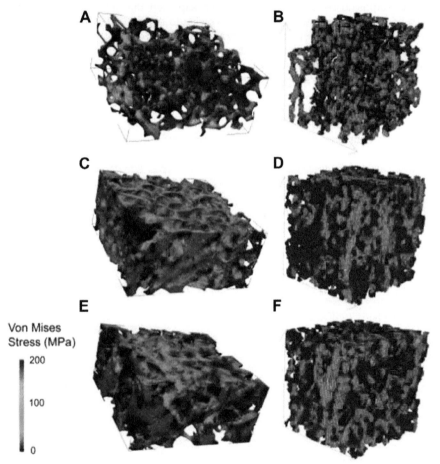

Fig. 5. Images showing tissue stress levels under axial loading generated by micro–finite element analysis based on µCT of the iliac crest bone biopsies (*A, C, E*) and high-resolution pQCT (*B, D, F*) of the radius in a premenopausal woman with idiopathic osteoporosis (*A, B*), a normal premenopausal control (*C, D*), and a patient with hypoparathyroidism (*E, F*). Dark blue indicates the regions with lowest stress, and dark red indicates the regions with highest stress. The lowest stress levels are seen in the subject with hypoparathyroidism. (*From* Cohen A, Dempster DW, Muller R, et al. Assessment of trabecular and cortical architecture and mechanical competence of bone by high-resolution peripheral computed tomography: comparison with transiliac bone biopsy. Osteoporos Int 2010;21:269; with permission.)

effects of PTH treatment in hypoparathyroidism have been investigated, both with the use of the foreshortened PTH (1–34) molecule[3,5,26–29] as well as with the full re-combinant human PTH(1-84) formulation.[2,4,12,30,31] Although conventional therapy for hypoparathyroidism is not able to alter the skeletal abnormalities in hypoparathy-roidism,[10] use of PTH has shown reversal of many of these abnormalities. In 2015, the Food and Drug Administration approved rhPTH (1–84) as an adjunct to calcium and vitamin D for the treatment of adults with hypoparathyroidism; in 2017, it was approved by the European Medicines Agency as well.

Effects of Parathyroid Hormone Treatment on Bone Turnover

Biochemical markers of bone turnover initially increase dramatically with PTH treat-ment.[3–5,28] In a cohort study by Gafni and colleagues[5] of 5 patients with hypoparathy-roidism treated with PTH (1–34) for 1.5 years, bone turnover markers increased 2- to 7-fold from baseline. In a longer and larger randomized parallel group study, 27 pa-tients with hypoparathyroidism (postsurgical n = 11, idiopathic n = 8, calcium recep-tor sensing mutation n = 6, polyglandular failure n = 2) were treated by Winer and colleagues[3] for 3 years with either calcitriol or PTH (1–34) titrated to serum calcium levels. Markers of bone turnover, including alkaline phosphatase, osteocalcin, urinary pyridinoline, and deoxypyridinoline, increased markedly above the normal range, although a slight downward trend was detectable beginning at 2.5 years.[3] More recently, Sikjaer and colleagues[4] found in a 6-month randomized double-blind pla-cebo-controlled study of PTH (1–84) administered to 62 patients with hypoparathy-roidism (postsurgical n = 58, idiopathic n = 4) at a dose of 100 µg/d that biochemical markers of bone turnover increased dramatically (procollagen type I amino-terminal propeptide by 1315% and s-CTx increased by 1209%), although the levels of osteocalcin and s-CTx seemed to plateau between 20 and 24 weeks. Simi-larly, in 33 subjects (postsurgical n=20, autoimmune n=12, DiGeorge n=1) treated by Rubin and colleagues[29] with PTH (1–84) for 6 years, bone turnover markers increased significantly, reaching a 3-fold peak from baseline values at 6 to 12 months and subsequently declining. Bone turnover markers increased significantly, reaching a 3-fold peak above baseline values at 1 year and subsequently declining but remaining higher than pretreatment values. Taken together, these data suggest that PTH has an initial exuberant effect to increase biochemical markers of bone turnover, with subse-quent tempering over time to a new, steady-state, more euparathyroid level. Notably, the skeletal effects of PTH injections seem to depend on the frequency of the dose. Once-daily or twice-daily PTH(1–34) injections[30,31] and alternate-day or once-daily rhPTH (1–84) injections produce persistently increased levels of bone turnover markers.[3,29] In contrast, continuous infusion of hPTH (1–34) by pump normalized the levels of bone turnover markers in a 12-week study[30]; but further studies of pump delivery of hPTH (1–34) are required to determine its long-term effects on bone.[31]

Effects of Parathyroid Hormone Treatment on Bone Mineral Density

Treatment with PTH (1–34) as titrated to serum calcium levels, when compared with calcitriol by Winer and colleagues,[3] did not result In a change in BMD over 3 years in adult patients with hypoparathyroidism, although there was a tendency for nonsig-nificant decreases at the lumbar spine and radius. In children, there was a significant decrease at radial BMD after 3 years of PTH (1–34).[32] When PTH(1–84) was given by Sikjaer and colleagues[4] to adults at 100 µg/d for 6 months, BMD decreased at the whole body, spine, hip, and femoral neck but not at the forearm; the BMD decreases correlated with the increases in biochemical markers of bone turnover.[4] Quantitative computed tomography analysis of this cohort showed that vBMD in cancellous bone increased, despite the decrease in aBMD at the lumbar spine, whereas cortical vBMD decreased.[4] In the 6-year treatment study of rhPTH(1–84), lumbar spine BMD increased (3.8 ±1%, P = .004) as did the total hip BMD (2.4 ±1%, P = .02), whereas femoral neck BMD remained stable and the distal one-third radius decreased (−4.4 ±1%, P<.0001). These data suggest that the relative distribution of trabecular and cortical bone might differ with PTH treatment at specific skeletal sites.

Effects of Parathyroid Hormone Treatment on Histomorphometric Indices

Iliac crest bone biopsies were performed by Sikjaer and colleagues[12] in 51 patients in the 6-month randomized controlled trial of PTH(1–84) treatment (PTH group n = 26; placebo group n = 25). μCT analysis demonstrated lower trabecular thickness with PTH treatment, with an increase in the bone surface and the presence of a more complex trabecular network, suggesting the development of thinner and better connected trabeculae.[12] Intratrabecular tunneling, or the longitudinal splitting of a single trabeculae into 2 thinner new trabeculae (**Fig. 6**), was observed in the PTH(1–84) group. The presence of intratrabecular tunneling was associated with greater calcium mobilization, as evidenced by higher bone turnover and a tendency toward a greater decrease in calcium and active vitamin D supplementation.[4,12] With regard to cortical bone, at 6 months more Haversian canals per unit area were observed, with a trend toward increased cortical porosity, although cortical bone tissue density was not different.[12] A similar pattern was observed in the open-label 1.5-year study of Gafni and colleagues,[5] with an increase in cancellous bone volume, trabecular number, and cortical porosity and a decrease in trabecular separation.

In an open-label study of rhPTH (1–84) treatment for 2 years, paired iliac crest bone biopsies were performed before and after rhPTH (1–84) treatment at 1 year (n = 14) and at 2 years (n = 16); a separate group had an early quadruple-label biopsy[33] at 3 months (n = 16).[2] An early anabolic effect was apparent, with an early increase in the mineralizing surface (MS), osteoid surface, and BFR at 3 months (MS at baseline: 0.39 ±0.6% vs MS at 3 months: 5.47 ±6.0%; P = .004), which peaked at 12 months (MS at baseline: 0.7 ±0.6% vs MS at 1 year: 7.1 ±6.0%, P = .001) and was similar to euparathyroid levels at 2 years (MS at baseline: 1.18 ±2.2% vs MS at 2 years: 3.34 ±0.8%; P = .04; MS in healthy controls: 4.33 ±3.2%). The remodeling changes were most pronounced in the cancellous envelope at 1 year; within 2 years, with the exception of osteoid surface, the differences were no longer significant at the endocortical and intracortical envelopes.[2] Structural changes after rhPTH (1–84) treatment included reduced trabecular width (144 ±34 μm to 128 ±34 μm, P = .03) and increases in trabecular number (1.74 ±0.34/mm to 2.07 ±0.50/mm, P = .02) at 2 years. As in the studies of Sikjaer and colleagues[12] and Gafni and colleagues,[5] intratrabecular tunneling was apparent (**Fig. 7**). Cortical porosity increased at 2 years (7.4% ±3.2% to 9.2% ±2.4%, P = .03; see **Fig. 7**), although cortical width did not change. Preliminary histomorphometric data suggest that restoration of remodeling indices persist after 8 years of rhPTH (1–84).[34] Longitudinal 3D analysis of the biopsies by μCT confirm that the microstructural changes, including decreased trabecular thickness and increased connectivity density, occur relatively early with PTH treatment and are detectable to a greater extent at 1 year than at 2 years.[35] Backscattered electron imaging of the biopsies showed that with rhPTH (1–84) treatment over 1 year there was a decrease in the degree of mineralization and an increase in the heterogeneity of mineralization.[36] After 2 years of rhPTH (1–84), the degree of mineralization was similar to baseline, although the greater heterogeneity in matrix mineralization persisted. These data suggest that the greatest effects on bone mineralization density

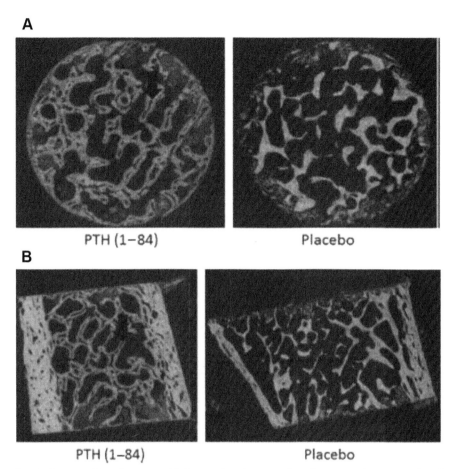

Fig. 6. Iliac crest biopsies, one with intratrabecular tunneling from a patient treated with PTH (1–84) 100 mg/d for 24 weeks and one without tunneling from a placebo-treated patient. (*A*) Cross-sectional view; (*B*) longitudinal sectional view. (*From* Sikjaer T, Rejnmark L, Thomsen JS, et al. Changes in 3-dimensional bone structure indices in hypoparathyroid patients treated with PTH (1–84): a randomized controlled study. J Bone Miner Res 2012;27:783; with permission.)

distribution occur early with PTH exposure to the hypoparathyroid skeleton. Overall, the histomorphometric data suggest that administration of PTH tends to improve abnormal dynamic and structural skeletal properties in hypoparathyroidism.

Effects of Parathyroid Hormone Treatment on Fractures

Data are not available on the effects of PTH treatment in hypoparathyroidism on fracture risk. Given the well-characterized improvements in skeletal properties, a decrease in fracture risk would be anticipated; but this expectation awaits confirmation from larger and longer studies.

Osteosarcoma Risk with Parathyroid Hormone Treatment

PTH (1–34) and rhPTH (1–84) were found to increase the osteosarcoma risk in rats.[37] However, the risk is dose related and the noncarcinogenic doses for both PTH (1–34)

A

Hypoparathyroidism Baseline

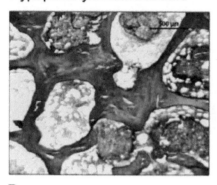

Hypoparathyroidism 1 Y PTH(1–84)

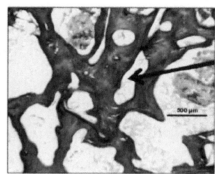

B

Hypoparathyroidism Baseline

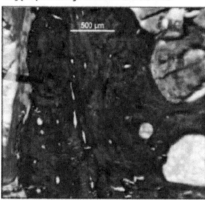

Hypoparathyroidism 1 Y PTH(1–84)

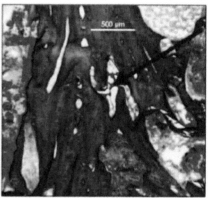

Fig. 7. Iliac crest biopsy illustrating changes in the trabecular (*A*) and cortical (*B*) structure before and after 1 year of PTH (1–84) treatment in a subject with hypoparathyroidism. Note the increases in trabecular tunneling and cortical porosity (*arrows*) in the posttreatment biopsy. (*From* Rubin MR, Dempster DW, Sliney J Jr, et al. PTH (1–84) administration reverses abnormal bone-remodeling dynamics and structure in hypoparathyroidism. J Bone Miner Res 2011;26:2734; with permission.)

(4.5 μg/kg/d) and rhPTH (1–84) (10 μg/kg/d) are markedly greater than those used to treat hypoparathyroidism.[38] Although this issue could be of particular concern in children with unfused epiphyses, the 3-year data of Winer and colleagues[32] in children and a 13-year case report[39] are reassuring in this regard. Moreover, long-standing hyperparathyroidism is not associated with the development of osteosarcomas despite chronically elevated PTH levels.[40] Furthermore, no increased rate of osteosarcoma has emerged despite extensive use of hPTH (1–34) in patients with hypoparathyroidism or osteoporosis since teriparatide (Forteo) was approved in 2002, although most of the latter were treated for only 2 years.[41]

SUMMARY

Hypoparathyroidism is associated with marked abnormalities in bone parameters. With PTH replacement, many of the altered indices begin to approximate normal bone. These skeletal findings speak to the fundamental importance of PTH in the maintenance of bone structure and function. Future work is needed to determine whether fractures rates are increased in hypoparathyroidism or reduced with PTH treatment.

REFERENCES

1. Langdahl BL, Mortensen L, Vesterby A, et al. Bone histomorphometry in hypoparathyroid patients treated with vitamin D. Bone 1996;18:103–8.
2. Rubin MR, Dempster DW, Sliney J Jr, et al. PTH(1-84) administration reverses abnormal bone-remodeling dynamics and structure in hypoparathyroidism. J Bone Miner Res 2011;26:2727–36.
3. Winer KK, Ko CW, Reynolds JC, et al. Long-term treatment of hypoparathyroidism: a randomized controlled study comparing parathyroid hormone-(1-34) versus calcitriol and calcium. J Clin Endocrinol Metab 2003;88:4214–20.
4. Sikjaer T, Rejnmark L, Rolighed L, et al. The effect of adding PTH(1-84) to conventional treatment of hypoparathyroidism: a randomized, placebo-controlled study. J Bone Miner Res 2011;26:2358–70.
5. Gafni RI, Brahim JS, Andreopoulou P, et al. Daily parathyroid hormone 1-34 replacement therapy for hypoparathyroidism induces marked changes in bone turnover and structure. J Bone Miner Res 2012;27:1811–20.
6. Abugassa S, Nordenstrom J, Eriksson S, et al. Bone mineral density in patients with chronic hypoparathyroidism. J Clin Endocrinol Metab 1993;76:1617–21.
7. Fujiyama K, Kiriyama T, Ito M, et al. Attenuation of postmenopausal high turnover bone loss in patients with hypoparathyroidism. J Clin Endocrinol Metab 1995;80:2135–8.
8. Seeman E, Wahner HW, Offord KP, et al. Differential effects of endocrine dysfunction on the axial and the appendicular skeleton. J Clin Invest 1982;69:1302–9.
9. Touliatos JS, Sebes JI, Hinton A, et al. Hypoparathyroidism counteracts risk factors for osteoporosis. Am J Med Sci 1995;310:56–60.
10. Rubin MR, Dempster DW, Zhou H, et al. Dynamic and structural properties of the skeleton in hypoparathyroidism. J Bone Miner Res 2008;23:2018–24.
11. Chen Q, Kaji H, Iu MF, et al. Effects of an excess and a deficiency of endogenous parathyroid hormone on volumetric bone mineral density and bone geometry determined by peripheral quantitative computed tomography in female subjects. J Clin Endocrinol Metab 2003;88:4655–8.
12. Sikjaer T, Rejnmark L, Thomsen JS, et al. Changes in 3-dimensional bone structure indices in hypoparathyroid patients treated with PTH(1-84): a randomized controlled study. J Bone Miner Res 2012;27:781–8.
13. Kruse K, Kracht U, Wohlfart K, et al. Biochemical markers of bone turnover, intact serum parathyroid horn and renal calcium excretion in patients with pseudohypoparathyroidism and hypoparathyroidism before and during vitamin D treatment. Eur J Pediatr 1989;148:535–9.
14. Mizunashi K, Furukawa Y, Miura R, et al. Effects of active vitamin D3 and parathyroid hormone on the serum osteocalcin in idiopathic hypoparathyroidism and pseudohypoparathyroidism. J Clin Invest 1988;82:861–5.
15. Rubin MR, Manavalan JS, Dempster DW, et al. Parathyroid hormone stimulates circulating osteogenic cells in hypoparathyroidism. J Clin Endocrinol Metab 2011;96:176–86.
16. Costa AG, Cremers S, Rubin MR, et al. Circulating sclerostin in disorders of parathyroid gland function. J Clin Endocrinol Metab 2011;96:3804–10.

17. Duan Y, De Luca V, Seeman E. Parathyroid hormone deficiency and excess: similar effects on trabecular bone but differing effects on cortical bone. J Clin Endocrinol Metab 1999;84:718–22.

18. Cusano NE, Nishiyama KK, Zhang C, et al. Noninvasive assessment of skeletal microstructure and estimated bone strength in hypoparathyroidism. J Bone Miner Res 2016;31:308–16.

19. Malluche HH, Matthews C, Faugere MC, et al. 1,25-Dihydroxyvitamin D maintains bone cell activity, and parathyroid hormone modulates bone cell number in dogs. Endocrinology 1986;119:1298–304.

20. Rubin MR, Dempster DW, Kohler T, et al. Three dimensional cancellous bone structure in hypoparathyroidism. Bone 2010;46:190–5.

21. Rubin MD, Dempster J, Sliney C, et al. Indices of bone quality are markedly abnormal in hypoparathyroidism. J Bone Miner Res 2006;(supp 21):1135.

22. Underbjerg L, Sikjaer T, Mosekilde L, et al. The epidemiology of nonsurgical hypoparathyroidism in denmark: a nationwide case finding study. J Bone Miner Res 2015;30:1738–44.

23. Underbjerg L, Sikjaer T, Mosekilde L, et al. Cardiovascular and renal complications to postsurgical hypoparathyroidism: a Danish nationwide controlled historic follow-up study. J Bone Miner Res 2013;28:2277–85.

24. Underbjerg L, Sikjaer T, Mosekilde L, et al. Post-surgical hypoparathyroidism - risk of fractures, psychiatric diseases, cancer, cataract, and infections. J Bone Miner Res 2014;29(11):2504–10.

25. Mitchell DM, Regan S, Cooley MR, et al. Long-term follow-up of patients with hypoparathyroidism. J Clin Endocrinol Metab 2012;97:4507–14.

26. Chawla H, Saha S, Kandasamy D, et al. Vertebral fractures and bone mineral density in patients with idiopathic hypoparathyroidism on long-term follow-up. J Clin Endocrinol Metab 2017;102:251–8.

27. Cohen A, Dempster DW, Muller R, et al. Assessment of trabecular and cortical architecture and mechanical competence of bone by high-resolution peripheral computed tomography: comparison with transiliac bone biopsy. Osteoporos Int 2010;21:263–73.

28. Cusano NE, Rubin MR, McMahon DJ, et al. Therapy of hypoparathyroidism with PTH(1-84): a prospective four-year investigation of efficacy and safety. J Clin Endocrinol Metab 2013;98:137–44.

29. Rubin MR, Cusano NE, Fan WW, et al. Therapy of hypoparathyroidism with PTH(1-84): a prospective six year investigation of efficacy and safety. J Clin Endocrinol Metab 2016;101:2742–50.

30. Winer KK, Zhang B, Shrader JA, et al. Synthetic human parathyroid hormone 1-34 replacement therapy: a randomized crossover trial comparing pump versus injections in the treatment of chronic hypoparathyroidism. J Clin Endocrinol Metab 2012;97:391–9.

31. Winer KK, Fulton KA, Albert PS, et al. Effects of pump versus twice-daily injection delivery of synthetic parathyroid hormone 1-34 in children with severe congenital hypoparathyroidism. J Pediatr 2014;165:556–63.e1..

32. Winer KK, Sinaii N, Reynolds J, et al. Long-term treatment of 12 children with chronic hypoparathyroidism: a randomized trial comparing synthetic human parathyroid hormone 1-34 versus calcitriol and calcium. J Clin Endocrinol Metab 2010;95:2680–8.

33. Lindsay R, Cosman F, Zhou H, et al. A novel tetracycline labeling schedule for longitudinal evaluation of the short-term effects of anabolic therapy with a single

iliac crest bone biopsy: early actions of teriparatide. J Bone Miner Res 2006;21: 366–73.

34. Long-term administration of rhPTH(1-84) results in marked and sustained improvements in skeletal indices by bone histomorphometry in hypoparathyroidism 2017. Available at: http://www.asbmr.org/education/AbstractDetail?aid= 0f96a6c1-6c8b-4af6-b8e3-ff9d3cec2b00. Accessed February 25, 2018.

35. Rubin MR, Zwahlen A, Dempster DW, et al. Effects of parathyroid hormone administration on bone strength in hypoparathyroidism. J Bone Miner Res 2016;31:1082–8.

36. Misof BM, Roschger P, Dempster DW, et al. PTH(1-84) administration in hypoparathyroidism transiently reduces bone matrix mineralization. J Bone Miner Res 2016;31:180–9.

37. Watanabe A, Yoneyama S, Nakajima M, et al. Osteosarcoma in Sprague-Dawley rats after long-term treatment with teriparatide (human parathyroid hormone (1-34)). J Toxicol Sci 2012;37:617–29.

38. Jolette J, Wilker CE, Smith SY, et al. Defining a noncarcinogenic dose of recombinant human parathyroid hormone 1-84 in a 2-year study in Fischer 344 rats. Toxicol Pathol 2006;34:929–40.

39. Theman TA, Collins MT, Dempster DW, et al. PTH(1-34) replacement therapy in a child with hypoparathyroidism caused by a sporadic calcium receptor mutation. J Bone Miner Res 2009;24:964–73.

40. Silverberg SJ, Shane E, Jacobs TP, et al. A 10-year prospective study of primary hyperparathyroidism with or without parathyroid surgery. N Engl J Med 1999;341: 1249–55.

41. Andrews EB, Gilsenan AW, Midkiff K, et al. The US postmarketing surveillance study of adult osteosarcoma and teriparatide: study design and findings from the first 7 years. J Bone Miner Res 2012;27:2429–37.

Hypoparathyroidism and the Kidney

Munro Peacock, DSc, FRCP

KEYWORDS

- Hypoparathyroidism • Kidney • Calcium homeostasis • Phosphate homeostasis
- Tubular reabsorption calcium • Tubular reabsorption phosphate • PTH
- 1,25 dihydroxy vitamin D

KEY POINTS

- Hypocalcemia and hyperphosphatemia are the pathognomonic biochemical features of hypoparathyroidism and result directly from the lack of parathyroid hormone (PTH) action on the kidney.
- Hypocalcemia is symptomatic causing a spectrum of neuromuscular disturbances ranging from epilepsy and tetany to paresthesia. Hyperphosphatemia is subclinical but chronically promotes ectopic mineralization disease.
- The renal tubule expresses PTHR and in the absence of PTH action, the mechanisms transporting calcium and phosphate reabsorption result in chronic hypocalcemia and hyperphosphatemia.
- Diagnosis of hypoparathyroidism requires essential biochemical measures, including serum concentrations of calcium, phosphate, and PTH and renal tubular reabsorption of calcium and phosphate.
- Vitamin D–thiazide treatment regimens lead to ectopic mineralization and renal damage. PTH treatment acting via renal tubular reabsorption may have fewer side effects.

INTRODUCTION

Hypocalcemia and hyperphosphatemia are the pathognomonic biochemical features of hypoparathyroidism. Both result directly from the lack of parathyroid hormone (PTH) action on the kidney, reflecting the major role the kidney plays in setting normal circulating levels of both calcium and phosphate, (inorganic phosphorus) (**Fig. 1**). A narrow physiologic range in serum calcium exists due to a tight negative feedback relationship between serum calcium concentration and PTH secretion. Hypocalcemia is usually symptomatic and manifests as a spectrum of neuromuscular disturbances ranging

Disclosure Statement: M. Peacock is the principal investigator on clinical trials supported by Shire Human Genetics Therapies, Inc studying the efficacy of recombinant human PTH 1 – 84 injections subcutaneously in the management of patients with hypoparathyroidism.
Department of Medicine, Division of Endocrinology, Indiana University School of Medicine, 1120 West Michigan Street Cl 365, Indianapolis, IN 46202, USA
E-mail address: mpeacock@iu.edu

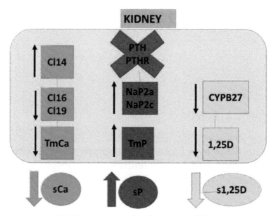

Fig. 1. The kidney is responsible for setting the level of calcium and phosphate in the circulation. In the absence of PTH (X PTH) or a failure of its action on the parathyroid receptor (X PTHR), there is a decrease in tubular reabsorption of calcium (↓TmCa), and an increase in the tubular reabsorption of phosphate (↑TmP). The decrease in TmCa is caused by an up-regulation of Claudin14 (↑ Cl14), which in turn downregulates Claudin16 (↓Cl16) and Claudin19 (↓Cl19) in the thick ascending tubule, resulting in hypocalcemia (↓sCa). The increase in TmP is caused by an increase in activity of the sodium phosphate transporters (↑ NaP2a, NaP2c) in the proximal tubule resulting in hyperphosphatemia (↑sP). The reduced activity of 1alpha hydroxylase enzyme (↓CYPB27) causes reduced production of 1,25 dihydroxy vitamin D (↓1,25D) and decreased serum 1,25 D (↓1,25D).

from epilepsy and tetany to mild paresthesia.[1] Circulating phosphate concentration, on the other hand, does not directly regulate PTH secretion and the normal range is relatively wide. Hyperphosphatemia is subclinical but chronically promotes ectopic mineralization disease.

The renal tubule is rich in parathyroid hormone receptor (PTH1R)[2] and in the absence of PTH action, the activity of the mechanisms transporting calcium and phosphate reabsorption deregulate resulting in chronic hypocalcemia and hyperphosphatemia (see **Fig. 1**). Hypoparathyroidism due to absence of PTH or a failure of PTH1R to respond has a wide range of etiologies and may present at any age.[1] Before birth, calcium and phosphate concentrations in the maternal circulation largely determine fetal circulating levels and genetic hypoparathyroidism only causes problems postnatally.[3] Immediately after birth, the kidney rapidly takes control of setting blood levels of calcium and phosphate using PTH, fibroblast growth factor 23 (FGF23), and 1, 25 dihydroxy vitamin D (1,25D), the 3 main hormones regulating mineral homeostasis and metabolism.[4] In conjunction with gut absorption, the kidney throughout the life span maintains tissue requirements for both minerals, particularly the requirements for bone, which has the highest requirement, especially during longitudinal growth.

Diagnosis and management of hypoparathyroidism rest on a platform of essential blood and urine measures. These include circulating concentrations of calcium, phosphate, and PTH and measures of renal tubular reabsorption of calcium and phosphate. The aim of clinical management is to maintain normocalcemia and normophosphatemia. Increasing calcium gut absorption using calcium supplements in combination with pharmacologic doses of vitamin D and its analogs and increasing renal calcium reabsorption with thiazide diuretics have been the mainstay of therapy. Until recently, PTH with its major action on renal tubular reabsorption of calcium and phosphate has not been readily available as treatment.[5,6]

Vitamin D treatment in hypoparathyroidism can lead to adverse effects by inducing episodes of hypercalcemia and/or hypercalciuria, leading to renal failure and ectopic mineralization. The product of calcium and phosphate concentration in extracellular fluid (ECF), in conjunction with mineral crystal inhibitors and promoters, is a major determinant of the propensity for calcium phosphate mineral to deposit in soft tissues.[7] In hypoparathyroidism, episodic hypercalcemia from therapy leads to ectopic mineralization. The kidney in hypoparathyroidism is particularly vulnerable to treatment-induced renal damage.[8–10]

RENAL TUBULAR REABSORPTION OF CALCIUM
Calcium Transport by Kidney

Serum calcium concentration in healthy adults and children is approximately 9.6 mg/dL, and of this, approximately 60% is ultrafilterable by the glomerulus. The adult kidney has a glomerular filtration rate (GFR) of approximately 100 mL/min and produces more than 8000 mg calcium in the glomerular filtrate (GF) every 24 hours.[4] The renal tubule reabsorbs approximately 97.5% with the unreabsorbed calcium, approximately 200 mg/24 hours, appearing in urine. The renal tubule has 3 distinct anatomic and functional segments involved in calcium reabsorption. The proximal tubule reabsorbs 65% of the luminal calcium, the thick ascending limb of the tubule (CTAL) reabsorbs a further 25%, and the distal tubule recovers a final 8%[11] (**Fig. 2**). The relationship between filtered load and tubular reabsorption is positive and linear and never reaches unity over the range of circulating calcium encountered in humans (**Fig. 3**A).[12] Unlike phosphate, there is no distinct maximal tubular reabsorption rate above which all the increase in filtered load is excreted.

Parathyroid Hormone Receptor 1 and Tubular Reabsorption of Calcium

The PTH1R, a member of the G protein–coupled transmembrane receptor family B,[13] is abundantly expressed throughout the renal tubule.[2] Reabsorption occurs both transcellularly via receptor potential cation channels, TRVP5[14] on the luminal membrane of the distal nephron, and paracellularly via claudins, a family of tight-junction membrane proteins, the proximal tubule, and the CTAL.[15] Allele variation of TRVP5 in humans may account for lower urine calcium in black individuals than white individuals[16] and TRVP5 mutations in mice decrease calcium reabsorption.[17] Claudin2 is involved in calcium transport in the proximal tubule; claudin14, 16, and 19 in the thick ascending limb; and claudin4, 7, and 8 in the distal tubule. Mutations in claudin16 and claudin19 cause decreased tubular reabsorption of calcium and magnesium.[18] Activity of claudin16 and claudin19 are unaffected by PTH, but in the absence of PTH action, claudin14 activity is upregulated, which in turn reduces claudin16 and 19 and results in decreased tubular reabsorption[19] (see **Fig. 1**). This contrasts with other disorders causing reduced calcium reabsorption, most of which result in secondary hyperparathyroidism in an attempt to maintain normocalcemia. The observation that some patients with hypoparathyroidism failed to increase serum calcium with injected PTH led to the concept of hormone receptor resistance and the classification of this form of hypoparathyroidism as pseudohypoparathyroidism type 1.[20] In this form of hypoparathyroidism, serum PTH is markedly increased in the face of hypocalcemia. In pseudohypoparathyroidism type1B, although PTH1R is nonresponsive in the proximal kidney, it is responsive in bone, resulting in hypocalcemia with secondary hyperparathyroid bone disease.[21] However, the increased net bone resorption is insufficient to offset hypocalcemia produced by the decreased generation of 1,25-dihydroxyvitamin D[21,22] until tertiary hyperparathyroidism with severe hyperparathyroid bone disease develops.[23]

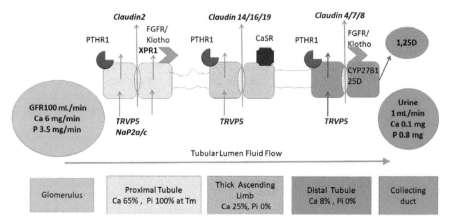

Fig. 2. *Calcium.* At a total serum calcium (Ca) of 10 mg/dL (6 mg/dL ultrafilterable), and a GFR of 100 mL/min, approximately 6 mg/min Ca enters the renal tubule. The proximal tubule reabsorbs 65% of the Ca both transcellularly by TRVP5 and paracellularly by Claudin2 down a sodium-induced concentration gradient. The thick ascending limb, which richly expresses PTH1R, reabsorbs approximately 25% of the filtered calcium transcellularly by TRVP5 and paracellularly by Claudin16/19. The presence of PTH suppresses Claudin 14, whereas its absence upregulates Claudin14, which inhibits Claudin16/19-induced calcium reabsorption. The thick ascending limb also expresses CaSR and independent of PTH but acting through the Claudin pathways, decreases tubular calcium reabsorption. The distal tubule reabsorbs approximately 8% of the filtered Ca using TRVP5 and Claudin4/7/8 transporters. Approximately 0.1 mg/mL per minute of the filtered Ca appears in urine. *Phosphate.* The glomerulus filters approximately 3.5 mg/min phosphate (P). The proximal tubule reabsorbs approximately 2.5 mg/100 mL per minute, the tubular maximum, and the remainder flows through the tubule unabsorbed and appears in urine at a rate of approximately 0.8 mg/min. Transport of P into the proximal tubule occurs via NaP2a and NaP2c and is secreted back to blood by transporters including XPR1. The proximal tubule expresses PTHR and in the absence of PTH action, phosphate reabsorption is increased. FGF23 also regulates NaP2a/2c transporters in the proximal tubule via an FGFR/Klotho receptor complex.

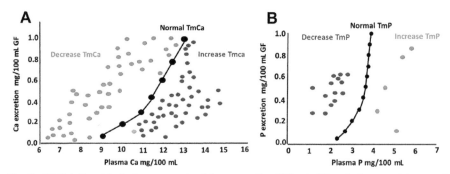

Fig. 3. (A) Relationship between renal calcium excretion/100 mL GF and plasma calcium mg/100 mL (GF = 60% plasma calcium mg/dL) established by intravenous calcium infusion in healthy subjects and (*black*, normal TmCa), in patients with hypoparathyroidism (*green*, decreased TmCa) and patients with primary hyperparathyroidism (*blue*, increased TmCa). (B) Relationship between renal phosphate excretion/100 mL GF and plasma phosphate mg/100 mL (GF = plasma phosphate mg/dL) in healthy subjects (*black*) and patients with hypoparathyroidism (*green*, increased TmP) and primary hyperparathyroidism (*blue*, decreased TmP). (*Data from* [A] Peacock M, Robertson WG, Nordin BE. Relation between serum and urinary calcium with particular reference to parathyroid activity. Lancet 1969;1(7591):384–6; and [B] Bijvoet OL, Morgan DB, Fourman P. The assessment of phosphate reabsorption. Clin Chim Acta 1969;26(1):15–24.)

Calcium Sensing Receptor

The renal tubule also abundantly expresses the calcium sensing receptor (CaSR), particularly in the thick ascending limb.[24] Activation of CaSR decreases calcium reabsorption and inactivation of CaSR increases calcium reabsorption.[25] CaSR in the thick ascending limb functions to prevent excess calcium reabsorption.[11] Activation mutations in CaSR cause autosomal dominant hypocalcemic hypercalciuria[26,27] and inactivation mutations cause familial hypocalciuric hypercalcemia.[28] CaSR acts on claudin14, which inhibits the actions of claudin16 and 19 on calcium tubular reabsorption, and claudin14 is a negative regulator of calcium reabsorption.[29,30] CaSR acts in the absence of PTH.[30–32] However, activation mutations of CaSR produce hypocalcemia because of the intrinsic abnormality of CaSR in the parathyroid gland, which reduces secretion of PTH.[33] Thus, although serum PTH is measurable in activating mutations of CaSR, it is inappropriately low for the level of hypocalcemia and lower than that occurring with pseudohypoparathyroidism. Notwithstanding, serum PTH is a key measure that helps clinically to separate hypocalcemic hypercalciuria from hypoparathyroid and pseudohypoparathryoid hypocalcemia.

Sodium

The effects of sodium on renal calcium transport are major and occur in hypoparathyroidism independently of PTH. The strong positive association between renal calcium and sodium excretion is extensively documented in the literature, and indeed has been frequently considered to be involved in the pathogenesis of common diseases, such as hypertension, renal stone disease, and osteoporosis. Sodium transport by the renal tubule has major effects on calcium reabsorption.[34–37] In the proximal tubule, calcium reabsorption is intimately dependent on the reabsorption of sodium and water. Increased reabsorption of sodium and water, as say from dehydration, results in a marked secondary increase in calcium reabsorption and may promote or aggravate hypercalcemia. On the other hand, sodium and osmotic loads in the proximal tubule cause both natriuria and calciuria by retarding the reabsorptive flow of both ions. In the thick ascending limb of Henle, loop diuretics, such as furosemide, simultaneously decrease sodium and calcium reabsorption causing rapid-onset calciuria.[37] In the distal tubule, the thiazide-sensitive sodium chloride cotransporter regulates reabsorption of sodium and chloride. Here, thiazide diuretics increase calcium reabsorption while decreasing sodium reabsorption.[37]

RENAL TUBULAR REABSORPTION OF PHOSPHATE
Phosphate Transport by Kidney

Serum phosphate (inorganic phosphorus) has a concentration of 2.5 to 4.9 mg/dL in healthy adults. In children, serum concentration has a higher reference range due to an intrinsic increase in maximum tubular reabsorption rate.[38] Serum phosphate decreases from a mean of approximately 6 mg/dL in the newborn to a value of 3.5 mg/dL by late puberty. Because some hypoparathyroid diseases appear in childhood, tubular reabsorption is an essential measurement for diagnosis and management. Approximately 20% of the phosphate in serum is protein bound, but because of Donnan membrane effects at the glomerulus, more than 95% of serum phosphate appears in the GF. Clinically, the phosphate concentration in the GF is taken as the same as that of serum. At a normal GFR of 100 mL/min, approximately 3.5 mg/min of phosphate appears in the filtrate at the Bowman capsule (see **Fig. 2**). The kidney has a tubular maximum capacity for phosphate reabsorption (TmP) of approximately 2.5 mg/100 mL GF. Less than this level, all phosphate is reabsorbed, and greater than this level, the excess is excreted (**Fig. 3**B). The relationship is unity, although there is a small splay extending over a range of 1 mg/100 mL GF. Western diets are rich in phosphorus (organic and inorganic) and well above the 700 mg recommended adult daily requirement. Thus, phosphate is always present in the urine and serum phosphate concentration is higher than TmP. At normal dietary intakes of phosphorus in an adult in phosphorus balance, the 24-hour urine contains more than 800 mg of phosphate.

Parathyroid Hormone/Parathyroid Hormone Receptor 1 and Tubular Reabsorption of Phosphate

The proximal tubule reabsorbs approximately 80% of the filtered phosphate when serum phosphate level is greater than the tubular maximum for reabsorption (see **Fig. 3**B). Transport is transcellular and occurs via luminal membrane sodium/phosphate transporters, mainly type NaP2a and NaP2c.[39] Phosphate moves from lumen to cell by cotransporting with sodium. Phosphate export from the basal membrane of the tubular cell to the ECF is poorly defined; however, in part it involves the xenotropic and polytropic retroviral receptor1 (XPR1). Inactivation of *Xpr1* in the renal tubule of mice leads to decreased tubular reabsorption of phosphate.[40]

Three Main Factors Regulate Tubular Phosphate Reabsorption in Hypoparathyroidism

PTH is the major regulator.[41] The absence of PTH increases NaP2a and NaP2c activity in the proximal tubule, causing increased phosphate reabsorption and hyperphosphatemia (see **Fig. 3**B).

A second phosphate-regulating hormone, FGF23 secreted by osteocytes, and acting via an FGFR/Klotho receptor complex[42] decreases NaP2a and NaP2c activity,[43] and in humans decreases serum phosphate and decreases tubular reabsorption.[44] Serum FGF23 is increased in hypoparathyroidism secondary to hyperphosphatemia.[45] However, the increase fails to offset the lack of the PTH effect on tubular reabsorption, suggesting the need for FGF23 to have PTH available either for its action or for its secretion by the osteocyte.

The third factor is serum calcium concentration. Infusions of calcium in patients with hypoparathyroidism decreases tubular phosphate reabsorption and produces normophosphatemia.[46] Similarly, in patients with hypoparathyroidism treated with a vitamin D regimen, as the plasma calcium normalizes, tubular reabsorption of phosphate decreases and serum phosphate falls to the normal range[47] (**Fig. 4**). The mechanism is not well understood but may involve calcium acting via the CaSR in the luminal membrane of the proximal tubule to decrease phosphate reabsorption.[11,35,48]

RENAL SECRETION OF 1,25 DIHYDROXY VITAMIN D

The renal tubule expresses the vitamin D receptor[49] and the enzymes CYP 27B1[50] and CYP24A1[51,52] (see **Figs. 1** and **2**). In the absence of PTH, CYP 27B1 activity decreases and 25 hydroxy vitamin D conversion to 1,25D is reduced and CYP24A1 activity increases and 25 hydroxy vitamin D is preferentially oxidized to 24,25 dihydroxyvitamin D.[53,54] In hypoparathyroidism, circulating levels of 1,25-dihydroxyvitamin D are in the low normal range.[55,56] There is malabsorption of calcium, which is reversible with 1,25-dihydroxyvitamin D or its analogs[47] (**Fig. 5**). The increased FGF23 in hypoparathyroidism[45] may also decrease production of 1,25-dihydroxyvitamin D.[43,57,58] PTH treatment of hypoparathyroidism substantially increases serum 1,25D.[59–61]

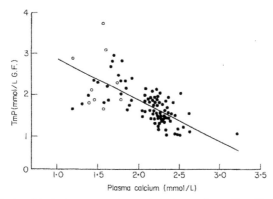

Fig. 4. Inverse relationship between maximum tubular reabsorption (TmP mmol/L GF) and plasma calcium mmol/L in 28 patients with hypoparathyroidism (19 postsurgical and 9 idiopathic), off (o) and on (•) treatment with a vitamin D regimen. As plasma calcium increased into the normal reference range with treatment, TmP decreased into the normal range. (*Data from* Heyburn PJ, Peacock M. The management of hypoparathyroidism with 1 alpha hydroxy vitamin D3. Clin Endocrinol 1977;7 Suppl:209S–14S.)

RENAL PHOSPHATE AND CALCIUM REABSORPTION: CLINICAL ASSESSMENT

Reabsorption of calcium and phosphate are essential measurements in the diagnosis and management of patients with hypoparathyroidism. Subjects should fast from the night before, discard the overnight urine in the morning, and drink water to remain hydrated. Urine is collected over 2 hours and blood drawn with minimal hemostasis after 1 hour. Calcium (Ca), phosphate (P), and creatinine (Cr) are measured in both blood (s) and urine (u) samples. From the concentrations in blood and urine measured in the same units, calcium excreted/100 mL GF (CaE) is uCa × sCr/uCr and calcium reabsorbed/100 GF (CaR) is sCa − CaE.[62] Maximal tubular reabsorption (TmCa) can be estimated from the graph (see **Fig. 3**A) or from the formula TmCa = CaR/1 − 0.08 $\log_e$ sCa/CaE. Phosphate is expressed in the same terms. Phosphate

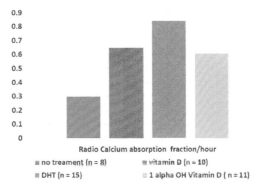

Fig. 5. Fractional rate of absorption of radio calcium from 20 mg stable calcium oral dose (normal mean = 0.55) in patients with hypoparathyroidism untreated (n = 8) and on treatment (vitamin D3 0.25–1.25 mg/d, n = 10), DHT (0.25–1.25 mg/d, n = 26), and 1-alpha hydroxyl vitamin D3 (1–3 μg/d, n = 20). (*Data from* Heyburn PJ, Peacock M. The management of hypoparathyroidism with 1 alpha hydroxy vitamin D3. Clin Endocrinol 1977;7 Suppl:209S–14S.)

excreted/100 mL GF (PE) is uP $\times$ sCr/uCr and phosphate reabsorbed/100 GF (PR) is sP $-$ PE. TmP= PR/1 $-$ 0.1 $\log_e$ sP/PE can be estimated from graph[63] or nomogram.[64] Reabsorption is also usefully expressed as calcium and phosphate creatinine clearance ratio (uCa $\times$ sCr/sCa $\times$ uCr, and uP $\times$ sCr/sP $\times$ uCr) but does not express reabsorption in units of 100 mL/GF and thus cannot be directly related to serum concentration.[34]

Fasting uCa/uCr and uP/uCr provide estimates of the calcium and phosphate input to the circulation from tissues, largely bone, that maintain serum calcium and phosphate concentration in the absence of absorbed dietary calcium. However, in hyperabsorptive states, such as occurs with high doses of oral calcium and vitamin D treatment regimens in patients with hypoparathyroidism, an overnight fast is insufficient time to clear absorbed calcium from the extracellular space. A 24-hour urine calcium and phosphate provide approximate estimates of daily absorption of calcium and phosphate from the diet. Neither the 24-hour urine nor the fasting urine provide measures of tubular reabsorption.

TREATMENT OF HYPOPARATHYROIDISM
Vitamin D, Calcium, and Thiazide

Pharmacologic doses of oral vitamin D, along with large dietary calcium supplements became established therapy for managing hypoparathyroidism during the first half of the twentieth century even as the various forms of the disease were being elucidated. Dihydrotachysterol (DHT), a potent vitamin D analog not requiring renal hydroxylation for activity, became the treatment of choice.[65] The regimen relieved hypocalcemic symptoms by increasing calcium absorption, while simultaneously producing normophosphatemia both by decreasing renal phosphate reabsorption and by decreasing phosphate absorption by binding dietary phosphate with calcium and reducing its bioavailability. PTH gland extracts were also available for parenteral use. They were shown to relieve tetany and reverse hypocalcemia and hyperphosphatemia largely by effects on tubular reabsorption.[66] However, their cost, variable potency, similar toxicity to DHT, and inconvenience of daily parenteral administration inhibited their clinical development. However, thiazide diuretics, which increase tubular reabsorption of calcium, also became part of the treatment regimen when studies showed that they produced a small but clinically significant rise in serum calcium concentration in patients with hypoparathyroidism (**Fig. 6**).[67] Calcitriol[68] and its analog 1-alpha vitamin

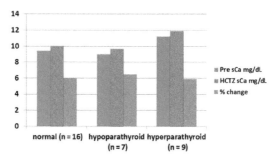

Fig. 6. Effect of oral hydrochlorothiazide (100 mg $\times$2/d) in healthy subjects (n = 16 subjects, 11 studies), patients with hypoparathyroidism (n = 7 patients, 10 studies), and patients with primary hyperparathyroidism (n = 9 patients, 13 studies) on serum calcium mg/dL. Serum calcium increased by approximately 6% in both the presence and absence of PTH. (*Data from* Brickman AS, Massry SG, Coburn JW. Changes in serum and urinary calcium during treatment with hydrochlorothiazide: studies on mechanisms. J Clin Invest 1972;51:945–54.)

D[47] with much shorter biological half-life have now largely replaced DHT. The therapeutic window for calcitriol and analogs is narrow, particularly in the presence of high dietary calcium supplements. Frequent hypercalcemic episodes occur producing high calcium phosphate serum product and promoting ectopic mineralization and renal failure, and such treatment is suboptimal. Further, in some patients, particularly those with comorbid disease of the bowel, it is sometimes impossible to achieve normocalcemia with a vitamin D, calcium, and thiazide regimen.

Parathyroid Hormone

With the availability of parenteral PTH preparations suitable for clinical use, there is renewed interest in treating hypoparathyroidism with exogenous PTH. Intervention studies in children with hypoparathyroidism using daily subcutaneous injections of PTH 1 – 34 demonstrated a long-term effect on normalizing serum calcium and phosphate levels by an action on renal calcium and phosphate tubular reabsorption.[59] When a constant infusion of PTH was compared with 2 daily injections, serum calcium and phosphate were similar with both treatments but tubular reabsorption of calcium was increased and tubular reabsorption of phosphate decreased more with constant infusion.[60] This study demonstrated that not only was PTH achieving normocalcemia by its action on the kidney, but also that a constant infusion was more physiologic than twice-daily injections (**Fig. 7**A). Constant infusion also produced lower 24-hour urine calcium due to less stimulation of 1,25 D secretion (**Fig. 7**B). Importantly, constant infusion of PTH did not stimulate bone resorption and required only approximately a third of the daily dose of PTH compared with daily injections (see **Fig. 7**B). These studies clearly showed that the effect of PTH on serum calcium and phosphate in hypoparathyroidism was completely due to renal actions and confirmed the central role

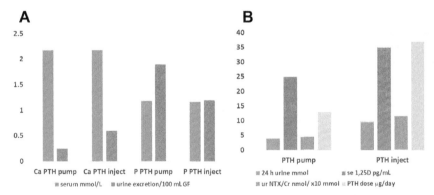

Fig. 7. Comparison of mean PTH dosage per day and biochemistry and in 8 patients with postsurgical hypoparathyroidism treated with PTH 1 – 34 delivered by pump (PTH pump) and by twice-daily injection (PTH inject) aimed at maintaining normocalcemia. (*A*) Serum calcium (Ca), phosphate (P) mmol/L and the corresponding renal calcium and phosphate excretion mmol/dL GF in the first morning 4-hour urine collection with blood drawn at the midpoint of collection. At similar filtered loads, urine calcium excretion was lower (that is, tubular reabsorption higher) and urine phosphate was higher (that is, tubular reabsorption lower) with pump than with injection. (*B*) Twenty-four-hour urine calcium mmol, mean serum 1,25 D pg/mL over 24 hours, 24-hour urine NTX/Cr ratio nmol/10× mmol and mean PTH dose µg/d over a 6-month study was lower with pump than with injection. (*Data from* Winer KK, Zhang B, Shrader JA, et al. Synthetic human parathyroid hormone 1–34 replacement therapy: a randomized crossover trial comparing pump vs injections in the treatment of chronic hypoparathyroidism. J Clin Endocrinol Metab 2012;97(2):391–9.)

the kidney plays in setting the circulating concentrations of calcium and phosphate in health and in parathyroid disorders[69,70]

HYPOPARATHYROIDISM AND KIDNEY FUNCTION
Genetic Disease of Kidney and Parathyroid

Many of the nonsurgical cases of hypoparathyroidism are due to genetic mutations.[71] In some, the mutation results in both hypoparathyroidism and renal disease. In hypoparathyroidism, occurring with sensorineural deafness and renal dysplasia (HDR syndrome), there is a mutation in GATA3.[72] The parathyroid, inner ear, and kidney express the gene during embryonic development. The disease presents as an autosomal recessive disease in which there is renal failure due to hypoplastic cystic kidneys, sensorineural deafness from development problems in the inner ear, and hypoparathyroidism due to failure to develop the parathyroid.

Vitamin D Treatment and Renal Function

Population studies from Europe indicate that the prevalence of hypoparathyroidism is approximately 30 per 100,000 and that surgical cases are more common than nonsurgical.[9,10] More than 70% of these patients with hypoparathyroidism had treatment with vitamin D regimens and had a significantly higher occurrence of renal diseases, renal failure, and kidney stones (**Fig. 8**). The cause of the chronic renal failure was not established. However, in early descriptions of the disease when treatment with vitamin D was less established, renal complications were not a prominent feature, strongly suggesting that renal disease is not an intrinsic consequence of lack of PTH action.[20] It is probable that management with a vitamin D regimen is suboptimal, causing episodes of increased calcium phosphate product in the ECF with resulting renal damage. Nephrocalcinosis and renal calcium stone disease are well-recognized complications of vitamin D intoxication. Even in specialized centers, patients managed with pharmacologic doses of vitamin D, DHT, or 1 alpha hydroxy vitamin D have frequent episodes of hypercalcemia and hyperphosphatemia (**Fig. 9**).[47] Chronicity of treatment also increases the risk of renal damage. Children with hypoparathyroidism who require lifelong treatment are at high risk of renal damage from nephrocalcinosis and kidney stones.[73]

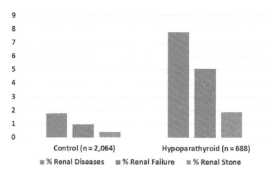

Fig. 8. Renal diseases, renal failure, and renal stone disease percentages in postsurgical hypoparathyroidism (n = 688) compared with controls (n = 2064) in an epidemiologic Danish study. (*Data from* Underbjerg L, Sikjaer T, Mosekilde L, et al. Cardiovascular and renal complications to postsurgical hypoparathyroidism: a Danish nationwide controlled historic follow-up study. J Bone Miner Res 2013;28(11):2277–85.)

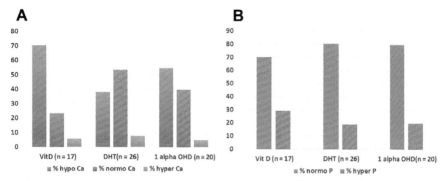

Fig. 9. Occurrence (%) of hypocalcemia, normocalcemia, and hypercalcemia (*A*) and normo-phosphatemia and hyperphosphatemia (*B*) in 63 patients with hypoparathyroidism followed clinically for variable times on pharmacologic doses of vitamin D (VitD, n = 17), dihydrotachysterol (DHT, n = 26), and 1 alpha hydroxy vitamin D (1 alpha OHD, n = 20). (*Data from* Heyburn PJ, Peacock M. The management of hypoparathyroidism with 1 alpha hydroxy vitamin D3. Clin Endocrinol 1977;7 Suppl:209S–14S.)

REFERENCES

1. Shoback DM, Bilezikian JP, Costa AG, et al. Presentation of hypoparathyroidism: etiologies and clinical features. J Clin Endocrinol Metab 2016;101(6):2300–12.

2. Lupp A, Klenk C, Rocken C, et al. Immunohistochemical identification of the PTHR1 parathyroid hormone receptor in normal and neoplastic human tissues. Eur J Endocrinol 2010;162(5):979–86.

3. Kovacs CS. Calcium, phosphorus, and bone metabolism in the fetus and newborn. Early Hum Dev 2015;91(11):623–8.

4. Peacock M. Calcium metabolism in health and disease. Clin J Am Soc Nephrol 2010;5(Suppl 1):S23–30.

5. Winer KK, Yanovski JA, Sarani B, et al. A randomized, cross-over trial of once-daily *versus* twice-daily parathyroid hormone 1-34 in treatment of hypoparathyroidism. J Clin Endocrinol Metab 1998;83(10):3480–6.

6. Cusano NE, Rubin MR, Irani D, et al. Use of parathyroid hormone in hypoparathyroidism. J Endocrinol Invest 2013;36(11):1121–7.

7. Margolis HC, Kwak SY, Yamazaki H. Role of mineralization inhibitors in the regulation of hard tissue biomineralization: relevance to initial enamel formation and maturation. Front Physiol 2014;5:339.

8. Underbjerg L, Sikjaer T, Mosekilde L, et al. Cardiovascular and renal complications to postsurgical hypoparathyroidism: a Danish nationwide controlled historic follow-up study. J Bone Miner Res 2013;28(11):2277–85.

9. Astor MC, Lovas K, Debowska A, et al. Epidemiology and health-related quality of life in hypoparathyroidism in Norway. J Clin Endocrinol Metab 2016;101(8): 3045–53.

10. Vadiveloo T, Donnan PT, Leese GP. A population-based study of the epidemiology of chronic hypoparathyroidism. J Bone Miner Res 2018;33(3):478–85.

11. Ba J, Friedman PA. Calcium-sensing receptor regulation of renal mineral ion transport. Cell Calcium 2004;35(3):229–37.

12. Peacock M, Robertson WG, Nordin BE. Relation between serum and urinary calcium with particular reference to parathyroid activity. Lancet 1969;1(7591):384–6.

13. Nagai S, Okazaki M, Segawa H, et al. Acute down-regulation of sodium-dependent phosphate transporter NPT2a involves predominantly the cAMP/PKA pathway as revealed by signaling-selective parathyroid hormone analogs. J Biol Chem 2011;286(2):1618–26.

14. Hoenderop JG, Nilius B, Bindels RJ. Epithelial calcium channels: from identification to function and regulation. Pflugers Arch 2003;446(3):304–8.

15. Hou J, Rajagopal M, Yu AS. Claudins and the kidney. Annu Rev Physiol 2013;75:479–501.

16. Wang L, Holmes RP, Peng JB. Molecular modeling of the structural and dynamical changes in calcium channel TRPV5 induced by the African-Specific A563T variation. Biochemistry 2016;55(8):1254–64.

17. Loh NY, Bentley L, Dimke H, et al. Autosomal dominant hypercalciuria in a mouse model due to a mutation of the epithelial calcium channel, TRPV5. PLoS One 2013;8(1):e55412.

18. Hou J. The role of claudin in hypercalciuric nephrolithiasis. Curr Urol Rep 2013;14(1):5–12.

19. Sato T, Courbebaisse M, Ide N, et al. Parathyroid hormone controls paracellular Ca(2+) transport in the thick ascending limb by regulating the tight-junction protein Claudin14. Proc Natl Acad Sci U S A 2017;114(16):E3344–53.

20. Albright F, Reifenstein EC. The parathyroid glands and metabolic bone disease. Baltimore (MD): Williams and Wilkins; 1948.

21. Murray TM, Rao LG, Wong MM, et al. Pseudohypoparathyroidism with osteitis fibrosa cystica: direct demonstration of skeletal responsiveness to parathyroid hormone in cells cultured from bone. J Bone Miner Res 1993;8(1):83–91.

22. Srivastava T, Krudys J, Mardis NJ, et al. Cinacalcet as adjunctive therapy in pseudohypoparathyroidism type 1b. Pediatr Nephrol 2016;31(5):795–800.

23. Neary NM, El-Maouche D, Hopkins R, et al. Development and treatment of tertiary hyperparathyroidism in patients with pseudohypoparathyroidism type 1B. J Clin Endocrinol Metab 2012;97(9):3025–30.

24. Riccardi D, Hall AE, Chattopadhyay N, et al. Localization of the extracellular Ca2+/polyvalent cation-sensing protein in rat kidney. Am J Physiol 1998;274(3 Pt 2):F611–22.

25. Riccardi D, Brown EM. Physiology and pathophysiology of the calcium-sensing receptor in the kidney. Am J Physiol Renal Physiol 2010;298(3):F485–99.

26. Pearce SH, Williamson C, Kifor O, et al. A familial syndrome of hypocalcemia with hypercalciuria due to mutations in the calcium-sensing receptor. N Engl J Med 1996;335(15):1115–22.

27. Baron J, Winer KK, Yanovski JA, et al. Mutations in the Ca(2+)-sensing receptor gene cause autosomal dominant and sporadic hypoparathyroidism. Hum Mol Genet 1996;5(5):601–6.

28. Brown EM. Familial hypocalciuric hypercalcemia and other disorders with resistance to extracellular calcium. Endocrinol Metab Clin North Am 2000;29(3):503–22.

29. Gong Y, Renigunta V, Himmerkus N, et al. Claudin-14 regulates renal Ca(+)(+) transport in response to CaSR signalling via a novel microRNA pathway. EMBO J 2012;31(8):1999–2012.

30. Toka HR, Al-Romaih K, Koshy JM, et al. Deficiency of the calcium-sensing receptor in the kidney causes parathyroid hormone-independent hypocalciuria. J Am Soc Nephrol 2012;23(11):1879–90.

31. Kos CH, Karaplis AC, Peng JB, et al. The calcium-sensing receptor is required for normal calcium homeostasis independent of parathyroid hormone. J Clin Invest 2003;111(7):1021–8.

32. Loupy A, Ramakrishnan SK, Wootla B, et al. PTH-independent regulation of blood calcium concentration by the calcium-sensing receptor. J Clin Invest 2012; 122(9):3355–67.

33. Brown EM. The calcium-sensing receptor: physiology, pathophysiology and CaR-based therapeutics. Subcell Biochem 2007;45:139–67.

34. Peacock M. Renal excretion of calcium. In: Nordin BEC, editor. Calcium in human biology. Berlin: Spriner Verlag; 1988. p. 125–69.

35. Ward DT. Calcium receptor-mediated intracellular signalling. Cell Calcium 2004; 35(3):217–28.

36. Moor MB, Bonny O. Ways of calcium reabsorption in the kidney. Am J Physiol Renal Physiol 2016;310(11):F1337–50.

37. Alexander RT, Dimke H. Effect of diuretics on renal tubular transport of calcium and magnesium. Am J Physiol Renal Physiol 2017;312(6):F998–1015.

38. Kruse K, Kracht U, Gopfert G. Renal threshold phosphate concentration (TmPO4/GFR). Arch Dis Child 1982;57(3):217–23.

39. Forster IC, Hernando N, Biber J, et al. Phosphate transporters of the SLC20 and SLC34 families. Mol Aspects Med 2013;34(2–3):386–95.

40. Ansermet C, Moor MB, Centeno G, et al. Renal Fanconi syndrome and hypophosphatemic rickets in the absence of xenotropic and polytropic retroviral receptor in the nephron. J Am Soc Nephrol 2017;28(4):1073–8.

41. Picard N, Capuano P, Stange G, et al. Acute parathyroid hormone differentially regulates renal brush border membrane phosphate cotransporters. Pflugers Arch 2010;460(3):677–87.

42. Urakawa I, Yamazaki Y, Shimada T, et al. Klotho converts canonical FGF receptor into a specific receptor for FGF23. Nature 2006;444(7120):770–4.

43. Shimada T, Hasegawa H, Yamazaki Y, et al. FGF-23 is a potent regulator of vitamin D metabolism and phosphate homeostasis. J Bone Miner Res 2004; 19(3):429–35.

44. Zhang X, Imel EA, Ruppe MD, et al. Pharmacokinetics and pharmacodynamics of a human monoclonal anti-FGF23 antibody (KRN23) in the first multiple ascending-dose trial treating adults with X-linked hypophosphatemia. J Clin Pharmacol 2016;56(2):176–85.

45. Gupta A, Winer K, Econs MJ, et al. FGF-23 is elevated by chronic hyperphosphatemia. J Clin Endocrinol Metab 2004;89(9):4489–92.

46. Eisenberg E. Effects of serum calcium level and parathyroid extracts on phosphate and calcium excretion in hypoparathyroid patients. J Clin Invest 1965;44: 942–6.

47. Heyburn PJ, Peacock M. The management of hypoparathyroidism with 1 alpha hydroxy vitamin D3. Clin Endocrinol 1977;7(Suppl):209S-14S.

48. Mathias RS, Brown EM. Divalent cations modulate PTH-dependent 3',5'-cyclic adenosine monophosphate production in renal proximal tubular cells. Endocrinology 1991;128(6):3005–12.

49. Iida K, Shinki T, Yamaguchi A, et al. A possible role of vitamin D receptors in regulating vitamin D activation in the kidney. Proc Natl Acad Sci U S A 1995;92: 6112–6.

50. Zehnder D, Bland R, Walker EA, et al. Expression of 25-hydroxyvitamin D3-1alpha-hydroxylase in the human kidney. J Am Soc Nephrol 1999;10(12): 2465–73.

51. Knutson JC, DeLuca HF. 25-Hydroxyvitamin D3-24-hydroxylase. Subcellular location and properties. Biochemistry 1974;13(7):1543–8.

52. Jones G, Prosser DE, Kaufmann M. 25-Hydroxyvitamin D-24-hydroxylase (CYP24A1): its important role in the degradation of vitamin D. Arch Biochem Biophys 2012;523(1):9–18.

53. Tanaka Y, DeLuca HF. Measurement of mammalian 25-hydroxyvitamin D3 24R- and 1 alpha-hydroxylase. Proc Natl Acad Sci U S A 1981;78(1):196–9.

54. Zierold C, Mings JA, DeLuca HF. Regulation of 25-hydroxyvitamin D3-24-hydroxylase mRNA by 1,25-dihydroxyvitamin D3 and parathyroid hormone. J Cell Biochem 2003;88(2):234–7.

55. Haussler MR, McCain TA. Vitamin D metabolism and action. N Eng J Med 1977; 297:974–83, 1041–50.

56. Lund B, Sorensen OH, Lund B, et al. Vitamin D metabolism in hypoparathyroidism. J Clin Endocrinol Metab 1980;51(3):606–10.

57. Shimada T, Kakitani M, Yamazaki Y, et al. Targeted ablation of Fgf23 demonstrates an essential physiological role of FGF23 in phosphate and vitamin D metabolism. J Clin Invest 2004;113(4):561–8.

58. Perwad F, Zhang MY, Tenenhouse HS, et al. Fibroblast growth factor 23 impairs phosphorus and vitamin D metabolism in vivo and suppresses 25-hydroxyvitamin D-1alpha-hydroxylase expression in vitro. Am J Physiol Renal Physiol 2007; 293(5):F1577–83.

59. Winer KK, Sinaii N, Reynolds J, et al. Long-term treatment of 12 children with chronic hypoparathyroidism: a randomized trial comparing synthetic human parathyroid hormone 1-34 versus calcitriol and calcium. J Clin Endocrinol Metab 2010;95(6):2680–8.

60. Winer KK, Zhang B, Shrader JA, et al. Synthetic human parathyroid hormone 1-34 replacement therapy: a randomized crossover trial comparing pump versus injections in the treatment of chronic hypoparathyroidism. J Clin Endocrinol Metab 2012;97(2):391–9.

61. Liu XX, Zhu XY, Mei GH. Parathyroid hormone replacement therapy in hypoparathyroidism: a meta-analysis. Horm Metab Res 2016;48(6):377–83.

62. Peacock M, Nordin BEC. Tubular reabsorption of calcium in normals and hypercalciuric subjects. J Clin Pathol 1968;21:353–8.

63. Bijvoet OL, Morgan DB, Fourman P. The assessment of phosphate reabsorption. Clin Chim Acta 1969;26(1):15–24.

64. Walton R, Bijvoet O. Nomogram for the derivation of renal threshold phosphate concentration. Lancet 1975;2(7929):309–10.

65. Albright F, Bloomberg E, Drake T, et al. A comparison of the effects of A.T. 10 (Dihydrotachysterol) and Vitamin D on calcium and phosphorus metabolism in hypoparathyroidism. J Clin Invest 1938;17(3):317–29.

66. Albright F, Sulkowitch HW. The effect of vitamin D on calcium and phosphorus metabolism; studies on four patients. J Clin Invest 1938;17(3):305–15.

67. Brickman AS, Massry SG, Coburn JW. Changes in serum and urinary calcium during treatment with hydrochlorothiazide: studies on mechanisms. J Clin Invest 1972;51:945–54.

68. Markowitz ME, Rosen JF, Smith C, et al. 1,25-dihydroxyvitamin D3-treated hypoparathyroidism: 35 patients years in 10 children. J Clin Endocrinol Metab 1982; 55(4):727–33.

69. Peacock M. Primary hyperparathyroidism and the kidney: biochemical and clinical spectrum. J Bone Miner Res 2002;17(Suppl 2):N87–94.

70. Peacock M. Primary hyperparathyroidism and the kidney. In: Bilizikain JP, Marcus R, Levine M, et al, editors. The parathyroids. New York: Elsevier, Inc; 2014. p. 455–67.
71. Grigorieva IV, Thakker RV. Transcription factors in parathyroid development: lessons from hypoparathyroid disorders. Ann N Y Acad Sci 2011;1237:24–38.
72. Nesbit MA, Bowl MR, Harding B, et al. Characterization of GATA3 mutations in the hypoparathyroidism, deafness, and renal dysplasia (HDR) syndrome. J Biol Chem 2004;279(21):22624–34.
73. Levy I, Licht C, Daneman A, et al. The impact of hypoparathyroidism treatment on the kidney in children: long-term retrospective follow-up study. J Clin Endocrinol Metab 2015;100(11):4106–13.

Quality of Life in Hypoparathyroidism

Tamara J. Vokes, MD

KEYWORDS

- Hypoparathyroidism • Quality of life • PTH therapy • PTH1-34 • PTH1-84
- Hypocalcemia

KEY POINTS

- Patients with hypoparathyroidism treated with conventional therapy often have symptoms consistent with decreased quality of life (QOL); the symptoms vary within, as well as between, patients.
- Different studies report different manifestations of reduced QOL in hypoparathyroidism.
- Treatment with parathyroid hormone (PTH) injections has been shown to improve QOL in several but not all studies.
- It is presently not clear whether improved QOL in response to PTH therapy is related to stabilization in serum calcium levels or to some other effect of PTH on patients' well-being.

INTRODUCTION

Physicians caring for patients with hypoparathyroidism have long known that these patients have complaints suggestive of poor quality of life (QOL). Systematic evaluation of these complaints is, however, relatively recent and coincides with the initial efforts to introduce parathyroid hormone (PTH) therapy into the care of hypoparathyroidism. Several challenges exist in evaluating QOL in hypoparathyroidism. Patients have variable symptoms with significant differences in the nature and severity of symptoms both within and between patients. In addition, there are no validated disease-specific instruments for assessing these complaints. Consequently, the instruments used are relatively crude and lack both the precision and the sensitivity to adequately quantify the QOL impairments. Finally, the same limitations are present and possibly magnified when assessing the QOL response to treatment with PTH and its analogues. These limitations are, at least in part, the reason for the inconsistencies and contradictory conclusions derived from different studies. These limitations notwithstanding, we now have a substantial body of literature that is at least starting to address QOL in hypoparathyroidism on conventional as well as on PTH-based therapy.[1]

Disclosure: Dr T.J. Vokes is a consultant, investigator, and speaker for Shire and Radius Health.
Section of Endocrinology, Department of Medicine, University of Chicago, 5841 S. Maryland, MC1027, Chicago, IL 60637, USA
E-mail address: tvokes@medicine.bsd.uchicago.edu

Endocrinol Metab Clin N Am 47 (2018) 855–864
https://doi.org/10.1016/j.ecl.2018.07.010
0889-8529/18/© 2018 Elsevier Inc. All rights reserved.

Because many of the studies cited later used the 36-Item Short-Form Health Survey (SF-36) questionnaire, it is important to mention how the scores are generated from this instrument.[2] SF-36 survey consists of 36 questions grouped into 8 domains of physical and mental health: physical functioning (PF), role physical (RP), bodily pain (BP), general health (GH), vitality (VT), social functioning (SF), role emotional (RE), and mental health (MH). These 8 domains are then summarized into a physical component summary (PCS) score and a MH summary (MCS) score. There is a limited range of responses to each survey question (between 2 and 6). These responses are then grouped and recalculated on a scale from 0 to 100. In some studies, the results are given as raw scores and in others expressed as a norm-based score relative to normal population whereby the mean is 50 and standard deviation is 10.

QUALITY OF LIFE IN PATIENTS WITH HYPOPARATHYROIDISM ON CONVENTIONAL THERAPY WITH CALCIUM AND ACTIVE VITAMIN D

Many patients with hypoparathyroidism describe a multitude of symptoms that make their quality of life suboptimal and at times simply intolerable.[3–5] These symptoms can be broadly grouped into physical, cognitive, and emotional categories (**Table 1**). It is presently unclear to what degree these symptoms are a function of serum calcium level (which undoubtedly plays an important role here), the rate of change in serum calcium or variability in the serum calcium level, and the interaction between these and the patients' underlying level of well-being and resilience. The fact that patients with surgical hypoparathyroidism have considerably more complaints compared with those with the idiopathic form suggests that long-term habituation to low serum calcium level has a significant influence on the signs and symptoms.

The information regarding QOL on conventional therapy can be derived from epidemiologic studies (disease registries and surveys), from case control studies, and from the baseline data on QOL from clinical trials with PTH.

Epidemiologic Studies

A study based on the Danish national registry reported that 688 patients with surgical hypoparathyroid had higher scores for depression and psychiatric symptoms when compared with 1752 controls.[6] The same authors also reported that 180 patients with nonsurgical hypoparathyroidism had higher risk of neuropsychiatric disorders than 540 controls.[7] A survey from Norway invited 522 patients with hypoparathyroidism, and 283 of them responded and completed the SF-36 survey and the Hospital Anxiety and Depression scale.[8] In this study, patients with hypoparathyroidism scored significantly worse than the normative population on both instruments, with surgical patients having worse scores than nonsurgical, particularly in physical health domains.[8] Finally, an Internet-based survey conducted in the United States (Paradox study) included 374 patients. Most of these patients reported fatigue as well as

Table 1		
Complaints of patients with hypoparathyroidism that suggest poor quality of life		
Physical	**Cognitive**	**Emotional**
Fatigue	Poor memory	Depression
Low energy	Poor concentration	Anxiety
Pain	Brain fog	Personality disorder
Cramping/tetany	Slow processing	
Paresthesia	Inability to multitask	
Seizures		

emotional and cognitive problems.[9] However, both the Norwegian and the US survey-based studies may have been subject to selection bias, as some studies have shown that patients who have minor somatic and psychological disorders are more likely to accept QOL measurement than both healthy and more seriously affected subjects. Possibly, these subjects whose condition is closely related to impaired QOL (ie, whose expression is mostly decreased QOL) find its assessment particularly relevant and are, therefore, more likely to respond and to do so more meticulously than average subjects.[10]

Case-Control Studies

The earliest study to examine QOL in hypoparathyroidism is actually a case-control study. Arlt and colleagues[11] compared 25 women who had postsurgical hypoparathyroidism to 25 women who had thyroid surgery but retained a normal parathyroid function. Despite their calcium being at what would be considered a target range for this condition, women with hypoparathyroidism had worse QOL with a higher global complaint score particularly in the subscale score for anxiety, phobic anxiety, and their physical equivalents.

A more recent study from Denmark compared 22 patients with both surgical hypoparathyroidism and hypothyroidism to 22 patients with just surgical hypothyroidism and 22 matched controls who had neither hormonal deficiency.[12] Patients who had hypoparathyroidism had lower scores on the physical domains of the SF-36 as well as lower objective tests of muscle function compared with the other two groups.

In an interesting study from the Harvard system in the United States, the investigators administered SF-36 surveys to 340 patients with postsurgical hypoparathyroidism.[13] A modified SF-36 was also administered to 102 experienced endocrine surgeons and to 200 healthy controls who were given the standard preoperative description of hypoparathyroidism and asked to imagine what it would be like to live with this disease. The patients had considerably lower SF-36 scores than the other two groups. This finding indicates not only that the preoperative description of hypoparathyroidism is inadequate but also that even experienced endocrine surgeons do not appreciate the difficulties that this complication inflicts on affected subjects. This observation is, however, consistent with the common report from patients with hypoparathyroidism that many physicians whom they encounter are not aware of how difficult it may be to live with this disease.

Baseline Quality of Life from Studies of Parathyroid Hormone Therapy for Hypoparathyroidism

There have been several studies that prospectively examined QOL during clinical trials of PTH and from which baseline data can be used to glean the level of QOL impairment in hypoparathyroidism. This information is particularly useful because the subjects of these studies are better characterized in terms of their biochemical control and because the QOL measurements are obtained systematically and consistently. However, these studies may also suffer from selection bias. One possible source of bias is if the most symptomatic subjects seek help that is not available in the routine clinical care. Such a bias would result in a lower QOL score than what would be expected in a random sample of patients with hypoparathyroidism. Alternatively, clinical trial participants may have a better overall control and clinical picture with higher baseline QOL scores if they are already under clinical care of physicians who are conducting the trials and who may be more experienced in the management of this disease. These limitations notwithstanding, the information from clinical trials is a useful addition to the body of knowledge about QOL impairments.

Cusano and colleagues[14] from Columbia University in New York reported that 69 patients with hypoparathyroid with acceptable biochemical control had lower SF-36 scores for all domains ranging between 0.8 and 1.4 standard deviations less than the normative reference range.

In a study from Denmark, Sikjaer and colleagues[15] reported that 62 patients with chronic hypoparathyroidism had lower SF-36 scores than the normal population for most subscales, including PF, RP, BP, GH, VT, RE, and SF. The PCS was also less than the population normal, whereas the MCS was not. In the same study, the World Health Organization's (WHO) WHO-5 Well-being Index was low at the level consistent with depression in 10% and at the level indicating poor emotional well-being in 24% and was normal in 66% of patients. In this study, 22% of patients reported feeling very tired and 37% reported that they had been tired most of the time for a prolonged period of time, whereas 22% did not report tiredness.

A study from Italy also found that 42 subjects with surgical hypoparathyroidism had low SF-36 scores, but the comparison with the normal population was not given for this study.[16] Finally, a multicenter international study showed that even after optimized conventional therapy, the SF-36 scores were still lower than the population norms for PF, GH, RP, BP, and SF.[17]

QUALITY OF LIFE IN RESPONSE TO THERAPY WITH PARATHYROID HORMONE

Several studies have examined the QOL response to PTH therapy. The results will be presented for open-label and placebo-controlled trials.

Open-Label Studies

Two groups have examined QOL during open-labeled studies. The aforementioned study from Columbia University in New York City examined SF-36 scores in 54 patients during treatment with PTH (1–84) given at 100 mcg every other day.[14] This dosage was selected because it was shown to restore bone turnover from markedly reduced to normal levels. The SF-36 was administered at baseline and at 1, 2, 6, and 12 months after the initiation of PTH (1–84) therapy. In response to treatment with PTH, serum calcium remained stable despite the significant reduction in requirements for calcium (52%) and calcitriol supplements (51%). QOL scores were low at baseline and for most domains improved significantly after 1 month of PTH therapy and remained well above than the baseline over the 1 year of the study.[14] The same group followed 69 patients with hypoparathyroidism for up to 5 years.[18] Although all patients were initially on the aforementioned regimen of 100 mcg of PTH (1–84) every other day, when lower doses (25, 50, and 75 mcg) became available, the doses of PTH (1–84) and the supplements were titrated according to individual needs based on biochemical evaluation. QOL was assessed with the SF-36 at months 2, 6, 12, 18, 24, 30, 36, 42, 48, 54, and 60. The improvements in QOL were seen at 2 months and persisted during the 5 years of the study (**Fig. 1**). It should be noted, however, that only 25 patients had data for all 5 years. The remainder either did not yet reach that time point or had discontinued their participation in the study. As compared with the patients who stayed in the study, the 27 patients who discontinued PTH before 5 years had significantly lower SF-36 scores for at least some domains as well as for the total and MCS scores. However, reanalyzing the data after excluding patients who had discontinued PTH (1–84) did not change conclusions of the study. These results suggest that there are individual differences in the QOL response to PTH. It should be noted that in both the 1-year and the 5-year studies from Columbia University, serum calcium was relatively stable

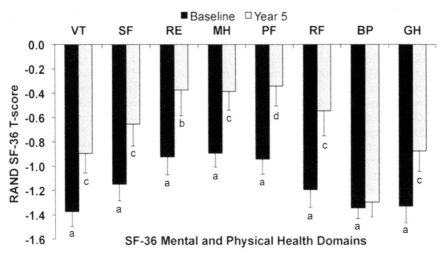

Fig. 1. SF-36 scores at baseline and after 5 years of treatment with PTH (1–84). Values are mean ±SE. RF is equivalent to RP. [a] *P*<.001 compared with normal population. [b] *P*<.05 compared with baseline. [c] *P*<.01 compared with baseline. [d] *P*<.001 compared with baseline. (*From* Cusano NE, Rubin MR, McMahon DJ, et al. PTH(1–84) is associated with improved quality of life in hypoparathyroidism through 5 years of therapy. J Clin Endocrinol Metabol 2014;99(10):3697; with permission.)

with no significant difference between levels before and during the administration of PTH (1–84).

QOL was also assessed in an Italian study where 42 subjects with surgical hypoparathyroidism received a twice-daily injection of 20 mcg of PTH (1–34) as PTH (1–84) was not available in Europe.[16] During the 6 months of the study, the SF-36 scores improved significantly for all domains and summary scores. However, it is important to point out that in this study serum calcium was low at baseline in many patients, in some less than the levels considered acceptable even for this disease. In response to treatment with PTH (1–34), serum calcium increased (from the mean of 7.6 to 8.9 mg/dL), whereas the dosages of supplements decreased from the mean of 4.0 to 1.7 g/d for calcium and from the mean of 0.8 mcg to 0.2 mcg/d for calcitriol. The same patients were followed for a total of 2 years during which time their serum calcium remained stable as did (for the most part) the dosages of calcium and vitamin D supplements.[19] The SF-36 scores also remained well above than the baseline, although, at least for some domains, the scores were lower at 2 years than at 6 months.[19]

Placebo-Controlled Studies

The first double-blind placebo-controlled study was conducted in Denmark and examined the effect of PTH (1–84) therapy on muscle function and QOL.[15] In this study, 62 adults with hypoparathyroidism were randomized to receive an injection of placebo (30 patients) or PTH (1–84) (32 patients) at a dose of 100 mcg daily. QOL was assessed by the SF-36 and by the WHO-5 Well-being Index survey. In this study, the doses of oral calcium and active vitamin D supplements were reduced only if patients developed hypercalcemia, which occurred in a significantly greater percentage of patients randomized to PTH (1–84) than those randomized to placebo. After 6 months of treatment, the SF-36 scores improved for 4 domains (RP, BP, VT, and RE) and for MCS in placebo-treated patients and only for the BP subscale in PTH-treated patients. The scores on the WHO-5 Well-being Index increased in both PTH (1–84)- and placebo-treated patients with no difference between the groups. The investigators concluded that the failure to demonstrate an improvement in QOL with PTH (1–84) in this study may have been due to higher rates of hypercalcemia in the group randomized to PTH.

QOL was also examined in REPLACE, the registration trial that lead to the Food and Drug Administration approval of recombinant human PTH (rhPTH) (1–84) for treatment of adults with chronic hypoparathyroidism.[17] The specifics of this multinational double-blind placebo-controlled study have been previously described.[20] It should be noted that the design of this study was different from all prior studies. Patients enrolled into the study first underwent a variable period (lasting 2–16 weeks) during which their doses of oral calcium and active vitamin D were adjusted to bring the serum calcium level as close to the target as possible with stable levels for 2 weeks. As a result of this optimization, serum calcium was higher by an average of 0.5 mg% at randomization than at enrollment. Patients were then randomized (2–1 ratio) to receive a daily injection of rhPTH (1–84) or matching placebo for 6 months. The starting dose was 50 mcg, and the dose could be increased during the 12-week titration phase to 75 and then 100 mcg per day, whereas the doses of the oral calcium and active vitamin D were reduced to maintain albumin-corrected serum calcium between 7.5 mg/dL and the upper limit of normal but ideally at the target level of 8 to 9 mg/dL. After week 12, during the maintenance phase, PTH doses could no longer be increased, whereas the calcium and vitamin D doses could be adjusted at the discretion of the investigators. QOL was assessed using the SF-36 at 0, 4, 12, and 24 weeks.

The SF-36 scores increased in 4 domains (BP, GH, VT, and PCS) in PTH (1–84)–treated patients and did not increase for any domains in the placebo-treated patients, whereas the between-group differences were not statistically significant. The authors also looked for possible predictors of QOL improvement that could explain the heterogeneity of the response and found that the baseline QOL was the strongest negative predictor of the QOL response to PTH (**Fig. 2**). As seen in **Fig. 2**, patients who had lower baseline scores had a greater response to treatment. It should also be noted that the slope of the relationship between the changes in PCS or MCS and the baseline scores (see **Fig. 2**) did not encompass zero in PTH (1–84)–treated patients but did so in placebo-treated patients (see the equations on **Fig. 2**). This finding indicates that patients who have poorer QOL on conventional therapy may derive greater benefit in response to rhPTH (1–84). Interestingly, there was no correlation between serum calcium and QOL either at baseline or in response to therapy. However, the design of the study (measuring serum calcium at each study visit) did not allow evaluation of whether minute-to-minute changes in serum calcium may affect patients' well-being.

REPLACE recruited subjects from North America, Western Europe, and Hungary, which afforded the opportunity to examine geographic differences in QOL and its response to PTH (1–84) therapy. Although the baseline scores were balanced between the PTH (1–84)– and placebo-treated groups for Western Europe and North America, the baseline scores tended to higher in Hungarian patients randomly assigned to PTH (1–84) than in those assigned to placebo. Furthermore, in response to rhPTH (1–84) treatment, there were no improvements in QOL scores in Hungarian patients. It is possible that this lack of improvement may be related to higher baseline scores, as the authors have seen that the response to PTH is negatively correlated to baseline QOL scores. Moreover, the Hungarian investigator who enrolled the patients from Hungary has also suggested that the patients may have misunderstood at least some of the questions on the SF-36 questionnaire (Dr Lakatos, personal communication, 2017) despite being given an appropriately translated form. Given these uncertainties about the validity of the data from Hungary, the investigators limited analysis to the patients from Western Europe and North America and found that this

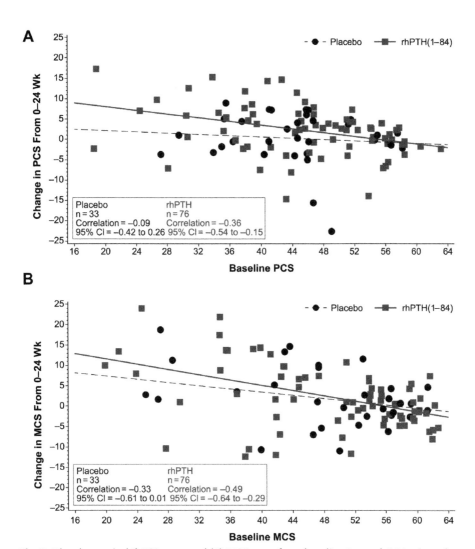

Fig. 2. The change in (*A*) PCS score and (*B*) MCS score from baseline to week 24 is plotted as a function of the baseline score in patients who received rhPTH (1–84) or placebo (*red squares* and *blue circles*, respectively). The regression line for rhPTH (1–84)–treated patients (*solid red line*) had a slope that did not encompass zero, whereas the slope of the line for placebo-treated patients (*broken blue line*) did. For all domains, the normal population has the mean of 50 and a standard deviation of 10. CI, confidence interval. (*From* Vokes TJ, Mannstadt M, Levine MA, et al. Recombinant human parathyroid hormone effect on health-related quality of life in adults with chronic hypoparathyroidism. J Clin Endocrinol Metabol 2018;103(2):727; with permission.)

subgroup showed a more robust QOL improvement to rhPTH (1–84) with statistically significant improvements seen for 6 domains and PCS scores in the PTH-treated patients. In contrast, there were no improvements in any domains in the placebo-treated group. The between group differences were statistically significant for RP, VT, and PCS.

REPLACE also enabled an analysis of the temporal pattern of QOL changes (**Fig. 3**). In response to PTH, QOL scores increased at 4 weeks and either varied over the

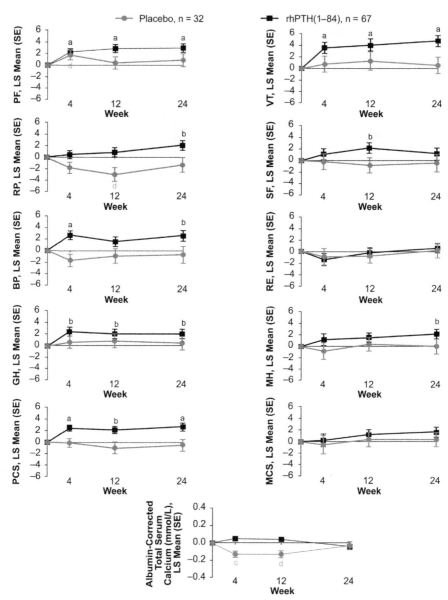

Fig. 3. Change in SF-36 scores and albumin-corrected total serum calcium levels. A time-course plot of the change from baseline to weeks 4, 12, and 24 in patients from North American and Western European sites who received rhPTH (1–84) or placebo (*black* and *gray symbols*, respectively). [a] $P<.001$ for rhPTH (1–84) versus baseline; [b] $P<.05$ for rhPTH (1–84) versus baseline; [c] $P<.001$ for placebo versus baseline; [d] $P<.05$ for placebo versus baseline. LS, least square; RP, role physical; SE, standard error. (*From* Vokes TJ, Mannstadt M, Levine MA, et al. Recombinant human parathyroid hormone effect on health-related quality of life in adults with chronic hypoparathyroidism. J Clin Endocrinol Metabol 2018;103(2):729; with permission.)

course of the study or remained at a higher level than in placebo. Of note, at the end of the study, when serum calcium levels were practically identical in the two groups, QOL scores were still higher in the rhPTH (1–84)–treated patients.

SUMMARY

There are now several published studies that demonstrated low QOL in patients with hypoparathyroidism who are treated conventionally with calcium and active vitamin D supplements. Although the studies that have examined the effect of PTH (1–84) therapy on QOL in hypoparathyroidism have some inconsistencies, there is some evidence that PTH (1–84) improves QOL more effectively than conventional therapy. Nevertheless, a significant limitation of these studies is the absence of a mechanism that explains what biological processes underlie the QOL impairments and how they can be assessed. It is not clear whether serum calcium is the sole determinant of the QOL impairments. Further, it is not clear whether it is the variability in serum calcium that may influence the patients' symptoms. Although it is possible that some salutatory effects of PTH (1–84) come from improved control of serum calcium, or taking fewer tablets each day, it is also possible that PTH (1–84) per se has effects that are not related to mineral metabolism. Further studies are needed with better instruments for assessing well-being. These instruments should have a more specific way of addressing cognitive, emotional, and physical aspects of patients' experience with the disease and its treatments. Although we have made great strides in documenting QOL impairments in hypoparathyroidism, the next decade is likely to bring about a much more granular understanding of these impairments, their biochemical underpinnings, and response to different therapeutic modalities.

REFERENCES

1. Buttner M, Musholt TJ, Singer S. Quality of life in patients with hypoparathyroidism receiving standard treatment: a systematic review. Endocrine 2017;58(1): 14–20.
2. Ware JE Jr, Sherbourne CD. The MOS 36-item short-form health survey (SF-36). I. Conceptual framework and item selection. Med Care 1992;30(6):473–83.
3. Bilezikian JP, Khan A, Potts JT Jr, et al. Hypoparathyroidism in the adult: epidemiology, diagnosis, pathophysiology, target-organ involvement, treatment, and challenges for future research. J Bone Miner Res 2011;26(10):2317–37.
4. Shoback D. Clinical practice. Hypoparathyroidism. N Engl J Med 2008;359(4): 391–403.
5. Shoback DM, Bilezikian JP, Costa AG, et al. Presentation of hypoparathyroidism: etiologies and clinical features. J Clin Endocrinol Metab 2016;101(6):2300–12.
6. Underbjerg L, Sikjaer T, Mosekilde L, et al. Postsurgical hypoparathyroidism–risk of fractures, psychiatric diseases, cancer, cataract, and infections. J Bone Miner Res 2014;29(11):2504–10.
7. Underbjerg L, Sikjaer T, Mosekilde L, et al. The epidemiology of nonsurgical hypoparathyroidism in Denmark: a nationwide case finding study. J Bone Minor Res 2015;30(9):1738–44.
8. Astor MC, Luvas K, Debowska A, et al. Epidemiology and health-related quality of life in hypoparathyroidism in Norway. J Clin Endocrinol Metab 2016;101(8): 3045–53.
9. Hadker N, Egan J, Sanders J, et al. Understanding the burden of illness associated with hypoparathyroidism reported among patients in the paradox study. Endocr Pract 2014;20(7):671–9.

10. Coste J, Quinquis L, Audureau E, et al. Non response, incomplete and inconsistent responses to self-administered health-related quality of life measures in the general population: patterns, determinants and impact on the validity of estimates — a population-based study in France using the MOS SF-36. Health Qual Life Outcomes 2013;11:44.

11. Arlt W, Fremerey C, Callies F, et al. Well-being, mood and calcium homeostasis in patients with hypoparathyroidism receiving standard treatment with calcium and vitamin D. Eur J Endocrinol 2002;146(2):215–22.

12. Sikjaer T, Moser E, Rolighed L, et al. Concurrent hypoparathyroidism is associated with impaired physical function and quality of life in hypothyroidism. J Bone Miner Res 2016;31(7):1440–8.

13. Cho NL, Moalem J, Chen L, et al. Surgeons and patients disagree on the potential consequences from hypoparathyroidism. Endocr Pract 2014;20(5):427–46.

14. Cusano NE, Rubin MR, McMahon DJ, et al. The effect of PTH(1-84) on quality of life in hypoparathyroidism. J Clin Endocrinol Metab 2013;98(6):2356–61.

15. Sikjaer T, Rolighed L, Hess A, et al. Effects of PTH(1-84) therapy on muscle function and quality of life in hypoparathyroidism: results from a randomized controlled trial. Osteoporos Int 2014;25(6):1717–26.

16. Santonati A, Palermo A, Maddaloni E, et al. PTH(1-34) for surgical hypoparathyroidism: a prospective, open-label investigation of efficacy and quality of life. J Clin Endocrinol Metab 2015;100(9):3590–7.

17. Vokes TJ, Mannstadt M, Levine MA, et al. Recombinant human parathyroid hormone effect on health-related quality of life in adults with chronic hypoparathyroidism. J Clin Endocrinol Metab 2018;103(2):722–31.

18. Cusano NE, Rubin MR, McMahon DJ, et al. PTH(1-84) is associated with improved quality of life in hypoparathyroidism through 5 years of therapy. J Clin Endocrinol Metab 2014;99(10):3694–9.

19. Palermo A, Santonati A, Tabacco G, et al. PTH(1-34) for surgical hypoparathyroidism: a 2-year prospective, open-label investigation of efficacy and quality of life. J Clin Endocrinol Metab 2018;103(1):271–80.

20. Mannstadt M, Clarke BL, Vokes T, et al. Efficacy and safety of recombinant human parathyroid hormone (1-84) in hypoparathyroidism (REPLACE): a double-blind, placebo-controlled, randomised, phase 3 study. Lancet Diabetes Endocrinol 2013;1(4):275–83.

Pseudohypoparathyroidism

Agnès Linglart, MD, PhD[a,b,c,]*, Michael A. Levine, MD[d,e],
Harald Jüppner, MD[f,g]

KEYWORDS

- GNAS • Pseudohypoparathyroidism • PTH resistance • Subcutaneous ossifications
- Brachydactyly • Early-onset obesity • Acrodysostosis

KEY POINTS

- Impaired parathyroid hormone (PTH)-dependent signaling at the PTH/PTHrP receptor is the principal feature of pseudohypoparathyroidism.
- Subcutaneous ossifications, brachydactyly, thyroid-stimulating hormone resistance, short stature, and early-onset obesity are common associated features of pseudohypoparathyroidism.
- Molecular genetic and/or epigenetic testing is advised.
- PTH resistance and secondary hyperparathyroidism should be managed to prevent hypocalcemia and increased bone resorption, respectively.
- Care is multidisciplinary for children and adults.

PATHOPHYSIOLOGY

On binding of parathyroid hormone (PTH) to its receptor, the heptahelical PTH/PTHrP receptor (PTH1R), leads to dissociation of Gsα (encoded by GNAS), the alpha-subunit of the heterotrimeric stimulatory G protein from the ßγ-subunits, with subsequent activation by Gsα of adenylyl cyclase and synthesis of the intracellular

Disclosure Statement: The authors have nothing to disclose.
[a] INSERM-U1185, Paris Sud Paris-Saclay University, Bicêtre Paris Sud Hospital, 64 Gabriel Péri Street, 94270 Le Kremlin Bicêtre, France; [b] APHP, Reference Center for Rare Disorders of the Calcium and Phosphate Metabolism, Network OSCAR and 'Platform of Expertise Paris Sud for Rare Diseases, Bicêtre Paris Sud Hospital, 64 Gabriel Péri Street, 94270 Le Kremlin Bicêtre, France; [c] APHP, Endocrinology and Diabetes for Children, Bicêtre Paris Sud Hospital, 64 Gabriel Péri Street, 94270 Le Kremlin Bicêtre, France; [d] Division of Endocrinology and Diabetes, Center for Bone Health, The Children's Hospital of Philadelphia, 3401 Civic Center Boulevard, Philadelphia, PA 19104, USA; [e] Department of Pediatrics, University of Pennsylvania Perelman, School of Medicine, 3615 Civic Center Boulevard, Philadelphia, PA 19104, USA; [f] Endocrine Unit, Massachusetts General Hospital, Harvard Medical School, 50 Blossom street, Boston, MA 02114, USA; [g] Pediatric Nephrology Unit, Massachusetts General Hospital, Harvard Medical School, 50 Blossom street, Boston, MA 02114, USA
* Corresponding author. Endocrinology and Diabetes for Children, Bicêtre Paris Sud Hospital, 64 Gabriel Péri Street, 94270 Le Kremlin Bicêtre, France.
E-mail address: agnes.linglart@aphp.fr

Endocrinol Metab Clin N Am 47 (2018) 865–888
https://doi.org/10.1016/j.ecl.2018.07.011
0889-8529/18/© 2018 Elsevier Inc. All rights reserved.

endo.theclinics.com

messenger cyclic AMP (cAMP) from ATP. Protein kinase A (PKA) is a primary target of cAMP, and binding of cAMP to regulatory subunits (eg, R1A encoded by *PRKAR1A*) unlocks the catalytic subunits, which unleashes a cascade of events that affect various cellular functions, including cell growth and differentiation, gene transcription, and protein expression. For example, PKA-dependent phosphorylation of intracellular enzymes either increases or decreases their activity, and phosphorylation of the transcription factor CREB (cAMP response element-binding protein) allows it to enter the cell nucleus where it regulates gene transcription. Among the many enzymes that are phosphorylated are phosphodiesterases (PDEs) such as PDE4D, which metabolize cAMP thereby terminating cAMP-dependent signaling events. Several additional cAMP targets have been identified, such as cyclic nucleotide-gated cation channels and the exchange proteins 1 and 2 (Epac 1 and 2) that are activated by cAMP.[1–3]

Renal resistance to PTH leads to impaired formation of $1,25(OH)_2D$, the fully active form of vitamin D, and reduces expression of sodium-dependent phosphate transporters in the renal tubules, thereby leading to hypocalcemia and hyperphosphatemia, with elevated serum PTH levels. PTH resistance can result from impaired cAMP generation, from accelerated cAMP degradation, or from impaired cAMP-dependent PKA activation. So far, most identified cases of PTH resistance are due to impaired generation of cAMP, and the defects are in the Gsα protein that couples the PTH1R to adenylyl cyclase rather than in the PTH1R itself. Because this post-receptor signal transduction pathway is used by many different G-protein–coupled receptors (GPCRs), it is not unusual to see reduced responsiveness to numerous other hormones, including thyroid-stimulating hormone (TSH), PTHrP (PTH-related peptide, a ligand that activates the PTH1R in chondrocytes thereby delaying their differentiation), growth hormone releasing hormone (GHRH), gonadotropins, catecholamines, and calcitonin, whose receptors couple to Gsα. Remarkably, even though the genetic defect that affects Gsα is present in all cells, hormonal resistance can vary with age and can affect tissues differently.[4–8]

PSEUDOHYPOPARATHYROIDISM FROM 1942 TO THE TWENTY-FIRST CENTURY

In 1942, Fuller Albright and colleagues[9] introduced the term pseudohypoparathyroidism (PHP) to describe PTH resistance in 3 patients with biochemical hypoparathyroidism (ie, hypocalcemia and hyperphosphatemia) and a constellation of unusual features that included short stature, obesity, round faces, brachydactyly, and heterotopic ossification (ie, Albright hereditary osteodystrophy [AHO]) who showed no change in their urinary phosphorous excretion after administration of parathyroid extract. A decade later, Albright and his colleagues[10] identified a variant of PHP, subsequently namely pseudo-PHP (PPHP), in a patient with AHO who had normal serum levels of calcium and phosphorus and showed an appropriate phosphaturic response to parathyroid extract. Since then, several related phenotypes have been described that resulted in the discovery of additional underlying disease mechanisms and/or genes, which provided novel insights into major biological functions like cAMP signaling, epigenetics, development, and cell differentiation, and thereby helped further refine the meaning of the term "pseudohypoparathyroidism."

In the 1960s, Aurbach and colleagues[11,12] discovered that kidney-derived and bone-derived tissues increase cAMP formation in response to parathyroid extract. They revealed that patients with PHP, diagnosed on the basis of hypocalcemia, hyperphosphatemia, and features of AHO, failed to increase urinary excretion of cAMP after administration of PTH, thereby linking the absent phosphaturic response to PTH to failure to generate cAMP in the kidney.[13] More than 20 years later, the introduction of sensitive immunometric PTH assays readily allowed establishing the diagnosis of PTH resistance in the setting of hypocalcemia and hyperphosphatemia.[14]

In 1980, the critical role of Gsα deficiency in the pathophysiology of PHP was independently demonstrated by Levine as well as Bourne and their respective collaborators. Both groups showed through the use of in vitro assays in which extracts from human erythrocyte membranes could reconstitute hormone-responsive adenylyl cyclase activity that patients with PHP with AHO have an approximately 50% reduction in Gsα bioactivity.[15,16] By contrast, patients with PHP without obvious AHO features had normal or only mildly impaired Gsα bioactivity. This led to a revised classification for PHP in which patients with PHP with AHO and reduced Gsα bioactivity were said to have PHP1A. Patients without AHO and largely normal Gsα bioactivity were said to have PHP1B.

Ten years later, the first mutations in *GNAS*, the gene encoding Gsα, were identified in PHP1A and PPHP, which stimulated a series of discoveries leading to a better understanding of this complex and heterogeneous group of diseases.[17,18] Particularly important was the observation that PHP1A occurs only in children of women affected by PHP1A or PPHP, whereas men with either condition have children affected by only PPHP.[19–22] This unusual mode of inheritance was confirmed in mouse models of PHP1A, that furthermore revealed first evidence for the tissue-specific reduction in paternal Gsα expression, namely an almost complete disappearance of Gsα protein in the renal cortex of animals with ablation of either *Gnas* exon 1 or 2 on the maternal allele.[23,24] In the early 2000s, Hayward and colleagues[25,26] discovered additional coding regions upstream of the *GNAS* exons encoding Gsα and demonstrated that the promoters of these exons undergo parent-specific methylation, namely methylation on the maternal allele for exons A/B, AS, and XL, methylation on the paternal allele for exon NESP.

Because patients affected by PHP1B typically show no evidence for AHO and normal Gsα activity, this PHP variant was initially thought to be caused by mutations in the PTH1R. However, after cloning the PTH1R in 1991,[27] several groups excluded mutations in this gene and its messenger RNA.[28–31] A few years later, it was demonstrated that PHP1B is associated with methylation defects at the *GNAS* A/B:TSS-DMR and frequently other differentially methylated regions (DMRs) within this complex locus.[32] The subsequent analyses of several large families in which numerous members are affected by PHP1B showed a dominant mode of inheritance and genetic studies revealed linkage to a region on chromosome 20q13.3 that comprises the *GNAS* locus; furthermore, PTH-resistant hypocalcemia occurred only when the disease-associated haplotype was inherited from a woman. Subsequent studies confirmed linkage to this chromosomal region in additional PHP1B families, but excluded most portions of the *GNAS* locus.[33] A loss of methylation restricted to the *GNAS* A/B:TSS-DMR was identified in the patients affected by this autosomal dominant (AD-PHP1B) form of the disease and a 3-kb deletion was eventually found 220 kb telomeric of the exon A/B that is located within the genomic region of the *STX16* gene; this deletion is the most frequent cause of AD-PHP1B.[34] Several other imprinting control regions were characterized through similar or related experimental approaches.[35–37] However, most PHP1B cases are sporadic and the underlying genetic defect has not yet been identified.

In recent years, it has become apparent that some AHO features, albeit less pronounced in most cases, can be encountered also in patients affected by PHP1B.[38–40] Furthermore, additional genes were identified as other causes of AHO-like abnormalities that occur in the absence or presence of PTH resistance.[41–46] These important advances in defining the molecular landscape of the different PHP and AHO variants, as well as the insights gained from different animal models raises the question whether a novel nomenclature is needed to more precisely define the clinical features of these related disorders. A European consortium therefore proposed a classification that is based on the underlying molecular diagnosis (see § "classifications"),[47] with a particular emphasis on PTH- and PTHrP-dependent signaling events. This led a group of 35 experts to produce the first consensus for the diagnosis and management of PHP and related disorders, which is a major advance to the field that will help guide health care professionals and patients.[48]

PSEUDOHYPOPARATHYROIDISM AND DIFFERENT CLASSIFICATION SYSTEMS

AHO features with or without hormonal resistance (particularly PTH, TSH, and GHRH resistance), and the presence of reduced or normal Gsα activity, measured by in vitro assays using patient-derived cells, is the basis of the first classification that was established in the early 1980s. According to this classification, cAMP response to exogenously administered PTH differentiates PHP1, in which blunted cAMP and phosphaturic responses are observed, from PHP2, in which the increase in urinary cAMP excretion is conserved but the phosphaturic response is deficient.[11] Because patients with PHP2 do not have other features of PHP, it is likely that in many cases these patients have undiagnosed vitamin D deficiency. In addition, PHP1A refers to the combination of AHO, hormonal resistances, and low Gsα activity, whereas PHP1C refers to the combination of AHO and hormonal resistances, yet normal Gsα activity. PHP1B refers to hormonal resistance and normal Gsα activity, typically in the absence of obvious AHO features, and PPHP refers to AHO features and reduced Gsα activity, in the absence of hormonal resistance.[13,49,50] **Table 1A** summarizes the first widely used, well-known classification, which is based on clinical and biochemical characteristics that can be readily assessed. On the other hand, this classification has several limitations that have been pointed out over the years, particularly the absence of disease-specific genetic mutations and the lack of inclusion of disorders that resemble AHO variants, for example, progressive osseous heteroplasia (POH), or that are caused by mutations in the PTH1R/Gsα/cAMP pathway, for example, different forms of acrodysostosis caused by mutations in *PTHLH*, *PRKAR1A*, *PDE4D*, *PDE3A*, and possibly other genes. Recently, several reviews including that of Haldeman-Englert and colleagues,[6] took advantage of the genetic and epigenetic discoveries, and proposed a modern overview of the spectrum of disorders of the *GNAS* inactivation (**Table 1B**).

In 2016, another classification was proposed by a European consortium through a methodological approach (**Table 1C**). This classification encompasses disorders that share a common mechanism responsible for clinical features, that is, «inactivating PTH/PTHrP signaling disorder» (iPPSD). Clinical and biochemical features that show minimal or no overlap with other conditions were defined as major criteria for the diagnosis of iPPSD, that is, PTH-resistance, subcutaneous ossifications, and brachydactyly type E, when associated with other features. The underlying genetic mutation has been incorporated into the classification through numbering; each gene with the disease-causing mutation is given a number, thus allowing patients to be assigned to a single genetically defined entity. However, this novel classification requires further validation, designation of the parental allele carrying the mutation, and the implication that impaired signaling at the PTH/PTHrP receptor is the "*sine qua non*" for the different forms of iPPSD can be misunderstood, as it excludes disease aspects that result from impaired cAMP-mediated signaling downstream of other Gsα-coupled receptors.[47] This latest classification (as well as the others) should be improved further, possibly by using another term that focuses on abnormal cAMP generation, metabolism, or action.

Table 1
Overview of the current classifications for pseudohypoparathyroidism

A: Classification Based on the cAMP Response to PTH and Gsα Functional Activity

	PHP1A	PHP1C	PPHP	PHP1B	PHP2
Clinical features	AHO	AHO	AHO		AHO
Additional features	Early-onset obesity Asthma Sleep apnea	Early-onset obesity		Early-onset obesity Lack of pubertal growth spurt	
Hormone resistance	Resistance to • PTH • TSH • Gonadotropins • Calcitonin	Resistance to • PTH • TSH		Resistance to • PTH • TSH (mild) • Calcitonin	Resistance to • PTH • TSH
In vitro activity of Gsα	≈50% of controls	Similar to controls	≈50% of controls	Similar or slightly below controls	Similar to controls
Molecular GNAS alteration	Mutation in the coding sequence of GNAS (maternal allele)	Mutation in the coding sequence of GNAS (maternal allele) (exon 13 preferentially)	Mutation in the coding sequence of GNAS (paternal allele)	Abnormal methylation at the GNAS A/B:TSS-DMR[a]	

B: GNAS Inactivation[6]

	GNAS Maternal Allele				GNAS Paternal Allele		
			PHP1B				Osteoma cutis
	PHP1A	PHP1C	AD-PHP1B	Spor-PHP1B	patUPD20q	PPHP	POH
Clinical features	AHO	AHO	Macrosomia	Macrosomia	Macrosomia	AHO IUGR Subcutaneous ossifications frequent	IUGR Subcutaneous ossifications	Subcutaneous ossifications

(continued on next page)

Table 1
(continued)

B: GNAS Inactivation[6]

| | GNAS Maternal Allele | | | | | GNAS Paternal Allele | | |
| | | | PHP1B | | | | | Osteoma |
	PHP1A	PHP1C	AD-PHP1B	Spor-PHP1B	patUPD20q	PPHP	POH	cutis
Hormonal features	Resistance to • PTH • TSH • Gonadotropins • Calcitonin	Resistance to • PTH • TSH • Gonadotropins • Calcitonin	Resistance to • PTH • TSH (mild)	Resistance to • PTH • TSH (mild)	Resistance to • PTH • TSH (mild)			
Gsα functional activity	≈ 50% of controls	Similar to controls	Similar or slightly below controls			≈ 50% of controls	≈ 50% of controls	?
GNAS inactivation	Mutation in the coding sequence of GNAS (maternal allele)		Abnormal methylation at the GNAS A/B:TSS-DMR And 3-kb deletion at the STX16 gene	Abnormal methylation at the GNAS A/B:TSS-DMR and at least at another GNAS DMR	Abnormal methylation at all GNAS DMRs Pat disomy of chromosome 20q	Mutation in the coding sequence of GNAS (maternal allele)		

C: Inactivating PTH/PTHrP Signaling Disorders[47]

iPPSD	Molecular Cause	Main Features
iPPSD1	Mutation in the coding sequence of PTH1R	PTH resistance and/or brachydactyly
iPPSD2	Mutation in the coding sequence of GNAS	PTH resistance and/or subcutaneous ossifications and/or brachydactyly
iPPSD3	Abnormal methylation at the GNAS A/B:TSS-DMR[a]	PTH resistance

iPPSD4	Mutation in the coding sequence of *PRKAR1A*	PTH resistance and/or brachydactyly
iPPSD5	Mutation in the coding sequence of *PDE4D*	Brachydactyly
iPPSD6	Mutation in the coding sequence of *PDE3D*	Brachydactyly +/− hypertension

Abbreviations: AD-P-IP1B, PHP type 1B with autosomal dominant inheritance; AHO, Albright hereditary osteodystrophy; BMI, body mass index; cAMP, cyclic AMP; DMR, differentially methylated region; GH, growth hormone; iPPSD, inactivating PTH/PTHrP signaling disorder; IUGR, intrauterine growth retardation; pat, paternal; patUPD2C, paternal disomy of chromosome 20; PHP, pseudohypoparathyroidism; POH, progressive osseous heteroplasia; PPHP, pseudo-pseudohypoparathyroidism; PTH, parathyroid hormone; PTH1R, PTH receptor type 1; Spor-PHP1B, sporadic PHP type 1B; Mat: maternal; TSH, thyroid-stimulating hormone.

[a] Patients with the autosomal dominant form of PHP1B display an abnormal methylation restricted to the GNAS *A/B*:TSS-DMR. In most cases, this loss of methylation is due to a recurrent deletion of about 3-kb in the genomic region of the *STX16* gene, 220-kb upstream of *GNAS*. In sporadic cases, the abnormal methylation at the GNAS *A/B*:TSS-DMR is associated with a loss of methylation involving at least another GNAS DMR. In patUPD20q patients, the methylation is abnormal at all GNAS DMRs, including the GNAS *A/B*:TSS-DMR.

Table 2
Clinical and biochemical features associated with the diagnosis of pseudohypoparathyroidism apart from PTH resistance, brachydactyly, and subcutaneous ossifications

Specific Features	Description	Mechanism	References
Impaired fetal growth	Mild IUGR in mat GNAS mutations Significant IUGR in pat GNAS mutations Increased birth weight and or length in mat GNAS LOI Significant IUGR in PRKAR1A and PDE4D mutations	Gsα and XLαs (and downstream signaling) contributes to fetal growth	59,87,119
Short stature	Short stature, z-score ≈ −2.5 in mat and pat GNAS mutations Lack of pubertal growth spurt in mat and pat GNAS mutations, and mat GNAS LOI	Gsα is crucial for the PTHrP signaling in the chondrocytes, especially during puberty	59,78
Obesity	Early-onset obesity in mat GNAS inactivation (mutations and LOI) Adult patients with a BMI >25 kg/m^2 ≈ 70% of those with a mat GNAS mutation ≈ 55% of those with a mat GNAS LOI	Gsα is crucial for the melanocortin signaling in the periventricular nucleus of the hypothalamus that regulates satiety. In addition, Gsα deficiency contributes to a low energy expenditure, decreased lipolysis and GHRH resistance	78 59,120,121
Metabolic syndrome	Decreased insulin sensitivity in children and adults with mat GNAS mutations	Gsα deficiency and obesity	122,123
Sleep apnea	Increased frequency in ≈ 45% of those with a mat GNAS mutation Likely increased in patients with PRKAR1A and PDE4D mutations as well	Not related to obesity, maybe to the mid-face hypoplasia	72
Cognitive impairment	≈ 70% of those with a mat GNAS mutation In small series: a subset of patients with PRKAR1A mutations and most patients with PDE4D mutations	cAMP is necessary for the neuronal development	43,56,73,74

(continued on next page)

Table 2
(*continued*)

Specific Features	Description	Mechanism	References
Asthma	Increased prevalence in Patients with a mat or pat *GNAS* mutation Patients with a mat *GNAS* LOI Patients with acrodysostosis		72,120,124
Dental symptoms	All descriptions in patients with mat *GNAS* mutations: enamel defects, blunted and shortened roots; hypodontia and oligodontia; failure of tooth eruption and tooth ankyloses	The defective signaling downstream of PTH1R in the tooth germ and cells may be involved	125
Cranial, skeletal, and neurologic anomalies	Craniosynostosis and Chiari 1 malformation may exist in patients with mat *GNAS* mutations and patients with acrodysostosis Carpal tunnel syndrome is as frequent as ≈ 70% of adults with a mat *GNAS* mutation Spinal stenosis has been described in case reports of patients with mat *GNAS* mutations and patients with acrodysostosis Sensorineural hearing loss in patients with mat *GNAS* mutations and patients with acrodysostosis		43,56,76,126
TSH resistance	Is present since infancy in Patients with a mat *GNAS* mutation (average TSH is ≈ 14 ± 10 mUI/L); some patients may have overt hypothyroidism at birth ≈ 30–100 patients with a mat *GNAS* LOI (average TSH is ≈ 5 mUI/L) Patients with a mutation in *PRKAR1A*	Excessive TSH response to TRH Partial resistance to TSH in the thyroid gland	48

(*continued on next page*)

Specific Features	Description	Mechanism	References
Calcitonin resistance	Is present in Patients with a mat GNAS mutation Patients with a mat GNAS LOI Patients with a mutation in PRKAR1A		48
Gonadotropin resistance	Delayed puberty, oligo- and amenorrhea in girls; cryptorchidism in boys with mat GNAS mutations Variable reports on elevated levels of FSH/ LH. Prolactin deficiency in patients with a mat GNAS mutation		22,79
GHRH resistance	GH deficiency: ≈ 50%–80% of children with a mat GNAS mutation	Defective Gsα signaling in the pituitary where Gsα is imprinted	69,70,92,127

Table 2
(continued)

Abbreviations: BMI, body mass index; cAMP, cyclic AMP; FSH, follicle-stimulating hormone; GH, growth hormone; GHRH, GH releasing hormone; IUGR, intrauterine growth retardation; LH, luteinizing hormone; LOI, Loss of imprinting; mat, maternal; pat, paternal; PTH1R, PTH receptor type 1; TRH, thyrotropin-releasing hormone; TSH, thyroid-stimulating hormone.

MAIN FEATURES LEADING TO THE DIAGNOSIS OF PSEUDOHYPOPARATHYROIDISM

We detail herein the main features leading to the diagnosis of PHP or triggering additional clinical, biochemical, and molecular investigations. Additional, less specific symptoms are also present in patients with pseudohypoparathyroidism. They are defined in **Table 2** and in the descriptions of the different diseases that follow.

Parathyroid Hormone Resistance

Resistance to PTH, the central hallmark of all forms of PHP, is defined by the association of hypocalcemia, hyperphosphatemia, and elevated serum PTH levels in the absence of vitamin D deficiency, abnormal magnesium levels, and renal insufficiency.[48] In the proper context, a patient may be suspected to have PHP, when very young, on the basis of hyperphosphatemia and elevated PTH levels, which usually precedes hypocalcemia.[6,51,52] As in all forms of hypoparathyroidism, hyperphosphatemia can lead to an elevated calcium-phosphorus product that induces ectopic calcifications (to be distinguished from heterotopic ossification) in certain tissues, notably the basal ganglia or ocular lens.[6]

Ectopic Ossifications

Ectopic ossification is a developmental defect that results from Gsα deficiency in mesenchymal stem cells, and is unrelated to serum levels of calcium or phosphorus. The Gsα deficiency leads to de novo differentiation of osteoblasts in extraskeletal connective tissues that produce islands of ectopic membranous bone, most commonly in the dermis and subcutaneous fat. They may present as small and asymptomatic nodules or as large, coalescent plaques of bone that evolve deeply into muscles and around joints. Subcutaneous ossifications preferentially affect the periarticular areas of the hands and feet and the feet plantar region[53] (**Fig. 1**). There is no evidence that environmental factors such as trauma or inflammation affect their progression. Some lesions occasionally extrude a chalky material.[6,48,53] Ectopic ossifications have been reported only so far in patients who have PHP1A or PPHP due to inactivating mutations involving *GNAS* exon 1 to 13 and are not observed in patients with mutations in *PRKAR1A, PDE4D, PTHLH,* or *PDE3A.*

Brachydactyly

Shortening of the metacarpals and metatarsals is the most common skeletal feature associated with PHP1A and PPHP, although some patients with PHP1B may also manifest this osteodystrophy.[38–40] Typically, brachydactyly involves the fourth and the fifth metacarpals/tarsals, that is, brachydactyly type E, and the distal phalanx of the thumb, that is, brachydactyly type D. Sometimes, brachydactyly E may be absent, yet there is always a short thumb and/or cone-shaped epiphyses.[54,55] Brachydactyly is the result of accelerated closure of growth plates, and is due to impaired PTHrP signaling in chondrocytes resulting from Gsα deficiency. This process also occurs in the long bones of the skeleton, and accounts in part for the short stature that is typical

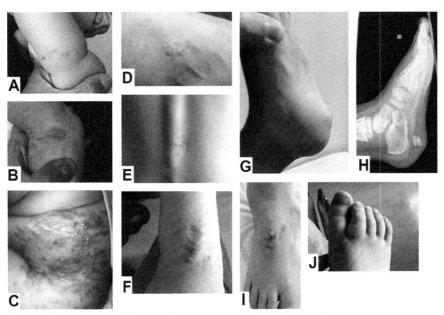

Fig. 1 Subcutaneous ossifications in patients with PHP1A or POH. All patients presented carry a loss-of-function mutation at the coding sequence of the *GNAS* gene. (*A–C*) Different features of subcutaneous ossifications in infants; note the red/purple color of the lesions. (*D–F*) Subcutaneous ossifications in children and adolescents. Small lesions become more pale. (*G, H*) Organized painful ossification below the heel; surgical excision was performed and the ossification did not recur. (*I*) Severe extended ossification of the foot and ankle, one part is extruding white material. (*J*) Painful ossification surrounding the metatarsal joint of the second toe.

of PHP1A and PPHP. In some patients, for example, acrodysostosis, all bones are affected and short.[54,56,57] In patients with *GNAS* inactivation, brachydactyly is not present at birth, and develops over time and is usually obvious by puberty. In patients with acrodysostosis, the shortening of the bones in the hands and feet is usually observed early in infancy.[41,43]

DIAGNOSIS OF PSEUDOHYPOPARATHYROIDISM

The diagnoses of PHP and AHO are based on the association of clinical and biochemical features that may vary depending on the age of the patient and on the family history. An infusion of PTH is rarely required to make a diagnosis.

Patients with a Coding Mutation on the Maternal GNAS Allele/PHP1A-1C/iPPSD2

These patients are born with moderate intrauterine growth retardation[58] yet develop early-onset obesity[59] (**Fig. 2**). An elevated TSH is often detected by neonatal screening and may be an initial feature of the disease,[8,51,60–63] which may be misdiagnosed as congenital hypothyroidism associated with a small thyroid gland.[64] Thirty percent to 80% of these patients may have subtle subcutaneous ossifications as early as in infancy that are not as severe as in POH.[65,66] PTH resistance, the hallmark of this disease, is usually not present at birth; it develops over time and hypocalcemia is present in most patients by the age of 7 to 8 years.[51,52,67] Interestingly, because brachydactyly and short stature represent the effect of premature cessation of long bone growth, these features also develop over time, and children are often normal statured

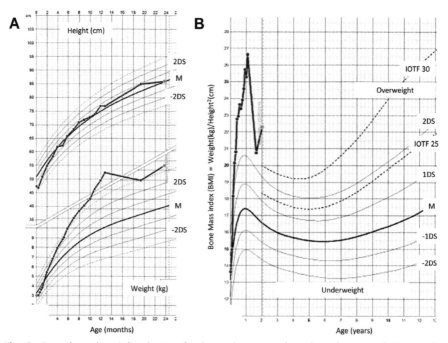

Fig. 2. Growth and weight charts of a boy who was referred at the age of 12 months because of an excessive weight gain. Elevated TSH and PTH at the time of referral led to genetic analyses that identified a *GNAS* mutation on exon 7. (*A*) growth and weight charts. (*B*) Body mass index chart.

during the first 5 to 7 years of life.[59] Growth hormone deficiency, due to impaired responsiveness of pituitary somatotropes to GHRH, also contributes to short stature.[68–71] These patients also have an increased risk of asthma, as well as sleep apnea, that is not solely explained by their obesity.[72]

Mild to moderate cognitive impairment is common in these patients, with a high degree of variability even within families. It is important to note that several psychiatric manifestations have been reported in these patients, which has been attributed to long-standing hypocalcemia.[73,74] Some patients may have structural central nervous system (CNS) findings, such as macrocephaly,[6,9] spinal stenosis, Chiari 1 malformation, and craniosynostosis, that may lead to neurologic abnormalities[75–77] (**Fig. 3**). The average final height of men and women with PHP1A is 158.1 ± 6.7 cm and 146.3 ± 8.0 cm, respectively.[59] As patients age, their mean body mass index tends to improve, although many patients remain obese in adulthood, especially women.[59,78] Resistance to other hormones has been described,[5,8] in particular to gonadotropins[22,79] and calcitonin.[80] Very few data are available on the gonadal function and fertility of these individuals.

Patients with a Coding Mutation on the Paternal GNAS Allele/PPHP-POH-Osteoma Cutis/iPPSD2

Patients with osteoma cutis, a variant of PPHP, manifest mild subcutaneous ossifications as the only feature of AHO. By contrast, patients with POH and PPHP are born with severe growth retardation.[58,59] In PPHP, prenatal growth retardation may be the only sign at birth; diagnosis may be delayed by several years. In newborns or infants, subcutaneous ossifications are highly suggestive of POH and osteoma cutis due to an inactivating mutation involving the paternal GNAS exons encoding Gsα.[53,81,82] Patients with PPHP present with an AHO phenotype and, in most cases, heterotopic ossifications. Patients with POH present with severe ossifications and mild or no other features of AHO. Osteoma cutis may present as an isolated plaque of ossification without any other clinical or biochemical features.[53] Mild elevations in PTH and TSH levels have been reported in occasional patients with PPHP.[83]

Patients with a GNAS Methylation Disorder/PHP1B/iPPSD3

The preeminent feature of PHP1B is resistance to PTH in proximal renal tubular cells. As in PHP1A, this biochemical phenotype develops progressively after birth[6,60,84] and

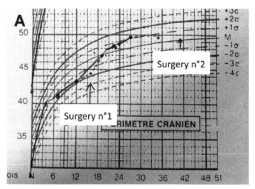
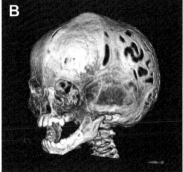

Fig. 3. Cranial circumference chart (*A*) and craniosynostosis (*B*) of a young girl with a maternally inherited GNAS deletion removing GNAS exons 1 and 2, and a severe PHP1A phenotype. The computed tomography scan was done at the time of the first surgery. Note the fusion of the coronal and sagittal sutures, and the cupper beaten aspect of the skull.

leads to the diagnosis on average by age of 13 years; note that many patients are diagnosed only during adulthood. Long-standing undiagnosed or insufficiently treated PTH resistance in patients with PHP1B is associated with increased bone resorption. In children, this may lead to bone pain, bone deformities, and "rickets"-like changes on radiographs.[84,85] In addition, children, as well as adults, may develop brown tumors and tertiary hyperparathyroidism.[86] Mild resistance to TSH is often present and characterized by TSH levels slightly above the upper level of normal (average 5.3 ± 4.7 mUI); free T4 levels are usually reported as normal.[48] Patients with PHP1B have significantly increased birth weights and/or lengths implying that maternally derived *GNAS* transcripts have an important role in fetal growth.[59,87] Possibly because of the defective Gsα signaling at the αMSH receptor in the CNS, these patients can show a dramatic weight gain in their first years of life, which is often not recognized by physicians.[59] The final height is similar to that of the reference population, that is, 160.4 ± 7.4 cm and 172.7 ± 8.4 cm for women and men with the autosomal form of PHP1B, and 160.7 ± 8.4 cm and 172.0 ± 6.2 cm for women and men with the sporadic form of PHP1B, respectively.[59] Most patients with PHP1B appear to have normal psychomotor development, gonadal function, and fertility.

Patients with Acrodysostosis/iPPSD4 and 5

The bone dysplasia is usually the first recognized sign in patients with acrodysostosis, in some cases as soon as the first months of life. In most patients, all bones of the hand and feet are short. Statural growth is impaired both prenatally and after birth. When acrodysostosis is caused by a *PRKAR1A* mutation, patients present with elevated levels of PTH and TSH, yet calcium and free T4 circulating levels remain within the normal range and do not appear to vary throughout life.[41,56,88,89] Some patients with *PDE4D* mutations also have evidence for PTH and TSH resistance, can have cognitive difficulties, and CNS complications, such as Chiari malformation.[42,43,56,90,91] Patients with *PDE3A* mutations have brachydactyly type E plus hypertension.

MOLECULAR DIAGNOSIS

The diagnosis of PHP is based on clinical characteristics and endocrine findings, but, whenever possible, should be confirmed through molecular genetic testing. The strategy for the molecular diagnosis of PHP has evolved considerably in the past decade thanks to the discovery of mutations in different genes involved in the Gsα/cAMP/PKA signaling pathway and to the implementation of new genomic techniques.

Analysis of the GNAS Locus in Patients with Distinctive Phenotypes

Patients affected with the specific phenotypes should undergo genetic testing targeted to the *GNAS* gene/locus.

Confirmatory sequencing of the *GNAS* locus should be performed in patients with suspected PHP1A, PPHP, POH, and osteoma cutis. Note that *GNAS* exon 1 is GC-rich and may be difficult to analyze through techniques involving DNA amplification by polymerase chain reaction (PCR).[17,22,38,58,92–97] Furthermore, microdeletions removing one or several *GNAS* exons may not be detected by Sanger or Next-Generation Sequencing, thus requiring techniques quantifying both parental alleles, such as multiplex ligation amplification probe (MLPA).[98]

Methylation analysis at the *GNAS* A/B:TSS-DMR should be performed in patients who present with PTH resistance with no or few signs of AHO, that is, PHP1B/iPPSD3, or in patients with PHP1A who do not have a mutation in those *GNAS* exons encoding Gsα.[34,38,99–102] Different techniques are available to screen for methylation defects including pyrosequencing or methyl-sensible MLPA (MS-MLPA). Once the epigenetic defect has been characterized at the GNAS A/B:TSS-DMR, it is of major importance to identify the genetic defect responsible for the disease.[103] Approximately 20% of the patients present with an inherited form of the disorder that is, in most cases, associated with a recurrent deletion removing 3 kb of the STX16 gene located upstream of GNAS.[34] In rare patients, the deletion is located elsewhere within the GNAS locus.[34–37,104–107] Approximately 10% of the patients present with epigenetic defects that involve all GNAS DMRs that are caused by a cytogenetic defect known as paternal uniparental disomy of chromosome 20q (patUPD20).[108–112] Therefore, in sporadic patients with PHP1B/iPPSD3 that display a broad GNAS methylation defect, experimental approaches to search for patUPD20, for example, single-nucleotide polymorphism array or microsatellite analysis, are recommended. Finally, approximately 70% of the patients with PHP1B/iPPSD3 are characterized by a methylation defect involving at least one GNAS DMR, in addition to the GNAS A/B:TSS-DMR, which establishes the diagnosis of sporadic PHP1B.

Exome Sequencing in Patients with Features of Pseudohypoparathyroidism

Patients who present with PTH resistance and/or features of AHO, especially in the absence of subcutaneous ossifications, may be preferentially investigated through targeted sequence analysis of different genes, for example, GNAS, PRKAR1A, PTHLH, PDE4D, and PDE3A. Patients with PHP for whom no molecular cause has been identified through these diagnostic approaches may benefit from exome and/or whole-genome sequencing.[8,56,96]

Genetic Counseling

Because of the variety of genes and molecular mechanisms involved in PHP, genetic counseling should be performed by physicians and/or geneticists trained for these rare disorders. Mutations in PRKAR1A, PTHLH, PDE4D, and PDE3D show an autosomal dominant mode of inheritance, that is, an approximately 50% risk of recurrence. In contrast, the phenotype associated with an inactivating defect in GNAS depends on the parent-of-origin. Maternally inherited mutations involving GNAS exons 1 to 13 lead to PHP1A/1C, whereas these mutations when paternally inherited may lead to PPHP, POH, or osteoma cutis. The transmission of the 3-kb STX16 deletion through the maternal lineage always leads to PTH resistance and thus the autosomal dominant form of PHP1B, whereas paternal transmission of such a mutation has no pathologic consequences. Patients who are affected with patUPD20q do not transmit their molecular defect, as imprints are erased and reset in the gametes. The mode of inheritance in patients with sporadic PHP1B with broad methylation defects at the GNAS locus remains unknown; the risk of recurrence is unknown, but it seems low.

MANAGEMENT

Once diagnosed, PTH resistance should be treated with activated forms of vitamin D, for example, calcitriol or alfacalcidol, to increase the serum calcium levels and to thereby reduce PTH levels. The authors recommend targeting a serum calcium level that is in the low-normal range and against normalizing the serum PTH concentration, to avoid the risk of hypercalcemia and/or hypercalciuria. PTH levels should be maintained at the upper limit or slightly above the reference range (eg, 50–150 pg/mL), as the distal renal nephron remains responsive to PTH and can reabsorb calcium, thereby reducing the risk of hypercalciuria. The vitamin D analogs may be started in infants when PTH rises (eg, 100–150 pg/mL), before hypocalcemia develops. The calcium intake should meet age-appropriate guidelines through regular diet or supplements. Severe hyperphosphatemia can be treated with oral phosphate binders other than CaCO3, if needed. Because cholecalciferol therapy helps increase calcium absorption in hypocalcemic patients,[113] we suggest maintaining serum levels of 25(OH) vitamin D within the normal range. Adequate management of PTH resistance to reduce the calcium-phosphate product to less than 55 may reduce the development or worsening of calcifications in the lens and brain, but will of course have no effect on heterotopic ossification (see previously). The treatment of PTH resistance and functional hypoparathyroidism requires regular monitoring of serum levels of calcium, phosphorus, PTH, monitoring of renal urinary excretion of calcium (<4 mg/kg per day in children) and renal function. Most patients with PHP1A are not at risk of developing renal calcifications[114] unless overtreated, thus increasing the risk of developing hypercalciuria.[115] Patients with hypothyroidism due to TSH resistance should receive oral thyroxine and undergo regular assessment of their thyroid function. Patients with PHP and short stature or decreased growth velocity should be evaluated for growth hormone (GH) deficiency. Although we lack long-term data to formally recommend GH therapy in patients with PHP and short stature, short-term results and small series have provided encouraging results for patients.[68,116] Dietary and lifestyle measures should be implemented at the time of diagnosis, irrespective of the body mass index, to prevent the development of obesity and metabolic complications. Weight control can be very challenging, as obesity is the result in part of decreased resting energy expenditure, and patients may not respond to standard approaches to caloric restriction. At present, there is no specific therapy for heterotopic ossifications. Small ossifications usually do not progress and do not require treatment. Ossifications that cause pain and/or irritations may be surgically removed, unless a large skin surface area is involved.[6,66] Nonsteroidal anti-inflammatory drugs, thiosulfate, or bisphosphonates have been sporadically reported for the treatment of extensive ossifications.[66,117] Large studies are, however, necessary to assess the efficacy of these drugs. Regular limb mobilization and physiotherapy are necessary when ossifications surround joints.[48] Future innovative therapies for patients with PHP may include phosphodiesterase inhibitors (eg, theophylline) aimed at increasing intracellular cAMP levels, and melanocortin receptor agonist (eg, setmelanotide).[118]

SUMMARY

PHP refers to rare clinical and endocrine manifestations that require additional investigations and molecular genetic testing to identify a defect in the Gsα/cAMP/PKA signaling pathway. Ectopic ossifications, TSH resistance, GH deficiency, and early-onset obesity are the most common associated features. Recognition of the causative genetic or epigenetic defect is of particular importance for predicting the natural history of the disorder as well as disease inheritance, and thus affording appropriate medical and genetic counseling to families. The signs and symptoms evolve throughout life and affect many organs; therefore, coordinated and multidisciplinary management is recommended for adult and pediatric patients.

REFERENCES

1. Spiegel AM. The molecular basis of disorders caused by defects in G proteins. Horm Res 1997;47:89–96.

2. Jarnaess E, Taskén K. Spatiotemporal control of cAMP signalling processes by anchored signalling complexes. Biochem Soc Trans 2007;35:931–7.

3. Weinstein LS, Yu S, Warner DR, et al. Endocrine manifestations of stimulatory G protein alpha-subunit mutations and the role of genomic imprinting. Endocr Rev 2001;22:675–705.

4. Levine MA, Germain-Lee E, Jan de Beur S. Genetic basis for resistance to parathyroid hormone. Horm Res 2003;60(Suppl 3):87–95.

5. Levine MA, Downs RW Jr, Moses AM, et al. Resistance to multiple hormones in patients with pseudohypoparathyroidism. Association with deficient activity of guanine nucleotide regulatory protein. Am J Med 1983;74:545–56.

6. Haldeman-Englert CR, Hurst ACE, Levine MA. Disorders of GNAS Inactivation. In: Adam MP, Ardinger HH, Pagon RA, et al, editors. GeneReviews®. Seattle (WA): University of Washington, Seattle; 1993-2018.

7. Turan S, Bastepe M. The GNAS complex locus and human diseases associated with loss-of-function mutations or epimutations within this imprinted gene. Horm Res Paediatr 2013;80:229–41.

8. Giovanna M, Francesca Marta E. Multiple hormone resistance and alterations of G-protein-coupled receptors signaling. Best Pract Res Clin Endocrinol Metab 2018;32:141–54.

9. Albright F, Burnett CH, Smith PH, et al. Pseudohypoparathyroidism—an example of 'Seabright-Bantam syndrome'. Endocrinology 1942;30:922–32.

10. Albright F, Forbes AP, Henneman PH. Pseudo-pseudohypoparathyroidism. Trans Assoc Am Physicians 1952;65:337–50.

11. Chase LR, Melson GL, Aurbach GD. Pseudohypoparathyroidism: defective excretion of 3′,5′-AMP in response to parathyroid hormone. J Clin Invest 1969; 48:1832–44.

12. Chase LR, Aurbach GD. Parathyroid function and the renal excretion of 3′5′-adenylic acid. Proc Natl Acad Sci U S A 1967;58:518–25.

13. Drezner M, Neelon FA, Lebovitz HE. Pseudohypoparathyroidism type II: a possible defect in the reception of the cyclic AMP signal. N Engl J Med 1973; 289:1056–60.

14. Nussbaum SR, Zahradnik RJ, Lavigne JR, et al. Highly sensitive two-site immunoradiometric assay of parathyrin, and its clinical utility in evaluating patients with hypercalcemia. Clin Chem 1987;33:1364–7.

15. Levine MA, Downs RW Jr, Singer M, et al. Deficient activity of guanine nucleotide regulatory protein in erythrocytes from patients with pseudohypoparathyroidism. Biochem Biophys Res Commun 1980;94:1319–24.

16. Farfel Z, Brickman AS, Kaslow HR, et al. Defect of receptor-cyclase coupling protein in psudohypoparathyroidism. N Engl J Med 1980;303:237–42.

17. Weinstein LS, Gejman PV, Friedman E, et al. Mutations of the Gs alpha-subunit gene in Albright hereditary osteodystrophy detected by denaturing gradient gel electrophoresis. Proc Natl Acad Sci U S A 1990;87:8287–90.

18. Patten JL, Johns DR, Valle D, et al. Mutation in the gene encoding the stimulatory G protein of adenylate cyclase in Albright's hereditary osteodystrophy. N Engl J Med 1990;322:1412–9.

19. Davies SJ, Hughes HE. Imprinting in Albright's hereditary osteodystrophy. J Med Genet 1993;30:101–3.

20. Wilson LC, Oude Luttikhuis ME, Clayton PT, et al. Parental origin of Gs alpha gene mutations in Albright's hereditary osteodystrophy. J Med Genet 1994;31: 835–9.

21. Campbell R, Gosden CM, Bonthron DT. Parental origin of transcription from the human GNAS1 gene. J Med Genet 1994;31:607–14.

22. Linglart A, Carel JC, Garabédian M, et al. GNAS1 lesions in pseudohypoparathyroidism Ia and Ic: genotype phenotype relationship and evidence of the maternal transmission of the hormonal resistance. J Clin Endocrinol Metab 2002;87:189–97.

23. Yu S, Yu D, Lee E, et al. Variable and tissue-specific hormone resistance in heterotrimeric Gs protein alpha-subunit (Gsalpha) knockout mice is due to tissue-specific imprinting of the gsalpha gene. Proc Natl Acad Sci U S A 1998;95: 8715–20.

24. Germain-Lee EL, Schwindinger W, Crane JL, et al. A mouse model of Albright hereditary osteodystrophy generated by targeted disruption of exon 1 of the Gnas gene. Endocrinology 2005;146:4697–709.

25. Hayward BE, Bonthron DT. An imprinted antisense transcript at the human GNAS1 locus. Hum Mol Genet 2000;9:835–41.

26. Hayward BE, Moran V, Strain L, et al. Bidirectional imprinting of a single gene: GNAS1 encodes maternally, paternally, and biallelically derived proteins. Proc Natl Acad Sci U S A 1998;95:15475–80.

27. Jüppner H, Abou-Samra AB, Freeman M, et al. A G protein-linked receptor for parathyroid hormone and parathyroid hormone-related peptide. Science 1991;254:1024–6.

28. Jan de Beur SM, Ding CL, LaBuda MC, et al. Pseudohypoparathyroidism 1b: exclusion of parathyroid hormone and its receptors as candidate disease genes. J Clin Endocrinol Metab 2000;85:2239–46.

29. Fukumoto S, Suzawa M, Kikuchi T, et al. Cloning and characterization of kidney-specific promoter of human PTH/PTHrP receptor gene: absence of mutation in patients with pseudohypoparathyroidism type Ib. Mol Cell Endocrinol 1998; 141:41–7.

30. Schipani E, Weinstein LS, Bergwitz C, et al. Pseudohypoparathyroidism type Ib is not caused by mutations in the coding exons of the human parathyroid hormone (PTH)/PTH-related peptide receptor gene. J Clin Endocrinol Metab 1995;80:1611–21.

31. Silve C, Santora A, Breslau N, et al. Selective resistance to parathyroid hormone in cultured skin fibroblasts from patients with pseudohypoparathyroidism type Ib. J Clin Endocrinol Metab 1986;62:640–4.

32. Liu J, Litman D, Rosenberg MJ, et al. A GNAS1 imprinting defect in pseudohypoparathyroidism type IB. J Clin Invest 2000;106:1167–74.

33. Bastepe M, Pincus JE, Sugimoto T, et al. Positional dissociation between the genetic mutation responsible for pseudohypoparathyroidism type Ib and the associated methylation defect at exon A/B: evidence for a long-range regulatory element within the imprinted GNAS1 locus. Hum Mol Genet 2001;10:1231–41.

34. Bastepe M, Fröhlich LF, Hendy GN, et al. Autosomal dominant pseudohypoparathyroidism type Ib is associated with a heterozygous microdeletion that likely disrupts a putative imprinting control element of GNAS. J Clin Invest 2003; 112:1255–63.

35. Chillambhi S, Turan S, Hwang DY, et al. Deletion of the noncoding GNAS antisense transcript causes pseudohypoparathyroidism type Ib and biparental defects of GNAS methylation in cis. J Clin Endocrinol Metab 2010;95:3993–4002.

36. Grigelioniene G, Nevalainen PI, Reyes M, et al. A large inversion involving GNAS exon A/B and all exons encoding Gsα is associated with autosomal dominant pseudohypoparathyroidism type Ib (PHP1B). J Bone Miner Res 2017;32(4): 776–83.

37. Richard N, Abeguilé G, Coudray N, et al. A new deletion ablating NESP55 causes loss of maternal imprint of A/B GNAS and autosomal dominant pseudo-hypoparathyroidism type Ib. J Clin Endocrinol Metab 2012;97:E863–7.
38. Elli FM, Linglart A, Garin I, et al. The prevalence of GNAS deficiency-related diseases in a large cohort of patients characterized by the EuroPHP network. J Clin Endocrinol Metab 2016;101:3657–68.
39. de Nanclares GP, Fernández-Rebollo E, Santin I, et al. Epigenetic defects of GNAS in patients with pseudohypoparathyroidism and mild features of Albright's hereditary osteodystrophy. J Clin Endocrinol Metab 2007;92:2370–3.
40. Mariot V, Maupetit-Méhouas S, Sinding C, et al. A maternal epimutation of GNAS leads to Albright osteodystrophy and parathyroid hormone resistance. J Clin Endocrinol Metab 2008;93:661–5.
41. Linglart A, Menguy C, Couvineau A, et al. Recurrent PRKAR1A mutation in acrodysostosis with hormone resistance. N Engl J Med 2011;364:2218–26.
42. Lee H, Graham JM Jr, Rimoin DL, et al. Exome sequencing identifies PDE4D mutations in acrodysostosis. Am J Hum Genet 2012;90:746–51.
43. Michot C, Le Goff C, Goldenberg A, et al. Exome sequencing identifies PDE4D mutations as another cause of acrodysostosis. Am J Hum Genet 2012;90:740–5.
44. Maass PG, Aydin A, Luft FC, et al. PDE3A mutations cause autosomal dominant hypertension with brachydactyly. Nat Genet 2015;47:647–53.
45. Klopocki E, Hennig BP, Dathe K, et al. Deletion and point mutations of PTHLH cause brachydactyly type E. Am J Hum Genet 2010;86:434–9.
46. Thomas-Teinturier C, Pereda A, Garin I, et al. Report of two novel mutations in PTHLH associated with brachydactyly type E and literature review. Am J Med Genet A 2016;170:734–42.
47. Thiele S, Mantovani G, Barlier A, et al. From pseudohypoparathyroidism to inactivating PTH/PTHrP signalling disorder (iPPSD), a novel classification proposed by the EuroPHP network. Eur J Endocrinol 2016;175:P1–17.
48. Mantovani G, Bastepe M, Monk D, et al. Diagnosis and management of pseudohypoparathyroidism and related disorders: first international consensus statement. Nat Rev Endocrinol 2018;14(8):476–500.
49. Mizunashi K, Furukawa Y, Sohn HE, et al. Heterogeneity of pseudohypoparathyroidism type I from the aspect of urinary excretion of calcium and serum levels of parathyroid hormone. Calcif Tissue Int 1990;46:227–32.
50. Patten JL, Levine MA. Immunochemical analysis of the alpha-subunit of the stimulatory G-protein of adenylyl cyclase in patients with Albright's hereditary osteodystrophy. J Clin Endocrinol Metab 1990;71:1208–14.
51. Usardi A, Mamoune A, Nattes E, et al. Progressive development of PTH resistance in patients with inactivating mutations on the maternal allele of GNAS. J Clin Endocrinol Metab 2017;102:1844–50.
52. Weinstein LS. The stimulatory G protein alpha-subunit gene: mutations and imprinting lead to complex phenotypes. J Clin Endocrinol Metab 2001;86:4622–6.
53. Pignolo RJ, Ramaswamy G, Fong JT, et al. Progressive osseous heteroplasia. diagnosis, treatment, and prognosis. Appl Clin Genet 2015;8:37–48.
54. Poznanski AK, Werder EA, Giedion A, et al. The pattern of shortening of the bones of the hand in PHP and PPHP—a comparison with brachydactyly E, Turner Syndrome, and acrodysostosis. Radiology 1977;123:707–18.
55. de Sanctis L, Vai S, Andreo MR, et al. Brachydactyly in 14 genetically characterized pseudohypoparathyroidism type Ia patients. J Clin Endocrinol Metab 2004;89:1650–5.

56. Linglart A, Fryssira H, Hiort O, et al. PRKAR1A and PDE4D mutations cause acrodysostosis but two distinct syndromes with or without GPCR-signaling hormone resistance. J Clin Endocrinol Metab 2012;97:E2328–38.

57. Robinow M, Pfeiffer RA, Gorlin RJ, et al. Acrodysostosis. A syndrome of peripheral dysostosis, nasal hypoplasia, and mental retardation. Am J Dis Child 1971; 121:195–203.

58. Richard N, Molin A, Coudray N, et al. Paternal GNAS mutations lead to severe intrauterine growth retardation (IUGR) and provide evidence for a role of XLαs in fetal development. J Clin Endocrinol Metab 2013;98:E1549–56.

59. Hanna P, Grybek V, Perez de Nanclares G, et al. Genetic and epigenetic defects at the GNAS locus lead to distinct patterns of skeletal growth but similar early-onset obesity. J Bone Miner Res 2018. https://doi.org/10.1002/jbmr.3450.

60. Romanet P, Osei L, Netchine I, et al. Case report of GNAS epigenetic defect revealed by a congenital hypothyroidism. Pediatrics 2015;135:e1079–83.

61. Lubell T, Garzon M, Anyane Yeboa K, et al. A novel mutation causing pseudohypoparathyroidism 1A with congenital hypothyroidism and osteoma cutis. J Clin Res Pediatr Endocrinol 2009;1:244–7.

62. Balavoine AS, Ladsous M, Velayoudom FL, et al. Hypothyroidism in patients with pseudohypoparathyroidism type Ia: clinical evidence of resistance to TSH and TRH. Eur J Endocrinol 2008;159:431–7.

63. Pinsker JE, Rogers W, McLean S, et al. Pseudohypoparathyroidism type 1a with congenital hypothyroidism. J Pediatr Endocrinol Metab 2006;19:1049–52.

64. Picard C, Decrequy A, Guenet D, et al. Diagnosis and management of congenital hypothyroidism associated with pseudohypoparathyroidism. Horm Res Paediatr 2015;83:111–7.

65. Shoemaker AH, Jüppner H. Nonclassic features of pseudohypoparathyroidism type 1A. Curr Opin Endocrinol Diabetes Obes 2016. https://doi.org/10.1097/MED.0000000000000306.

66. Salemi P, Skalamera Olson JM, Dickson LE, et al. Ossifications in Albright hereditary osteodystrophy: role of genotype, inheritance, sex, age, hormonal status, and BMI. J Clin Endocrinol Metab 2018;103:158–68.

67. Turan S, Fernandez-Rebollo E, Aydin C, et al. Postnatal establishment of allelic Gαs silencing as a plausible explanation for delayed onset of parathyroid hormone resistance owing to heterozygous Gαs disruption. J Bone Miner Res 2014;29:749–60.

68. Mantovani G, Ferrante E, Giavoli C, et al. Recombinant human GH replacement therapy in children with pseudohypoparathyroidism type Ia: first study on the effect on growth. J Clin Endocrinol Metab 2010;95:5011–7.

69. Germain-Lee EL. Short stature, obesity, and growth hormone deficiency in pseudohypoparathyroidism type 1a. Pediatr Endocrinol Rev 2006;3(Suppl 2):318–27.

70. de Sanctis L, Bellone J, Salerno M, et al. GH secretion in a cohort of children with pseudohypoparathyroidism type Ia. J Endocrinol Invest 2007;30:97–103.

71. Mantovani G, Spada A. Resistance to growth hormone releasing hormone and gonadotropins in Albright's hereditary osteodystrophy. J Pediatr Endocrinol Metab 2006;19(Suppl 2):663–70.

72. Landreth H, Malow BA, Shoemaker AH. Increased prevalence of sleep apnea in children with pseudohypoparathyroidism type 1a. Horm Res Paediatr 2015;84: 1–5.

73. Farfel Z, Friedman E. Mental deficiency in pseudohypoparathyroidism type I is associated with Ns-protein deficiency. Ann Intern Med 1986;105:197–9.

74. Mouallem M, Shaharabany M, Weintrob N, et al. Cognitive impairment is prevalent in pseudohypoparathyroidism type Ia, but not in pseudopseudohypoparathyroidism: possible cerebral imprinting of Gsalpha. Clin Endocrinol (Oxf) 2008;68:233–9.

75. Graul-Neumann LM, Bach A, Albani M, et al. Boy with pseudohypoparathyroidism type 1a caused by GNAS gene mutation (deltaN377), Crouzon-like craniosynostosis, and severe trauma-induced bleeding. Am J Med Genet A 2009; 149A:1487–93.

76. Martínez-Lage JF, Guillén-Navarro E, López-Guerrero AL, et al. Chiari type 1 anomaly in pseudohypoparathyroidism type Ia: pathogenetic hypothesis. Childs Nerv Syst 2011;27:2035–9.

77. Visconti P, Posar A, Scaduto MC, et al. Neuropsychiatric phenotype in a child with pseudohypoparathyroidism. J Pediatr Neurosci 2016;11:267–70.

78. Long DN, McGuire S, Levine MA, et al. Body mass index differences in pseudohypoparathyroidism type 1a versus pseudopseudohypoparathyroidism may implicate paternal imprinting of Galpha(s) in the development of human obesity. J Clin Endocrinol Metab 2007;92:1073–9.

79. Namnoum AB, Merriam GR, Moses AM, et al. Reproductive dysfunction in women with Albright's hereditary osteodystrophy. J Clin Endocrinol Metab 1998;83:824–9.

80. Vlaeminck-Guillem V, D'herbomez M, Pigny P, et al. Pseudohypoparathyroidism Ia and hypercalcitoninemia. J Clin Endocrinol Metab 2001;86:3091–6.

81. Kaplan FS, Shore EM. Progressive osseous heteroplasia. J Bone Miner Res 2000;15:2084–94.

82. Shore EM, Ahn J, Jan de Beur S, et al. Paternally inherited inactivating mutations of the GNAS1 gene in progressive osseous heteroplasia. N Engl J Med 2002; 346:99–106.

83. Turan S, Thiele S, Tafaj O, et al. Evidence of hormone resistance in a pseudopseudohypoparathyroidism patient with a novel paternal mutation in GNAS. Bone 2015;71:53–7.

84. Linglart A, Maupetit-Méhouas S, Silve C. GNAS-related loss-of-function disorders and the role of imprinting. Horm Res Paediatr 2013;79:119–29.

85. Burnstein MI, Kottamasu SR, Pettifor JM, et al. Metabolic bone disease in pseudohypoparathyroidism: radiologic features. Radiology 1985;155:351–6.

86. Neary NM, El-Maouche D, Hopkins R, et al. Development and treatment of tertiary hyperparathyroidism in patients with pseudohypoparathyroidism type 1B. J Clin Endocrinol Metab 2012;97:3025–30.

87. Bréhin A-C, Colson C, Maupetit-Méhouas S, et al. Loss of methylation at GNAS exon A/B is associated with increased intrauterine growth. J Clin Endocrinol Metab 2015;100:E623–31.

88. Nagasaki K, Iida T, Sato H, et al. PRKAR1A mutation affecting cAMP-mediated G protein-coupled receptor signaling in a patient with acrodysostosis and hormone resistance. J Clin Endocrinol Metab 2012;97.E1808–13.

89. Muhn F, Klopocki E, Graul-Neumann L, et al. Novel mutations of the PRKAR1A gene in patients with acrodysostosis. Clin Genet 2013;84:531–8.

90. Kaname T, Ki CS, Niikawa N, et al. Heterozygous mutations in cyclic AMP phosphodiesterase-4D (PDE4D) and protein kinase A (PKA) provide new insights into the molecular pathology of acrodysostosis. Cell Signal 2014;26: 2446–59.

91. Lindstrand A, Grigelioniene G, Nilsson D, et al. Different mutations in PDE4D associated with developmental disorders with mirror phenotypes. J Med Genet 2014;51:45–54.

92. de Sanctis L, Giachero F, Mantovani G, et al. Genetic and epigenetic alterations in the GNAS locus and clinical consequences in pseudohypoparathyroidism: Italian common healthcare pathways adoption. Ital J Pediatr 2016;42:101.

93. Thiele S, Werner R, Grötzinger J, et al. A positive genotype-phenotype correlation in a large cohort of patients with pseudohypoparathyroidism type Ia and pseudo-pseudohypoparathyroidism and 33 newly identified mutations in the GNAS gene. Mol Genet Genomic Med 2015;3:111–20.

94. Lemos MC, Thakker RV. GNAS mutations in pseudohypoparathyroidism type 1a and related disorders. Hum Mutat 2015;36:11–9.

95. Elli FM, deSanctis L, Ceoloni B, et al. Pseudohypoparathyroidism type Ia and pseudo-pseudohypoparathyroidism: the growing spectrum of GNAS inactivating mutations. Hum Mutat 2013;34:411–6.

96. Weinstein LS, Xie T, Zhang Q-H, et al. Studies of the regulation and function of the Gs alpha gene Gnas using gene targeting technology. Pharmacol Ther 2007;115:271–91.

97. Ahrens W, Hiort O, Staedt P, et al. Analysis of the GNAS1 gene in Albright's hereditary osteodystrophy. J Clin Endocrinol Metab 2001;86:4630–4.

98. Garin I, Elli FM, Linglart A, et al. Novel microdeletions affecting the GNAS locus in pseudohypoparathyroidism: characterization of the underlying mechanisms. J Clin Endocrinol Metab 2015;100:E681–7.

99. Mantovani G, de Sanctis L, Barbieri AM, et al. Pseudohypoparathyroidism and GNAS epigenetic defects: clinical evaluation of Albright hereditary osteodystrophy and molecular analysis in 40 patients. J Clin Endocrinol Metab 2010;95: 651–8.

100. Maupetit-Méhouas S, Mariot V, Reynès C, et al. Quantification of the methylation at the GNAS locus identifies subtypes of sporadic pseudohypoparathyroidism type Ib. J Med Genet 2011;48:55–63.

101. Court F, Martin-Trujillo A, Romanelli V, et al. Genome-wide allelic methylation analysis reveals disease-specific susceptibility to multiple methylation defects in imprinting syndromes. Hum Mutat 2013;34:595–602.

102. Brix B, Werner R, Staedt P, et al. Different pattern of epigenetic changes of the GNAS gene locus in patients with pseudohypoparathyroidism type Ic confirm the heterogeneity of underlying pathomechanisms in this subgroup of pseudohypoparathyroidism and the demand for a new classification of GNAS-related disorders. J Clin Endocrinol Metab 2014;99:E1564–70.

103. Garin I, Mantovani G, Aguirre U, et al. European guidance for the molecular diagnosis of pseudohypoparathyroidism not caused by point genetic variants at GNAS: an EQA study. Eur J Hum Genet 2015;23:438–44.

104. Takatani R, Molinaro A, Grigelioniene G, et al. Analysis of multiple families with single individuals affected by pseudohypoparathyroidism type Ib (PHP1B) reveals only one novel maternally inherited GNAS deletion. J Bone Miner Res 2015;31:796–805.

105. Elli FM, de Sanctis L, Peverelli E, et al. Autosomal dominant pseudohypoparathyroidism type Ib: a novel inherited deletion ablating STX16 causes loss of imprinting at the A/B DMR. J Clin Endocrinol Metab 2014;99:E724–8.

106. Fernandez-Rebollo E, García-Cuartero B, Garin I, et al. Intragenic GNAS deletion involving exon A/B in pseudohypoparathyroidism type 1A resulting in an

apparent loss of exon A/B methylation: potential for misdiagnosis of pseudohypoparathyroidism type 1B. J Clin Endocrinol Metab 2010;95:765–71.

107. Linglart A, Gensure RC, Olney RC, et al. A novel STX16 deletion in autosomal dominant pseudohypoparathyroidism type Ib redefines the boundaries of a cis-acting imprinting control element of GNAS. Am J Hum Genet 2005;76: 804–14.

108. Takatani R, Minagawa M, Molinaro A, et al. Similar frequency of paternal uniparental disomy involving chromosome 20q (patUPD20q) in Japanese and Caucasian patients affected by sporadic pseudohypoparathyroidism type Ib (sporPHP1B). Bone 2015;79:15–20.

109. Dixit A, Chandler KE, Lever M, et al. Pseudohypoparathyroidism type 1b due to paternal uniparental disomy of chromosome 20q. J Clin Endocrinol Metab 2013; 98:E103–8.

110. Bastepe M, Altug-Teber O, Agarwal C, et al. Paternal uniparental isodisomy of the entire chromosome 20 as a molecular cause of pseudohypoparathyroidism type Ib (PHP-Ib). Bone 2011;48:659–62.

111. Fernández-Rebollo E, Lecumberri B, Garin I, et al. New mechanisms involved in paternal 20q disomy associated with pseudohypoparathyroidism. Eur J Endocrinol 2010;163:953–62.

112. Bastepe M, Lane AH, Jüppner H. Paternal uniparental isodisomy of chromosome 20q—and the resulting changes in GNAS1 methylation—as a plausible cause of pseudohypoparathyroidism. Am J Hum Genet 2001;68:1283–9.

113. Heaney RP, Barger-Lux MJ, Dowell MS, et al. Calcium absorptive effects of vitamin D and its major metabolites. J Clin Endocrinol Metab 1997;82:4111–6.

114. Hansen DW, Nebesio TD, DiMeglio LA, et al. Prevalence of nephrocalcinosis in pseudohypoparathyroidism: is screening necessary? J Pediatr 2018. https://doi.org/10.1016/j.jpeds.2018.03.003.

115. Matos V, van Melle G, Boulat O, et al. Urinary phosphate/creatinine, calcium/creatinine, and magnesium/creatinine ratios in a healthy pediatric population. J Pediatr 1997;131:252–7.

116. Albright hereditary osteodystrophy: natural history, growth, and cognitive/behavioral assessments - Full Text View - ClinicalTrials.gov. Available at: https://clinicaltrials.gov/ct2/show/NCT00209235. Accessed May 20, 2018.

117. Macfarlane RJ, Ng BH, Gamie Z, et al. Pharmacological treatment of heterotopic ossification following hip and acetabular surgery. Expert Opin Pharmacother 2008;9:767–86.

118. Srivastava G, Apovian C. Future pharmacotherapy for obesity: new anti-obesity drugs on the horizon. Curr Obes Rep 2018;7:147–61.

119. Lebrun M, Richard N, Abeguilé G, et al. Progressive osseous heteroplasia: a model for the imprinting effects of GNAS inactivating mutations in humans. J Clin Endocrinol Metab 2010;95:3028–38.

120. Roizen JD, Danzig J, Groleau V, et al. Resting energy expenditure is decreased in pseudohypoparathyroidism type 1A. J Clin Endocrinol Metab 2016;101: 880–8.

121. Carel JC, Le Stunff C, Condamine L, et al. Resistance to the lipolytic action of epinephrine: a new feature of protein Gs deficiency. J Clin Endocrinol Metab 1999;84:4127–31.

122. Shoemaker AH, Lomenick JP, Saville BR, et al. Energy expenditure in obese children with pseudohypoparathyroidism type 1a. Int J Obes (Lond) 2013;37: 1147–53.

123. Muniyappa R, Warren MA, Zhao X, et al. Reduced insulin sensitivity in adults with pseudohypoparathyroidism type 1a. J Clin Endocrinol Metab 2013;98: E1796–801.
124. Lynch DC, Dyment DA, Huang L, et al. Identification of novel mutations confirms PDE4D as a major gene causing acrodysostosis. Hum Mutat 2013;34:97–102.
125. Reis MTA, Matias DT, Faria M E J de, et al. Failure of tooth eruption and brachydactyly in pseudohypoparathyroidism are not related to plasma parathyroid hormone-related protein levels. Bone 2016;85:138–41.
126. Kashani P, Roy M, Gillis L, et al. The association of pseudohypoparathyroidism type Ia with chiari malformation type I: a coincidence or a common link? Case Rep Med 2016;2016:7645938.
127. Mantovani G, Maghnie M, Weber G, et al. Growth hormone-releasing hormone resistance in pseudohypoparathyroidism type Ia: new evidence for imprinting of the Gs alpha gene. J Clin Endocrinol Metab 2003;88:4070–4.

Conventional Treatment of Hypoparathyroidism

Muriel Babey, MD[a], Maria-Luisa Brandi, MD, PhD[b], Dolores Shoback, MD[c],*

KEYWORDS

- Hypoparathyroidism • Hypocalcemia • Serum calcium • PTH • Calcitriol
- Serum phosphate

KEY POINTS

- Conventional therapy of hypoparathyroidism consists of oral calcium and activated vitamin D or vitamin D supplements at doses adjusted to meet the needs of the patient.
- Therapeutic goals are to prevent symptoms and signs of hypocalcemia; to maintain low normal calcium and normal phosphate levels and a calcium-phosphate product less than 55 mg^2/dL^2; and to avoid hypercalciuria, hypercalcemia, and end-organ complications such as renal and other extraskeletal calcifications.
- Calcium carbonate is better absorbed at a low gastric pH level achieved at meal times. Calcium citrate is a better choice for patients taking proton pump inhibitors or H2 agonists and can be taken with or without meals.
- Calcitriol or alfacalcidol, both activated forms of vitamin D, are considered the treatments of choice for most patients with hypoparathyroidism.
- Diets rich in calcium may reduce the amount of calcium supplements needed, but phosphate intake needs to be considered carefully.

INTRODUCTION

Hypoparathyroidism leads to hypocalcemia, hyperphosphatemia, and elevated fractional excretion of calcium in the urine, due to either absent or inadequately low circulating concentrations of parathyroid hormone (PTH). Conventional therapy of hypoparathyroidism consists of oral calcium and activated vitamin D or vitamin D

Disclosure Statement: Dr D. Shoback has received consulting fees from Shire Pharmaceuticals and Ascendis Pharmaceuticals. Dr M.L. Brandi has received consulting fees and grant support from Alexion, Abiogen, Amgen, Eli Lilly, and Shire Pharmaceuticals. Dr M. Babey has nothing to disclose.
[a] Department of Medicine, Highland Hospital, 1411 East 31st Street, Oakland, CA 94602, USA;
[b] Department of Surgery and Translational Medicine, University of Florence, Viale Pieraccini 6, 50139 Florence, Italy; [c] Endocrine Research Unit, Department of Medicine, San Francisco Department of Veterans Affairs Medical Center, University of California, San Francisco, 111N, 1700 Owens Street, 3rd Floor Room 369, San Francisco, CA 94158, USA
* Corresponding author.
E-mail address: Dolores.shoback@ucsf.edu

supplementation at varying doses. Calcium levels are usually restored to the low normal range with conventional treatment, but several effects of PTH in bone and kidney and possibly in the central nervous system are likely not adequately addressed with conventional management.

THERAPEUTIC GOALS, PREVENTION OF COMPLICATIONS, AND MONITORING DURING TREATMENT OF HYPOPARATHYROIDISM

There are several therapeutic goals in the management of chronic hypocalcemia due to hypoparathyroidism, summarized by the First International Conference on the Management of Hypoparathyroidism as discussed later (**Box 1**).[1,2]

First, hypocalcemia should be avoided to prevent complications such as tetany, seizures, painful muscle cramps, paresthesias, and other neuromuscular manifestations and to minimize chronic fatigue, poor concentration, reduced memory, and cognitive function, which are often connected to the impaired quality of life that patients with hypoparathyroidism report.[3–7] Clinical symptoms and signs of hypocalcemia by history, physical examination, and laboratory tests should be monitored every 6 months, once stable therapeutic dosing of calcium supplements and vitamin D analogues has been achieved.

Second, serum calcium levels should be maintained slightly below the normal range (ie, no more than 0.5 mg/dL below normal) or in the low normal range. While adjusting treatment with calcium and activated vitamin D or vitamin D, clinical and laboratory assessment (serum calcium, albumin, and phosphate levels) should be done frequently, up to a few times per week, weekly, or monthly, depending on the clinical circumstances and the treatment being adjusted.

Third, the calcium-phosphate product should be kept at less than 55 mg^2/dL^2 (4.4 $mmol^2/L^2$) in an effort to prevent ectopic calcifications in the brain, kidneys, vascular system, and other soft tissues. If a patient is very stable, laboratory tests (serum calcium, phosphate, creatinine levels) may be obtained every 6 or 12 months. The same parameters should be reassessed with any changes of medications.

Fourth, hypercalciuria should be prevented or minimized to avoid kidney stone formation, nephrocalcinosis, renal dysfunction, and end-stage renal disease. Twenty-four–hour urinary calcium excretion and serum creatinine level and estimated glomerular filtration rate should be measured at least once yearly and after adjustments in medication doses. If a patient with hypoparathyroidism is taking thiazide diuretic, serum sodium, potassium, magnesium, and urea nitrogen levels should be added to the abovementioned measurements. Volume status can be monitored by clinical assessment and physical examination.

Box 1
Summary of therapeutic goals

1. Prevention of hypocalcemia

2. Maintenance of low normal serum calcium level

3. Maintenance of calcium-phosphate product less than 55 mg^2/dL^2

4. Prevention of hypercalciuria

5. Avoidance of hypercalcemia

6. Maintenance of normal phosphate level

7. Avoidance of renal and other extraskeletal calcifications

Fifth, hypercalcemia can lead to symptoms (eg, weakness, altered mental status, nausea, constipation, dehydration, and abdominal pain), increased risk of renal and soft tissue calcification, and renal dysfunction. Laboratory tests including serum calcium, phosphate, urea nitrogen, creatinine, and electrolyte levels should be obtained twice a year or yearly if very stable. During active management and medication titration, clinical assessment and serum biochemical determinations should occur more frequently.

Sixth, serum phosphate should be maintained within the normal range or at levels only slightly greater than that to prevent extraskeletal calcifications. Serum phosphate levels should be obtained every 6 months or more often during dose adjustments. Following a low-phosphate diet is recommended if this target is not reached, and oral phosphate binders may even be used, if serum phosphate levels are very high and do not respond to dietary measures alone.

Seventh, the risk of renal and other extraskeletal calcifications should be addressed to prevent renal dysfunction and ultimately the progression to chronic kidney disease; central nervous system calcifications with possible dysfunction contributing to seizures, altered mental status, and movement disorder; and visual loss due to cataracts. Renal imaging (ultrasonography or computed tomography) should be obtained at baseline and considered every 5 years or more frequently as the clinical circumstances demand, which would be the presence of renal stones or development of impaired renal function or any other renal complication. Monitoring for the development and progression of cataracts is to be considered. No specific monitoring for brain calcifications could be made in the absence of prospective data, but such testing can be considered on a case by case basis.

TREATMENT WITH CALCIUM AND VITAMIN D AND ITS ANALOGUES

Calcium supplements combined with activated vitamin D are routinely prescribed for the initial management of chronic hypoparathyroidism (**Fig. 1**). Different dosing approaches have been used to achieve serum calcium levels slightly lower or in the lower portion of the reference range (8.0–8.5 mg/dL; 2.0–2.12 mM) by increasing intestinal calcium content and absorption. Twenty-four–hour urinary calcium should remain within sex-specific reference ranges (men, <300 mg/d or 7.49 mmol/d; women, <250 mg/d or 6.24 mmol/d) to avoid the complications of renal stone formation, calcification, and dysfunction. A variety of regimens have been used, tailoring the treatment to the individual patient's circumstances. In some situations, a lower dose of calcium salt (providing 800–1200 mg elemental calcium per day in divided doses) is given with a relatively higher dose of activated vitamin D (calcitriol or alfacalcidol). Alternatively, a high dose of calcium (2–3 g of elemental calcium per day in divided doses) is combined with a relatively low dose of activated vitamin D and proves successful for a given patient. Different treatment approaches have not been rigorously compared, and no one treatment plan is clearly more effective or safer than another over time or prevents complications. The goal of treatment is to avoid ongoing symptoms and signs of hypocalcemia and long-term complications of hypocalcemia, hypercalcemia, and hyperphosphatemia. Patients with chronic hypoparathyroidism will require lifelong supplementation and careful clinical and biochemical monitoring throughout.

CALCIUM SUPPLEMENTS

In patients with chronic hypocalcemia due to hypoparathyroidism, oral calcium supplementation is almost always needed (see **Fig. 1**). Approximately 1 to 2 g of elemental calcium (including total diet plus supplement) is recommended on a daily basis in

Calcium supplements
1 to 2 grams of elemental calcium including total diet

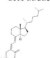

Calcium carbonate (40% elemental calcium)
- better absorbed with low pH level with meals
- binds phosphate

Calcium citrate (21 % elemental calcium)
- given with or without meals,
- ok in combination with PPI or H2 agonists

Vitamin D and its Analogs

Calcitriol
- activated Vitamin D analog
- treatment of choice in most patients
- dose titration every 2 to 3 d

Vitamin D3 (Cholecalciferol)
- dose titration every 2–3 mo
- very high doses required

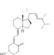

Alfacalcidol
- synthetic activated Vitamin D analog
- average dose twice the level of calcitriol

Vitamin D2 (Ergocalciferol)
- half-life approximately 3 wk
- consider vitamin D2 or D3 with recurrent hypocalcemia while on calcitriol

Fig. 1. Conventional management with calcium and activated vitamin D supplementation illustrated. The most commonly used calcium supplements are calcium carbonate (40% elemental calcium) and calcium citrate (21% elemental calcium) depicted on the left. Calcium carbonate is best absorbed with meals, while calcium citrate can be taken in combination with proton pump inhibitors or H2 agonists and without food. Activated vitamin D, either calcitriol or alfacalcidol shown on the right, is usually prescribed in patients with chronic hypoparathyroidism. Vitamin D3 (cholecalciferol) or vitamin D2 (ergocalciferol) can be considered with recurrent hypocalcemia while on activated vitamin D therapy.

divided doses. The bioavailability seems similar between calcium from dairy products and calcium supplements, particularly calcium carbonate or calcium citrate.[8] High intake of dairy calcium is better avoided, because dairy products are rich in phosphate as well as calcium, and renal phosphate clearance is impaired in hypoparathyroidism. Calcium carbonate (40% elemental calcium by weight) binds phosphate and is better absorbed at a low pH level with meals.[9] Calcium citrate (21% elemental calcium by weight) is better absorbed in patients taking proton pump inhibitors (PPIs) or H2 agonists and can be taken with or without meals.[9] The dose of elemental calcium can be found on most supplement labels. Doses can be adjusted to control symptoms and maintain a low normal serum calcium concentration. If symptoms of hypocalcemia occur intermittently, oral calcium supplementation can be taken on an as-needed basis to improve serum calcium levels promptly.

The effects of calcium supplementation on cardiovascular events in euparathyroid individuals have been studied with conflicting results reported in reviews and meta-analyses.[10–14] The risk of cardiovascular disease, however, was not found to be increased in adults with chronic hypoparathyroidism in a retrospective cohort study.[15]

Common side effects of calcium supplementation consist of constipation and bloating. Concomitant use of magnesium supplementation and intake with food might be beneficial under those circumstances.

Calcium supplements may interfere with the absorption of other drugs such as levothyroxine,[16] ciprofloxacin, and tetracycline.[17] Patients with postsurgical hypoparathyroidism are often on thyroid hormone replacement and need to be instructed to take their levothyroxine in the early morning on an empty stomach and separated from calcium supplements.

VITAMIN D TREATMENT

Different forms of vitamin D are available for the treatment of hypocalcemia due to hypoparathyroidism, and they differ in onset and duration of action and overall potency (see **Fig. 1**). PTH drives the renal conversion of calcidiol (25-hydroxyvitamin D) to the active metabolite calcitriol (1,25-dihydroxyvitamin D). Calcitriol is, therefore, considered the treatment of choice in most patients with hypoparathyroidism, and by extension, so is alfacalcidol (or 1-alpha hydroxycholecalciferol), which is converted to calcitriol by hepatic 25-hydroxylation. Both calcitriol and alfacalcidol are considered activated vitamin D analogues or metabolites.[18] The serum half-lives of these activated forms of vitamin D range between 4 and 6 hours (once alfacalcidol is activated by liver), compared with the biological half-life of vitamin D2 or D3 of approximately 3 weeks.[19–21] Dose titration can occur every 2 to 3 days with activated vitamin D metabolites and every 2 to 3 months with calciferol, either given as cholecalciferol (vitamin D3) or ergocalciferol (vitamin D2). Calcitriol is usually administered in a daily dose of 0.5 to 1.5 μg, whereas the average dose of alfacalcidol is about twice that level, depending on individual patient needs. The dose required to maintain serum calcium in the desired range, within or slightly less than the lower limit of normal, may vary over time in the same patient. Very high doses of vitamin D2 or D3, on the order of 25,000 to 200,000 international unit (IU) daily, may be needed to achieve normocalcemia in some patients.[19,22]

Hypercalcemia can occur during the treatment with calcitriol or with vitamin D2 or D3. However, hypercalcemia due to calcitriol or alfacalcidol may only take a few days to resolve rather than a few weeks after cessation of treatment with vitamin D2 or D3.

In patients with hypoparathyroidism and especially with recurrent hypocalcemia, treatment with high-dose vitamin D2 or D3 can be considered. One study reported no differences in renal function or morbidity from hypercalcemia and less morbidity from hypocalcemia in patients treated with high-dose vitamin D, compared with those treated with calcitriol, in a retrospective study.[23]

Alfacalcidol and dihydrotachysterol (the latter no longer available in the United States) are synthetic analogues of vitamin D and are converted in the liver to the active metabolite 1,25-dihydroxyvitamin D. There are no studies available comparing the long-term treatment of the various activated vitamin D metabolites in patients with hypoparathyroidism. However, resolution of hypercalcemia following treatment with dihydrotachysterol, for example, may take slightly longer (3–14 days) compared with treatment with calcitriol (2–10 days) or alfacalcidol (5–10 days). Higher 25-hydroxyvitamin D levels 30 ng/mL or greater (>75 nmol/L) are a reasonable target to aim for, given the importance of calciferol to the production of 1,25-dihydroxyvitamin D in multiple extrarenal target organs.[24–26]

DIET AND IMPLEMENTATION OF HIGH CALCIUM AND LOW PHOSPHATE INTAKE

A diet rich in calcium is recommended, but phosphate intake must be considered. One way to control phosphate intake in patients with hyperphosphatemia is to avoid commercially produced foods.

A diet tailored to the needs of patients with hypoparathyroidism is not usually suggested to patients. This strategy could potentially be useful in their management. At most, patients are sometimes told to introduce foods rich in calcium and at times told to reduce their consumption of foods containing phosphorus (ie, sodas, eggs, and meat products).[27] It is recommended for patients with hypoparathyroidism to plan an optimal calcium-containing diet (1000–1500 mg calcium daily), with attention to the phosphorus content. Because milk and dairy products derived from it have high phosphorus content, these foods should be ingested in moderation.

All patients benefit from adequate water intake to decrease the risk of forming concentrated urine in the setting of hypercalciuria so as to prevent the deposition of calcium salts in the renal parenchyma and stone formation.

MANAGEMENT OF ACUTE HYPOCALCEMIA

A rapid decrease in serum calcium levels, resulting in acute symptomatic hypocalcemia, needs to be promptly addressed. This can be encountered immediately after anterior neck surgery, if there has been removal or devascularization of the parathyroid glands. This can occur if there is an unanticipated change in calcium and vitamin D requirements due to gastrointestinal symptoms or if there is poor compliance in a previously diagnosed and treated patient with chronic hypoparathyroidism.[4,28,29] If moderate to severe symptoms and signs of acute hypocalcemia are present, such as tetany, seizures, laryngospasm, or bronchospasm, intravenous infusion of calcium should be promptly administered in a two-step approach to address the clinically urgent situation. First, 1 or 2 ampules of a 10% calcium gluconate solution in 50 mL of 5% dextrose can be given intravenously slowly over 10 to 20 min with continuous electrocardiographic monitoring. Second, a slower intravenous infusion of calcium gluconate at the rate of 0.5 to 1.5 mg calcium per kilogram body weight per hour over an 8- to 10-hour period (or longer) can be prescribed along with continuous electrocardiographic monitoring. During intravenous calcium infusion, serum total calcium and albumin and/or serum ionized calcium levels should be measured every 4 to 6 hours. Any other electrolyte abnormalities including those of magnesium, potassium, and sodium should be trended and corrected as well.[30,31] Because they may contribute to the neurologic, muscular, and cardiac complications of severe symptomatic hypocalcemia.

Patients should be monitored on telemetry because arrhythmias may occur with rapid correction of acute hypocalcemia, especially in patients on a cardiac glycoside such as digoxin.

THERAPEUTIC APPROACH TO TRANSIENT HYPERCALCEMIA

Episodes of hypercalcemia may sometimes occur unpredictably, without changes in calcium supplementation or vitamin D analogue dosing, in patients with hypoparathyroidism. Most often hypercalcemia is due to vitamin D intoxication. Serum calcium levels are usually mildly elevated with no or only mild symptoms of hypercalcemia. The dose of calcium supplements and active vitamin D can be reduced by 25% to 50% in mild hypercalcemia while encouraging a high oral fluid intake. If renal impairment is present and hypercalcemia moderate to severe, calcium supplements and activated vitamin D should be discontinued temporarily, and the patient should receive intravenous isotonic saline infusion (3–4 L/d) for rehydration and to promote calcium excretion.

Loop diuretic administration is not strongly supported by clinical evidence, even though renal calcium excretion can be increased by these agents. Forced diuresis is reserved for managing patients with fluid overload, given the risk of precipitating calcium-phosphate crystals in the kidneys and causing hypokalemia and hypomagnesemia.[32]

If serum calcium needs to be rapidly reduced, salmon calcitonin (4 IU/kg) injections can be considered and administered intramuscularly or subcutaneously every 12 hours.[33,34] Calcitonin inhibits osteoclastic bone resorption and increases renal calcium excretion.[35] Calcitonin doses can be increased up to 8 IU/kg every 6 to 8 hours as needed. Hypocalcemic effect of calcitonin diminishes as early as after 24 to 48 hours likely because of receptor downregulation.[36,37]

In addition, glucocorticoids have been prescribed to treat hypercalcemia associated with vitamin D intoxication. It may take 2 to 3 days before the hypocalcemic effect is fully apparent. Glucocorticoids partly work to antagonize actions of vitamin D by decreasing intestinal calcium absorption and increasing renal calcium excretion. Duration of glucocorticoid treatment should be as short as possible due to potential for side effects.

Patients with hypoparathyroidism should be monitored for symptoms of hypercalcemia, such as lethargy, poor memory and concentration, generalized malaise and drowsiness, constipation, nausea, vomiting, diarrhea, and dry mouth with polydipsia and polyuria. After an episode of hypercalcemia, less vitamin D may be required according to case series.[38]

THERAPEUTIC APPROACH TO HYPERCALCIURIA

Urinary calcium is positively correlated with serum calcium in patients with hypoparathyroidism.[18,39] To maintain an acceptable urinary calcium, serum calcium should be targeted slightly below or in the lower part of the normal reference range. High levels of dietary sodium can induce calcium excretion, so salt intake should be restricted to address this.[40] Thiazide diuretics lower urinary calcium by enhancing the renal tubular reabsorption of calcium.[41,42] If an individual with hypoparathyroidism is ingesting a high salt diet, the hypocalciuric effect of thiazide diuretics is diminished. Thiazide diuretic treatment lowers the risk of renal stones in idiopathic hypercalciuria.[43] No studies exist on the long-term effects of chronic treatment with thiazide diuretics in patients with hypoparathyroidism. Hydrochlorothiazide and bendroflumethiazide can be prescribed twice a day. Chlorthalidone has a longer half-life and is usually given once a day.[41] The hypocalciuric effect of thiazide diuretic depends on the dose, and relatively high doses can be administered to try to achieve these effects, if tolerated. The effects of thiazide diuretic on 24-hour urinary calcium should be checked 2 to 3 weeks after starting treatment or changing dosage. While a patient is taking thiazide diuretics, blood pressure and serum potassium levels need to be monitored. Often the patient will need potassium supplementation or the addition of a potassium-sparing diuretic. Hypokalemia should be avoided because it is associated with contraction metabolic alkalosis, which is unfavorable in patients with hypocalcemia. Approximately half of the serum total calcium is protein-bound, specifically to albumin. Binding of calcium to albumin is pH dependent, and that binding increases with an increase in pH. Greater binding of calcium to albumin leads to a decrease in the free ionized calcium fraction, potentiating symptoms of hypocalcemia.[44] Often serum calcium levels will increase slightly with thiazide diuretic treatment. However, the increase does not necessarily reflect an increase in the serum-free fraction of calcium, if metabolic alkalosis has occurred. Serum ionized calcium measurements are usually adjusted to a pH value of 7.4 and not reported at the actual pH level.

Often magnesium supplements are prescribed due to increased renal magnesium excretion caused by thiazide diuretics. Loop diuretics increase renal calcium excretion and should not be administered to patients with hypoparathyroidism.[45,46]

THERAPEUTIC APPROACH TO HYPERPHOSPHATEMIA

Extraskeletal calcifications (renal stones and calcifications, cataracts, and basal ganglia calcifications) are often present in patients with longstanding hypoparathyroidism.[47–49]

A high calcium-phosphate product likely increases the risk of extraskeletal calcifications, and it is, therefore, reasonable to decrease the serum phosphate level by prescribing and adhering to a low phosphate diet.[50] In a case series, the progression of basal ganglia calcification in patients with idiopathic hypoparathyroidism was positively associated with the calcium-phosphate product.[49] Up to now, no clinical trials have looked into lowering phosphate levels with phosphate binders to prevent extraskeletal calcifications.

THERAPEUTIC APPROACH TO HYPOMAGNESEMIA

It is critical to treat low serum magnesium levels while treating hypocalcemia.[51] Magnesium is needed for maintaining robust rates of PTH secretion and for signal transduction by PTH receptors. In hypomagnesemia, PTH actions in kidney and bone are inadequate for defending the serum calcium level, and hypocalcemia can result. This phenomenon is known as "functional hypoparathyroidism."[31,52] Patients with hypomagnesemia and hypoparathyroidism often demonstrate symptoms similar to hypocalcemia and do not respond as well to conventional treatment with calcium supplements and vitamin D.[53–55]

In chronic hypoparathyroidism, often mildly reduced serum magnesium levels are detected during conventional treatment. Handling of magnesium in the kidney as well as in the intestine is altered in hypoparathyroidism. Normal actions of PTH are to increase magnesium reabsorption in the distal renal tubule.[56,57] PPI should be discontinued in patients with hypomagnesemia, if this is possible.[58] Magnesium supplements can be given to treat hypomagnesemia and do not change serum calcium levels.[59] Gastric irritation, nausea, and diarrhea are reported as common side effects of magnesium supplements. If magnesium supplementation is not tolerated, one could consider prescribing a potassium-sparing diuretic because it lowers renal magnesium excretion.[60] Amiloride, but not spironolactone, is associated with a dose-related increase in serum magnesium levels in patients with normal parathyroid function and on the diuretic hydrochlorothiazide.[61]

THERAPEUTIC CHALLENGES

Patients on established regimens may sometimes abruptly exhibit an altered set of serum calcium values (either hyper- or hypocalcemia) due to different actions and potency of their vitamin D or activated vitamin D therapy, sometimes without clear explanation.[19,24,38] Importantly, conventional treatment does not make up for the lack of PTH effects in bone, the kidneys, and central nervous system. Reduced quality of life in patients with hypoparathyroidism is likely related to it.[7,15,62–64]

The use of recombinant human (rh)PTH (1–84) is indicated in patient with hypoparathyroidism who cannot be well controlled on conventional treatment according to the Prescribing Information.[63] There are several additional indications that may be considered, based on expert opinion formulated by the First International Conference on the Management of Hypoparathyroidism.[2] Such situations for consideration include inadequate control of serum calcium; increased doses of either supplemental calcium (>2.5 g) and/or activated vitamin D (>1.5 μg calcitriol or >3 μg alfacalcidol); evidence of renal involvement; hyperphosphatemia or calcium-phosphate product of greater than 55 mg^2 per dL^2 (or >4.4 mmol^2 per L^2); a gastrointestinal disorder or postbariatric surgery associated with malabsorption; and reduced quality of life on conventional therapy.

SUMMARY

Hypoparathyroidism is a rare disease with limited treatment options. The overarching goal is to control symptoms, while minimizing complications. The authors recommend assessing the patient's current circumstances including symptoms and signs of hypoparathyroidism, his/her ability to manage the current regimen, and his/her quality of life on the current regimen. Recent laboratory tests and past history need to be reviewed, and immediate and long-term end organ complications should be evaluated.

Conventional management primarily consists of calcium supplementation and activated vitamin D. Calcium supplements are usually given 3 to 4 times per day and start at 0.5 to 1.0 g of elemental calcium. Calcium carbonate is taken with meals and calcium citrate is prescribed if patient has achlorhydria or takes a PPI. Activated vitamin D (calcitriol or alfacalcidol) is administered in a daily dose of 0.5 to 1.5 μg. Furthermore, magnesium needs to be replaced if serum magnesium levels are low. Vitamin D3 should be given to correct low serum 25-dihydroxyvitamin D levels also. To lower urinary calcium excretion, a thiazide diuretic can be prescribed, combined with potassium supplementation or a potassium-sparing diuretic, while adhering to a low salt diet. If vascular and soft-tissue calcifications are present in the setting of a high calcium-phosphate product greater than 55 mg^2/dL^2, a low phosphate diet with or without phosphate binders is recommended. Conventional therapy with calcium/calcitriol supplementation has limitations given the negative impact on quality of life, renal complications, and brain calcification. rhPTH(1–84) shows promise in those patients for whom treatment is appropriate.

REFERENCES

1. Bilezikian JP, Brandi ML, Cusano NE, et al. Management of hypoparathyroidism: present and future. J Clin Endocrinol Metab 2016;101(6):2313–24.

2. Brandi ML, Bilezikian JP, Shoback D, et al. Management of hypoparathyroidism: summary statement and guidelines. J Clin Endocrinol Metab 2016;101(6): 2273–83.

3. Bilezikian JP, Khan A, Potts JT Jr, et al. Hypoparathyroidism in the adult: epidemiology, diagnosis, pathophysiology, target-organ involvement, treatment, and challenges for future research. J Bone Miner Res 2011;26(10):2317–37.

4. Shoback D. Clinical practice. Hypoparathyroidism. N Engl J Med 2008;359(4): 391–403.

5. Clarke BL, Brown EM, Collins MT, et al. Epidemiology and Diagnosis of Hypoparathyroidism. J Clin Endocrinol Metab 2016;101(6):2284–99.

6. Shoback DM, Bilezikian JP, Costa AG, et al. Presentation of hypoparathyroidism: etiologies and clinical features. J Clin Endocrinol Metab 2016;101(6):2300–12.

7. Arlt W, Fremerey C, Callies F, et al. Well-being, mood and calcium homeostasis in patients with hypoparathyroidism receiving standard treatment with calcium and vitamin D. Eur J Endocrinol 2002;146(2):215–22.

8. Mortensen L, Charles P. Bioavailability of calcium supplements and the effect of Vitamin D: comparisons between milk, calcium carbonate, and calcium carbonate plus vitamin D. Am J Clin Nutr 1996;63(3):354–7.

9. Heaney RP, Smith KT, Recker RR, et al. Meal effects on calcium absorption. Am J Clin Nutr 1989;49(2):372–6.

10. Hsia J, Heiss G, Ren H, et al. Calcium/vitamin D supplementation and cardiovascular events. Circulation 2007;115(7):846–54.

11. Bolland MJ, Avenell A, Baron JA, et al. Effect of calcium supplements on risk of myocardial infarction and cardiovascular events: meta-analysis. BMJ 2010;341: c3691.

12. Bolland MJ, Grey A, Avenell A, et al. Calcium supplements with or without vitamin D and risk of cardiovascular events: reanalysis of the women's health initiative limited access dataset and meta-analysis. BMJ 2011;342:d2040.

13. Chung M, Tang AM, Fu Z, et al. Calcium intake and cardiovascular disease risk: an updated systematic review and meta-analysis. Ann Intern Med 2016;165(12): 856–66.

14. Lewis JR, Calver J, Zhu K, et al. Calcium supplementation and the risks of atherosclerotic vascular disease in older women: results of a 5-year RCT and a 4.5-year follow-up. J Bone Miner Res 2011;26(1):35–41.

15. Underbjerg L, Sikjaer T, Mosekilde L, et al. Cardiovascular and renal complications to postsurgical hypoparathyroidism: a Danish nationwide controlled historic follow-up study. J Bone Miner Res 2013;28(11):2277–85.

16. Singh N, Singh PN, Hershman JM. Effect of calcium carbonate on the absorption of levothyroxine. JAMA 2000;283(21):2822–5.

17. Frost RW, Lasseter KC, Noe AJ, et al. Effects of aluminum hydroxide and calcium carbonate antacids on the bioavailability of ciprofloxacin. Antimicrob Agents Chemother 1992;36(4):830–2.

18. Davies M, Taylor CM, Hill LF, et al. 1,25-dihydroxycholecalciferol in hypoparathyroidism. Lancet 1977;1(8002):55–9.

19. Lund B, Sorensen OH, Lund B, et al. Vitamin D metabolism in hypoparathyroidism. J Clin Endocrinol Metab 1980;51(3):606–10.

20. Neer RM, Holick MF, DeLuca HF, et al. Effects of 1alpha-hydroxy-vitamin D3 and 1,25-dihydroxy-vitamin D3 on calcium and phosphorus metabolism in hypoparathyroidism. Metabolism 1975;24(12):1403–13.

21. Russell RG, Smith R, Walton RJ, et al. 1,25-dihydroxycholecalciferol and 1alpha-hydroxycholecalciferol in hypoparathyroidism. Lancet 1974;2(7871):14–7.

22. Sikjaer T, Rejnmark L, Rolighed L, et al. The effect of adding PTH(1-84) to conventional treatment of hypoparathyroidism: a randomized, placebo-controlled study. J Bone Miner Res 2011;26(10):2358–70.

23. Streeten EA, Mohtasebi Y, Konig M, et al. Hypoparathyroidism: less severe hypocalcemia with treatment with Vitamin D2 compared with calcitriol. J Clin Endocrinol Metab 2017;102(5):1505–10.

24. Holick MF. Vitamin D deficiency. N Engl J Med 2007;357(3):266–81.

25. Hewison M, Burke F, Evans KN, et al. Extra-renal 25-hydroxyvitamin D3-1alpha-hydroxylase in human health and disease. J Steroid Biochem Mol Biol 2007; 103(3–5):316–21.

26. Daniel D, Bikle SP, Wang Y. Physiologic and pathophysiologic roles of extra renal CYP27b1: case report and review. Bone Rep 2018;8:255–67.

27. Guarnotta V, Riela S, Massaro M, et al. The daily consumption of cola can determine hypocalcemia: a case report of postsurgical hypoparathyroidism-related hypocalcemia refractory to supplemental therapy with high doses of oral calcium. Front Endocrinol (Lausanne) 2017;8:7.

28. Cooper MS, Gittoes NJ. Diagnosis and management of hypocalcaemia. BMJ 2008;336(7656):1298–302.

29. Tohme JF, Bilezikian JP. Hypocalcemic emergencies. Endocrinol Metab Clin North Am 1993;22(2):363–75.

30. Mortensen L, Hyldstrup L, Charles P. Effect of vitamin D treatment in hypoparathyroid patients: a study on calcium, phosphate and magnesium homeostasis. Eur J Endocrinol 1997;136(1):52–60.
31. Rude RK, Oldham SB, Singer FR. Functional hypoparathyroidism and parathyroid hormone end-organ resistance in human magnesium deficiency. Clin Endocrinol (Oxf) 1976;5(3):209–24.
32. LeGrand SB, Leskuski D, Zama I. Narrative review: furosemide for hypercalcemia: an unproven yet common practice. Ann Intern Med 2008;149(4):259–63.
33. Wisneski LA. Salmon calcitonin in the acute management of hypercalcemia. Calcif Tissue Int 1990;46(Suppl):S26–30.
34. Deftos LJ, First BP. Calcitonin as a drug. Ann Intern Med 1981;95(2):192–7.
35. Austin LA, Heath H 3rd. Calcitonin: physiology and pathophysiology. N Engl J Med 1981;304(5):269–78.
36. Bilezikian JP. Clinical review 51: management of hypercalcemia. J Clin Endocrinol Metab 1993;77(6):1445–9.
37. Nilsson O, Almqvist S, Karlberg BE. Salmon calcitonin in the acute treatment of moderate and severe hypercalcemia in man. Acta Med Scand 1978;204(4): 249–52.
38. Hossain M. Vitamin-D intoxication during treatment of hypoparathyroidism. Lancet 1970;1(7657):1149–51.
39. Mitchell DM, Regan S, Cooley MR, et al. Long-term follow-up of patients with hypoparathyroidism. J Clin Endocrinol Metab 2012;97(12):4507–14.
40. Massey LK, Whiting SJ. Dietary salt, urinary calcium, and bone loss. J Bone Miner Res 1996;11(6):731–6.
41. Porter RH, Cox BG, Heaney D, et al. Treatment of hypoparathyroid patients with chlorthalidone. N Engl J Med 1978;298(11):577–81.
42. Santos F, Smith MJ, Chan JC. Hypercalciuria associated with long-term administration of calcitriol (1,25-dihydroxyvitamin D3). Action of hydrochlorothiazide. Am J Dis Child 1986;140(2):139–42.
43. Xu H, Zisman AL, Coe FL, et al. Kidney stones: an update on current pharmacological management and future directions. Expert Opin Pharmacother 2013; 14(4):435–47.
44. Rejnmark L, Vestergaard P, Heickendorff L, et al. Effects of thiazide- and loop-diuretics, alone or in combination, on calcitropic hormones and biochemical bone markers: a randomized controlled study. J Intern Med 2001;250(2):144–53.
45. Rejnmark L, Vestergaard P, Heickendorff L, et al. Loop diuretics increase bone turnover and decrease BMD in osteopenic postmenopausal women: results from a randomized controlled study with bumetanide. J Bone Miner Res 2006; 21(1):163–70.
46. Rejnmark L, Vestergaard P, Pedersen AR, et al. Dose-effect relations of loop- and thiazide-diuretics on calcium homeostasis: a randomized, double-blinded Latin-square multiple cross-over study in postmenopausal osteopenic women. Eur J Clin Invest 2003;33(1):41–50.
47. Tambyah PA, Ong BK, Lee KO. Reversible parkinsonism and asymptomatic hypocalcemia with basal ganglia calcification from hypoparathyroidism 26 years after thyroid surgery. Am J Med 1993;94(4):444–5.
48. Pohjola S. Ocular manifestations of idiopathic hypoparathyroidism. Acta Ophthalmol (Copenh) 1962;40:255–65.
49. Goswami R, Sharma R, Sreenivas V, et al. Prevalence and progression of basal ganglia calcification and its pathogenic mechanism in patients with idiopathic hypoparathyroidism. Clin Endocrinol (Oxf) 2012;77(2):200–6.

50. Malberti F. Hyperphosphataemia: treatment options. Drugs 2013;73(7):673–88.
51. Cholst IN, Steinberg SF, Tropper PJ, et al. The influence of hypermagnesemia on serum calcium and parathyroid hormone levels in human subjects. N Engl J Med 1984;310(19):1221–5.
52. Levi J, Massry SG, Coburn JW, et al. Hypocalcemia in magnesium-depleted dogs: evidence for reduced responsiveness to parathyroid hormone and relative failure of parathyroid gland function. Metabolism 1974;23(4):323–35.
53. Rosler A, Rabinowitz D. Magnesium-induced reversal of vitamin-D resistance in hypoparathyroidism. Lancet 1973;1(7807):803–4.
54. Jones KH, Fourman P. Effects of infusions of magnesium and of calcium in parathyroid insufficiency. Clin Sci 1966;30(1):139–50.
55. Dent CE, Harper CM, Morgans ME, et al. Insensitivity of vitamin D developing during the treatment of postoperative tetany; its specificity as regards the form of vitamin D taken. Lancet 1955;269(6892):687–90.
56. Quamme GA, Carney SL, Wong NL, et al. Effect of parathyroid hormone on renal calcium and magnesium reabsorption in magnesium deficient rats. Pflugers Arch 1980;386(1):59–65.
57. Quamme GA. Renal magnesium handling: new insights in understanding old problems. Kidney Int 1997;52(5):1180–95.
58. Hoorn EJ, van der Hoek J, de Man RA, et al. A case series of proton pump inhibitor-induced hypomagnesemia. Am J Kidney Dis 2010;56(1):112–6.
59. Lubi M, Tammiksaar K, Matjus S, et al. Magnesium supplementation does not affect blood calcium level in treated hypoparathyroid patients. J Clin Endocrinol Metab 2012;97(11):E2090–2.
60. Ryan MP. Magnesium and potassium-sparing diuretics. Magnesium 1986;5(5–6):282–92.
61. Murdoch DL, Forrest G, Davies DL, et al. A comparison of the potassium and magnesium-sparing properties of amiloride and spironolactone in diuretic-treated normal subjects. Br J Clin Pharmacol 1993;35(4):373–8.
62. Sikjaer T, Moser E, Rolighed L, et al. Concurrent hypoparathyroidism is associated with impaired physical function and quality of life in hypothyroidism. J Bone Miner Res 2016;31(7):1440–8.
63. Cusano NE, Rubin MR, McMahon DJ, et al. The effect of PTH(1-84) on quality of life in hypoparathyroidism. J Clin Endocrinol Metab 2013;98(6):2356–61.
64. Sikjaer T, Rolighed L, Hess A, et al. Effects of PTH(1-84) therapy on muscle function and quality of life in hypoparathyroidism: results from a randomized controlled trial. Osteoporos Int 2014;25(6):1717–26.

New Directions in Treatment of Hypoparathyroidism

Gaia Tabacco, MD[a,b], John P. Bilezikian, MD[a,*]

KEYWORDS

- Hypoparathyroidism • Treatment • rhPTH (1–84) • PTH (1–34)
- Bone mineral density • Bone turnover markers • Urinary calcium excretion

KEY POINTS

- The availability of replacement therapy with recombinant human parathyroid hormone (1–84) [rhPTH(1–84)] for hypoparathyroidism has improved the prospects of adequate control of calcium metabolism for many patients suffering with this disease.
- The data demonstrating efficacy and safety of rhPTH(1–84) are now available in both short-term and long-term studies.
- Although there is need to further improve the single daily dose protocol with other administration regimens or with different formulations of parathyroid hormone, it is clear that the therapeutic landscape of hypoparathyroidism has been permanently changed, giving physicians and their patients a wider set of options.

METHODS OF LITERATURE SEARCH FOR THIS ARTICLE

PubMed, MEDLINE, and DARE were searched according to PRISMA guidelines to identify published original articles and reviews concerning hypoparathyroidism, recombinant human parathyroid hormone (1–84) [rhPTH(1–84)], and PTH (1–34) treatment. In particular, the authors searched for articles that directly or indirectly investigated PTH and its analogues as a treatment for hypoparathyroidism with particular reference to their effects on calcium metabolism, bone mineral density (BMD), bone resorption and bone formation markers, static and dynamic histomorphometric changes by bone biopsy, urinary calcium excretion, and quality of life (QoL). The terms rhPTH(1–84) and PTH(1–34) were matched with the following terms: hypoparathyroidism, treatment, bone, BMD, calcium, QoL, bone turnover markers, urinary calcium excretion, and autosomal dominant hypocalcemia (ADH). Only publications written in English were included in this search (**Table 1**).

Disclosure: This article includes original research funded, in part, by the NIH (DK069350), Shire Pharmaceuticals and the FDA (02525).
[a] Division of Endocrinology, Department of Medicine, College of Physicians and Surgeons, Columbia University, 630 West 168th Street, New York, NY 10032, USA; [b] Unit of Endocrinology and Diabetes, Department of Medicine, Campus Bio-Medico University of Rome, Via Alvaro del Portillo 21, Rome 00128, Italy
* Corresponding author.
E-mail address: jpb2@columbia.edu

Endocrinol Metab Clin N Am 47 (2018) 901–915
https://doi.org/10.1016/j.ecl.2018.07.013
0889-8529/18/© 2018 Elsevier Inc. All rights reserved.

Table 1
A summary of clinical therapeutic trials in hypoparathyroidism

Study, Year	Number of Patients	Clinical Trial Design	Duration of Study	Therapeutic Regimen	Results	Urinary Calcium Excretion	Bone Mineral Density	Bone Formation and Resorption Markers	Quality of Life
Rubin et al,[6] 2010	30	Open-label	24 mo	100 µg of rhPTH(1–84) every other day; fixed dose	Calcium and vitamin D supplementation decreased significantly. Serum calcium concentration remained stable.	Stable	Spine increased, femoral neck unchanged 1/3 radius decreased	NA	NA
Sikjaer et al,[8] 2011; Sikjaer et al,[29] 2014	62	Double-blind, placebo-controlled, randomized	24 wk	100 µg of PTH(1–84) daily or placebo; fixed dose	Calcium and active vitamin D reduced by 75% and 73%, respectively. Hypercalcemia was frequent.	Transient increase	Spine decreased, femoral neck decreased 1/3 radius unchanged	Increased	Not improved
Mannstadt et al,[5] 2013 (REPLACE)	134	Double-blind, placebo-controlled, randomized phase 3	24 wk	50, 75, or 100 µg rhPTH(1–84) daily (n = 90) or placebo (n = 40); titration of dose	Treatment group vs placebo: 53% vs 2% achieved a 50% or greater reduction in calcium and active vitamin D. Serum calcium concentration remained stable.	Stable	NA	NA	NA
Cusano et al,[10] 2013	27	Open-label	4 y	100 µg of PTH(1–84) every other day; fixed	Supplemental calcium reduced by 37%; active vitamin D reduced by 45%. Serum calcium concentration remained stable.	Decrease at 1 and 3 y	Spine increased, femoral neck unchanged 1/3 radius decreased	Increased	NA

Study	N	Design	Duration	Dose	Outcome				
Lakatos et al,[9] (REPEAT) 2016	24	Open-label	24 wk	50, 75, or 100 μg rhPTH(1–84) daily	53% of patients achieved a 50% or greater reduction in calcium and active vitamin D. Serum calcium concentration remained stable.	Decrease	Spine unchanged femoral neck decreased 1/3 radius unchanged	Increased	NA
Rubin et al,[11] 2016	33	Open-label	6 y	50, 75, or 100 μg rhPTH(1–84) daily; titration	Calcium and vitamin D reduced. Serum calcium concentration remained stable.	Decrease at 1, 3, and 6 y	Spine increased, femoral neck unchanged 1/3 radius decreased at 2 y	Increased	NA
Rubin et al,[20] 2011	48	Open-label	24 mo	100 μg of PTH(1–84) every other day	Bone metabolism restored toward normal: reduced trabecular separation, increased trabecular number, and cortical porosity.	NA	NA	Increased	NA
Sikjaer et al,[19] 2012	44	Double-blind, placebo-controlled, randomized	24 wk	100 μg of PTH(1–84) daily or placebo; fixed	By μCT, number of Haversian canals increased; trabecular thickness and bone tissue density decreased.	NA	NA	Increased	NA
Rubin et al,[21] 2016	58	Open-label	24 mo	100 μg of PTH(1–84) every other day	Transient increase in trabecular bone strength.	NA	NA	NA	NA
Bilezikian et al,[15] 2017 (RELAY)	42	Dose-blinded	8 wk	25 or 50 μg of PTH(1–84) daily	Both doses were effective for a subset of patients.	NA	NA	NA	NA

(continued on next page)

Table 1
(continued)

Study, Year	Number of Patients	Clinical Trial Design	Duration of Study	Therapeutic Regimen	Results	Urinary Calcium Excretion	Bone Mineral Density	Bone Formation and Resorption Markers	Quality of Life
Cipriani et al,[22] 2017	52	Open-label	24 wk	50, 75, or 100 µg rhPTH(1–84) daily	TBS: increase after 18 mo, followed by a decrease at 24 mo.	NA	NA	NA	NA
Cusano et al,[28] 2013	44	Open-label	12 mo	100 µg of PTH(1–84) every other day	PTH(1–84) improves physical and mental functioning.	NA	NA	NA	Improved
Cusano et al,[27] 2014	69	Open-label	5 y	50, 75, or 100 µg rhPTH(1–84)	PTH(1–84) improves physical and mental functioning.	NA	NA	NA	Improved
Vokes et al,[26] 2018	122	Double-blind, placebo-controlled, randomized	24 wk	50, 75, or 100 µg rhPTH(1–84) daily (n = 83) or placebo (n = 39)	See QoL results.	NA	NA	NA	Treatment group improved: physical component, bodily pain, general health, and vitality scores
Winer et al,[3] 1996	10	Randomized, open-label crossover	20 wk	PTH(1–34) once daily vs calcitriol and calcium	PTH treatment maintains eucalcemia.	Decrease	NA	Increase	NA

Study	N	Design	Duration	Intervention	Findings				
Winer et al,[30] 1998	17	Randomized, open-label crossover	28 wk	PTH(1–34) once daily vs twice daily	Twice daily PTH treatment reduces the variability in serum calcium.	Trend to reduction	NA	increase i	NA
Winer et al,[31] 2003	27	Randomized, open-label parallel group	3 y	PTH(1–34) twice daily vs calcitriol and calcium	Serum calcium stable and equivalent between groups.	Stable	Femoral neck increased, spine and radius unchanged	Increased	Less fatigue and greater endurance with PTH treatment
Winer et al,[24] 2012	8	Randomized, open-label crossover	24 wk	PTH(1–34) delivered by pump vs twice daily	Pump delivery: less fluctuation of calcium and 65% reduction in PTH dose.	50% reduction with pump	NA	Increased: pump < twice daily	NA
Gafni et al,[37] 2012	5	Open-label	18 mo	PTH(1–34) twice or thrice daily	Increased cancellous bone volume and trabecular number; decreased trabecular separation.	NA	Spine femoral neck unchanged 1/3 radius decreased	Increased	NA
Santonati et al,[35] 2015	42	Open-label	6 mo	20 μg of PTH(1–34) twice daily	Improvement in calcium metabolism despite decrease of calcium and calcitriol supplementation.	Stable	NA	NA	Improved
Palermo et al,[36] 2018	42	Open-label	24 mo	20 μg of PTH(1–34) twice daily	Improvement in calcium metabolism despite decrease of calcium and calcitriol supplementation.	Increase	NA	NA	Improved

Abbreviation: TBS, trabecular bone score.

HISTORY

Not surprisingly, Fuller Albright was the first person, in 1929, to use PTH as replacement therapy for hypoparathyroidism. In a young hypoparathyroid patient, he showed the effect of a bovine extract of PTH to increase serum calcium and decrease serum phosphorous levels.[1] This prescient report was not followed-up in earnest until 1967. At that time, Melick and associates demonstrated the development of anti-PTH antibodies after short-term replacement therapy with bovine parathyroid extract.[2] This postponed further significant progress for another 30 years, by which time pure forms of hPTH became available.

In a series of ground-breaking studies, Winer and colleagues[3] in 1996 demonstrated, for the first time, the efficacy of hPTH (1–34) as a treatment for hypoparathyroidism. Her work is summarized later in this article. In the early 2000s, rhPTH(1–84) became a focus of therapeutic interest in hypoparathyroidism, culminating in the approval by the Food and Drug Administration (FDA) in 2015 of this full-length peptide as a replacement therapy for hypoparathyroidism.[4] The pivotal study of rhPTH(1–84) was called REPLACE,[5] a 24-week, randomized, double-blind, placebo-controlled, multicenter trial. In 2017 the European Commission granted Conditional Marketing Authorization for rhPTH(1–84) in Europe.

PARATHYROID HORMONE (1–84)
Effect on Calcium Metabolism

Work preceding the REPLACE trial, but leading the way toward it, began with rhPTH(1–84) as replacement therapy for hypoparathyroidism in an open-label study of 30 hypoparathyroid subjects treated with a dose of 100 μg every other day for 24 months. This study demonstrated the efficacy of rhPTH(1–84) to reduce supplemental calcium and 1,25-dihydroxyvitamin D requirements without substantially altering serum and urinary calcium levels.[6] Two different double-blind, placebo-controlled trials then followed.

The first one, called REPLACE,[5] is the pivotal trial that led to approval and registration of rhPTH(1–84). In this trial, patients with established hypoparathyroidism were first stabilized by a run-in period on a regimen of calcium and active forms of vitamin D and then randomized to rhPTH(1–84) (n = 90) or placebo (n = 44). The first endpoint required subjects to meet 3 goals by week 24: a 50% or greater reduction from baseline in their daily dose of oral calcium (goal 1) and active vitamin D (goal 2) while maintaining a serum calcium concentration greater than or the same as baseline concentration (goal 3). The starting dose of rhPTH(1–84) was 50 mcg/d or placebo, with titration upward to 75 or 100 mcg/d. At the end of the 24-week period, 53% patients in the rhPTH(1–84) group achieved the primary endpoint compared with only 2% (1 subject) in the placebo group ($P<.001$). A secondary endpoint of this study was the proportion of subjects who could reduce their calcium supplementation to 500 mg/d or less while entirely eliminating their need for active vitamin D. This endpoint was reached with 43% of those receiving rhPTH(1–84) meeting this goal versus only 5% of the placebo group ($P<.001$). Other observations in this trial included the serum phosphorus levels that fell to the mid-normal range, a calcium–phosphate product that also declined, and serum 1,25(OH)2D levels that were maintained within normal limits.[7]

The second, and smaller, double-blind, placebo-controlled trial enrolled 62 hypoparathyroid subjects. Patients were randomly assigned to daily subcutaneous rhPTH(1–84) in a fixed dose of 100 mcg or placebo.[8] Similar to the REPLACE study, there was a significant reduction in calcium supplements and activated vitamin D analogues and a lowering of phosphorus levels. The study design did not include titration of rhPTH(1–84), likely accounting, as a result, for more frequent episodes of hypercalcemia.

REPLACE was followed by the REPEAT study, a phase III, 24-week open-label extension that included patients who had completed the original REPLACE trial (n = 16) or who were newly recruited and previously untreated (n = 8). The aim of the study was to assess the ongoing safety and extended benefits of rhPTH(1–84) in patients with hypoparathyroidism.[9] At the end of the 24-week period, 75% of patients achieved the study endpoint, namely a reduction in oral calcium supplements and vitamin D analogues and maintenance or normalization of total serum calcium concentration along with a reduction in serum phosphorous concentration.

These studies all confirmed the efficacy of rhPTH(1–84) to improve the clinical management of hypoparathyroidism by reducing calcium and active vitamin D requirements while maintaining acceptable levels of the serum calcium. The efficacious aspects of rhPTH(1–84) have been confirmed in long-term studies that have been extended through 4[10] and 6 years of continuous therapy.[11] In short, long-term administration of rhPTH(1–84) leads to sustained and, in some cases, progressive reductions in supplemental calcium and 1,25-dihydroxyvitamin D requirements. The 6-year study is the longest clinical experience with PTH treatment available to date for the management of hypoparathyroidism or for any metabolic bone disease.

Dosage and Use of rhPTH(1–84)

The current approved dose rhPTH(1–84) is a once daily injection with dose ranging options from 25 to 100 mcg. The rationale for the daily administration regimen, in the context of variable dosing, comes from limited pharmacokinetics and pharmacodynamics studies. They have demonstrated that rhPTH(1–84), administered once daily, improves mineral metabolism of calcium, magnesium, and phosphate and hormonal metabolism of vitamin D toward normal in patients with hypoparathyroidism.[12] Plasma calcium levels return to baseline values 24 hours after injection,[13] thus supporting the rationale for once daily injection of the drug. Thigh injections are recommended for the treatment of hypoparathyroidism, because this site provides for slower absorption and more-prolonged PTH exposure and a larger and longer serum calcium response compared with the abdomen.[14] Experience has now been gained with a range of rhPTH(1–84) doses from 25 to 100 mcg daily.[15] In the RELAY trial, 42 patients were randomized to fixed 25 or 50 μg/d doses of subcutaneous rhPTH(1–84). At week 8, the primary endpoint (reductions in calcium to ≤500 mg/d and in calcitriol to ≤0.25 μg/d) was achieved by 21% and 26% of the patients receiving 25 and 50 μg/d of rhPTH(1–84), respectively. The secondary endpoint (≥50% reduction in calcium and calcitriol doses) was achieved by 11% and 26% of the patients receiving 25 and 50 μg/d of rhPTH(1–84), respectively.

The First International Workshop on the Management of Hypoparathyroidism suggested a series of guidelines to help practitioners in their decision to use rhPTH(1–84) in hypoparathyroidism.[16] The panel of experts in this report suggested that rhPTH(1–84) could be considered in any patient with well-established chronic hypoparathyroidism of any cause, except for ADH, who met any one of the following criteria: (1) variable and inconstant control of the serum calcium with frequent episodes of hypo- and hypercalcemia; (2) nephrolithiasis, nephrocalcinosis, or reduced creatinine clearance or estimated glomerular filtration rate to less than 60 mL/min; (3) hypercalciuria and/or other biochemical indices of renal stone risk; (4) persistently elevated serum phosphorus and/or calcium-phosphate product (>55 mg^2/dL^2 or 4.4 $mmol^2/L^2$); (5) excessive amounts of oral medications required to control symptoms such as greater than 2.5 g of calcium or greater than 1.5 μg of calcitriol (or >3.0 ug of the 1-alpha analogue), or both, and a gastrointestinal tract disorder that might lead to variable calcium and vitamin D absorption; or (6) reduced QoL.

Skeletal Metabolism with rhPTH(1–84)

Markers of bone formation and bone resorption are typically reduced along with higher bone density due to increased trabecular and cortical bone volume, in individuals with hypoparathyroidism.[17] After treatment, bone turnover markers increase quickly and markedly with the administration of rhPTH(1–84).[8-11] Both bone formation and bone resorption markers reach a peak approximately 3-fold above baseline values within approximately 1 year and then decline to levels that represent a new baseline that is higher than pretreatment baseline values.[18]

When compared with controls, patients with hypoparathyroidism tend to have increased BMD. Sikjaer and colleagues[8] showed that following 24 weeks of rhPTH(1–84) treatment, BMD decreased significantly at the whole body, the spine, the hip, and the femoral neck but not at the forearm. In the REPEAT trial,[9] after the same treatment period, BMD values trended downward in the hip (total and femoral neck) but not in the lumbar spine or distal one-third of the radius. However, when comparing patients who had been previously treated with rhPTH(1–84) in REPLACE with patients who were rhPTH(1–84)-naïve at the start of REPEAT, a trend toward decreased BMD values was observed among rhPTH(1–84)-naïve patients at all locations except the distal one-third radius, as also shown by Sikjaer and colleagues. In contrast, patients who had received rhPTH(1–84) in the REPLACE trial had increased BMD values at all locations except the distal one-third radius as shown in other long-term trials. To this point, Rubin and colleagues showed that after 6 years, bone density increased significantly by $3.8 \pm 1\%$ at the lumbar spine and by $2.4 \pm 1\%$ at the total hip. Femoral neck BMD was stable over this period of time, whereas the distal 1/3 radius BMD decreased by $4.4 \pm 1\%$. The pattern of changes in BMD is very similar to findings in patients who are treated with teriparatide [PTH(1–34)] for osteoporosis. They are also compatible with the differential effects of PTH at sites that are predominantly cortical (distal one-third radius) or trabecular (lumbar spine) bone.[11]

Histomorphometric changes were investigated by Sikjaer and colleagues[19] after 24 weeks of treatment and by Rubin and colleagues[20] after 24 months of rhPTH(1–84) treatment. Twenty-four weeks of rhPTH(1–84) treatment led to an increase in the number of Haversian canals per unit area in cortical bone and reduced trabecular thickness and trabecular bone tissue density.[19]

Structural changes were seen as early as 1 year after rhPTH(1–84) treatment, with reduced trabecular separation and increased trabecular number and cortical porosity. These structural changes are consistent with an increase in bone-remodeling rate in both the trabecular and cortical compartments and with a restoration of bone metabolism toward normal euparathyroid levels.[20] These histomorphometric 2-dimensional (2D) results were further explored using direct 3D microcomputed analysis with μFE. rhPTH(1–84) in hypoparathyroidism was associated with early but transient increases in trabecular bone strength.[21] Cipriani and colleagues[22] evaluated bone quality by trabecular bone score (TBS), during 24 months of PTH treatment, showing a significant increase of TBS from baseline after 18 months of treatment, followed by a decrease at 24 months. Misof and colleagues[23] studied cortical and cancellous bone mineralization density distribution (BMDD) by quantitative back-scattered electron microscopy after 2 years of treatment with rhPTH(1–84). Higher BMDD was reduced transiently at 1 year consistent with the early and exuberant increase in bone turnover markers at this time point.

Urinary Calcium Excretion

Many of the clinical trials, cited earlier, have not clearly demonstrated an effect of PTH treatment to reduce urinary calcium excretion, which is somewhat surprising, given the physiologic actions of PTH to conserve renal tubular calcium. The results, however, have been variable. Fixed or relatively high initial doses of rhPTH(1–84) have tended not to show reductions in urinary calcium excretion.[6,8] The higher incidence of hypercalcemia in the study of Sikjaer and colleagues[8] could account for the lack of effect in that trial. In contrast, other studies[5,9–11] have shown a decrease in calcium excretion, but only at specified time points (eg, 1, 3, and 6 years of treatment). Interpretation of these data are confounded by the fact that these studies have used 24-hour treatment protocols in which the urinary calcium is reflecting a relatively long period, well beyond the renal physiologic actions of PTH would be expected to be sustained. In fact, Clark and colleagues[12] showed that the greatest effect of rhPTH(1–84) to reduce the fractional excretion of calcium was within 3 to 6 hours of dosing. This suggests that the continued presence of PTH at the renal tubule is necessary for a sustained reduction in urinary calcium excretion. This proof of concept was substantiated further by the work of Winer and colleagues[24] in which an infusion pump protocol of PTH(1–34) administration was associated with a marked 60% to 70% reduction in urinary calcium excretion. Future efforts to substantially reduce urinary calcium excretion in hypoparathyroidism are likely to take advantage of these observations.

Quality of Life

Most studies that have attempted to quantitate QoL in hypoparathyroidism have shown uniform reductions in the metrics as defined by the RAND 36-item Short form (SF-36) scale.[25] Guidelines that recommend the use of rhPTH(1–84) in those whose QoL is reduced are based on studies that have shown improvements when these patients are treated with replacement hormone.[26–28] Using the SF-36 QoL tool, Cusano and colleagues[28] showed an improvement in the overall score after 1 year of rhPTH(1–84) treatment. This improvement could be demonstrated through 5 years of continuous therapy.[27] Vokes and colleagues[26] analyzed QoL in the REPLACE study. Although between-group differences were not statistically significant (treatment group vs placebo), there were significant improvements in all physical domains as well as the physical component summary score as compared with baseline values in those treated with rhPTH(1–84) but not in the placebo arm of the study. Two of the four mental health domains were also significantly improved over baseline in the treatment arm of the study. The magnitude of change was negatively correlated with baseline scores, such that patients with lower QoL at baseline were more likely to experience improvement in response to treatment. These results differ from the Danish randomized control trial in which rhPTH(1–84) did not improve QoL compared with placebo at 6 months.[29] One possible explanation for this difference is that hypercalcemia occurred more frequently in this study and may have hidden the positive effect of rhPTH(1–84) treatment. It is recognized that the SF-36 is a standard, validated tool for measuring QoL in general but it is not a validated, disease-specific tool for hypoparathyroidism. This limitation should be taken into account when evaluating QoL studies that used this tool. At this point, there is no disease-specific QoL tool for hypoparathyroidism.

PARATHYROID HORMONE (1–34)

PTH(1–34), the N-terminal fragment of the full-length peptide, contains all the classic biological activities of PTH. It binds equivalently well to the PTH receptor and, similarly, activates all the known downstream signaling pathways of PTH.[25]

Effect on Calcium Metabolism

Although PTH(1–34), also known as teriparatide, is not approved for the therapy of hypoparathyroidism, it is instructive to review the classical work of Winer and colleagues with this peptide because it preceded the experience with rhPTH(1–84). The initial study of Winer and colleagues[3] was short term (10 weeks) comparing daily teriparatide with a calcitriol/calcium control group. Although promising, single daily dosing was insufficient for 24-hour control, thus leading to a multiple daily dosing regimen in subsequent studies.[30] A 3-year open-label clinical trial, comparing twice daily PTH(1–34) with a calcium/calcitriol control,[31] showed acceptable serum calcium levels in both treatment groups. Winer and colleagues[32–34] showed similar results also in children. Other studies[35,36] have confirmed the results reported by Winer and colleagues,[3,30,31] showing in an open-label trial of 42 patients with postsurgical hypoparathyroidism for 6 and then 24 months, that calcium levels can be maintained while reducing the need for calcium and calcitriol supplements.

Bone Health

PTH(1–34) administration is associated with a significant early increase in bone formation markers (osteocalcin and alkaline phosphatase activity)[3,30] followed later by increases in both bone resorption and formation markers.[31] In the same study, BMD of the lumbar spine, femoral neck, radius, and whole body showed no significant difference between PTH(1-34) treatment and conventional therapy. Gafni's 18-month study yielded similar results.[37]

Urinary Calcium Excretion

As for rhPTH(1–84), the clinical trials with teriparatide failed to clearly demonstrate a sustained or consistent effect of PTH(1–34) treatment on urinary calcium excretion.

Quality of Life

Santonati and colleagues[35] and Palermo and colleagues[36] evaluated QoL in 42 subjects after 6 and then 24 months of PTH(1–34) treatment. All 8 domains of the SF-36 survey improved after 6 months of PTH(1–34) treatment. In addition, both the physical and the mental component summary scores significantly increased after 6 months of treatment and the improvement persists through 24 months.

SAFETY OF PARATHYROID HORMONE AND ITS PEPTIDES

All active PTH molecules, to date, when tested in high doses for 18 to 24 months in rats, will cause osteosarcoma.[38,39] For this reason, all PTHs and analogues approved for human use [teriparatide, abaloparatide, and rhPTH(1–84)] carry the FDA-mandated "black box" warning. The longest surveillance period that is available is the 16-year experience with teriparatide. During this period, well more than 2 million human subjects have been exposed and, as of the last report, no osteosarcoma toxicity signals have emerged. The animal toxicity studies using the nonhuman primate cynomolgus monkey have also been free of any suggestion of osteosarcoma.[40] The Osteosarcoma Surveillance Study, an ongoing 15-year surveillance study initiated in 2003, is a postmarketing commitment to the United States Food and Drug Administration to evaluate a potential association between teriparatide and osteosarcoma. After 7 years of the study, there were no osteosarcoma patients who had a prior history of teriparatide treatment.[41]

The most common adverse events related to the use of rhPTH(1–84) in hypoparathyroidism are muscle spasm, hypocalcemia, paresthesia, headache, and nausea.

These adverse events are also commonly seen in patients not treated with rhPTH(1–84). Long-term data on the safety and efficacy of PTH are available up through 6 years of continuous exposure.[17]

FUTURE DIRECTIONS

Administration of PTH by infusion pump. Clearly the dosage regimens of single or multiple daily doses of PTH do not mimic physiologic replacement of PTH. A more physiologic approach to the administration of PTH is a means by which the hormone can be continuously provided, such as is the case with the insulin pump in diabetes mellitus. To test the hypothesis that pump delivery of PTH(1–34) more closely mimics endogenous secretion, Winer and colleagues[24] compared pump versus twice-daily PTH(1–34) delivery in a randomized crossover trial on 8 adult patients with postsurgical hypoparathyroidism. Pump versus twice-daily delivery of PTH(1–34) produced less fluctuation in serum calcium and a 65% reduction in the PTH dose to maintain eucalcemia. Moreover, in this study, daily urinary calcium excretion was remarkably more than 50% lower with the pump.[24]

Different formulations of PTH. Pegylated PTH. Another approach to the goal of making PTH constantly available in hypoparathyroidism could take advantage of pegylated PTH,[42] a formulation that is created by attaching a polyethylene glycol chain to the PTH(1–34) peptide. By virtue of a larger molecular size, the pharmacodynamics and pharmacokinetic properties of the molecule are extended. In mice, pegylated PTH increased serum calcium with a peak after 24 hours. Calcium levels, which were still elevated at the 48-hour time point, did not return to baseline values until 96 hours postinjection. Pegylated PTH can be detected in the circulation for at least 24 hours as compared with the 4-hour circulatory life of PTH(1–34).

Different formulations of PTH. Long-Acting Analogues of PTH. Shimizu and colleagues[43] tested the pharmacologic properties of a long-acting PTH analogue (LA–PTH) in thyroparathyroidectomized (TPTX) rats, an acute model of hypoparathyroidism. Relative to the unmodified peptides, PTH(1–34) and PTH(1–84), LA-PTH was associated with enhanced and prolonged effects on blood calcium and phosphate levels. The pharmacokinetic profile of LA-PTH was found to be very comparable with that of PTH(1–34) and PTH(1–84), so another mechanism has to account for the long-lived actions of this PTH. The most current explanation is that the analogue binds to PTHR1 R^0 conformation with high affinity, leading to a prolonged cAMP signaling response. At an optimal dose of 1.8 nmol/kg, LA-PTH increased serum calcium levels in TPTX rats to near normal levels without increasing urinary calcium excretion. These findings were confirmed in moderate and severe forms of acquired hypoparathyroid mouse models. In each model, a single subcutaneous injection of LA-PTH increased serum calcium levels more effectively and for a longer duration (>24 hours) than did a 10-fold higher dose of PTH(1–34), without causing excessive urinary calcium excretion.[44]

Different formulations of PTH. "TransCon" PTH. TransCon PTH is a prodrug inactive form of PTH(1–34). It is bound to a polymer carrier that is slowly cleaved releasing fully active PTH(1–34) in a controlled manner over time. The conditions of the carrier are adjusted to provide active PTH continuously for more than 24 hours. Preliminary data from a phase 1, randomized, placebo-controlled trial in 10 adults showed that single injections up to 100 µg of TransCon PTH determine dose-dependent increases in albumin-adjusted calcium sustained for more than or equal to 72 hours. Under the conditions of the reported trial, fractional excretion of calcium did not change.[45]

AUTOSOMAL DOMINANT HYPOCALCEMIA

An inherited form of hypoparathyroidism, autosomal dominant hypocalcemia, is caused by gain of function mutations in the calcium-sensing receptor (CaR, ADH1) or the alpha subunit of the heterotrimeric G protein (GNA11, ADH2) that couples the receptor to intracellular signal generating pathways. When symptomatic, these patients are commonly managed with calcium and active vitamin D preparations. However, this treatment predisposes patients to the development of hypercalciuria, nephrocalcinosis, nephrolithiasis, and renal impairment.[46] Limited experience with this form of hypoparathyroidism using recombinant PTH(1–34) has been successful in controlling serum calcium level and reducing hypercalciuria. These patients, however, require higher doses of PTH to achieve a similar calcemic response compared with patients with postsurgical and/or idiopathic hypoparathyroidism.[30] Long-term PTH replacement in a child with ADH increased bone mass without negatively affecting mineralization and improved serum calcium overall. It did not prevent nephrocalcinosis but was otherwise well-tolerated without any other safety issues.[47]

Calcilytic compounds, negative modulators of the CaR have the potential to correct the underlying pathophysiologic alterations in parathyroid and kidney function caused by gain-of-function mutations affecting this receptor or the transmembrane G protein, G11.[48] By reducing the sensitivity of the CaR to Ca2+, calcilytics have potential as a therapy for these forms of hypoparathyroidism.[49] Calcilytics comprise 2 main classes of orally active compounds: amino alcohols (eg, NPS 2143, ronacaleret, NPSP795 [also known as SB-423562] and JTT-305/MK-5442 [also known as encaleret]) and quinazolinones (eg, ATF 936 and AXT 914).[49] In mouse models of ADH1 and ADH2, calcilytics can correct hypocalcaemia and hypercalciuria. NPS 2143 increases plasma calcium concentrations without inducing hypercalciuria.[50–52] JTT-305/MK-5442 treatment in mice improved serum and urinary calcium and phosphate levels by stimulating endogenous PTH secretion and prevented renal calcification.[53] Finally, NPSP795 has been administered to 5 adults with ADH1. NPSP795 increased plasma PTH levels and decreased urinary calcium excretion in an apparent dose-dependent manner, while maintaining blood calcium levels during fasting.[54] Although the optimal dose and dosing regimen are not yet determined, NPSP795 seems to represent a potential treatment for ADH.

SUMMARY

The availability of replacement therapy for hypoparathyroidism has improved the prospects of adequate control of calcium metabolism for many patients suffering with this disease. The data demonstrating efficacy and safety are now available in both short-term and long-term studies. Although there is need to further improve the single daily dose protocol with other administration regimens or with different formulations of PTH, it is clear that the therapeutic landscape of hypoparathyroidism has been permanently changed, giving physicians and their patients a wider set of options.

REFERENCES

1. Albright F, Ellsworth R. Studies on the physiology of the parathyroid glands. J Clin Invest 1929;7(2):183–201.
2. Melick RA, Gill JR, Berson SA, et al. Antibodies and clinical resistance to parathyroid hormone. N Engl J Med 1967;276(3):144–7.
3. Winer KK, Yanovski JA, Cutler GB. Synthetic human parathyroid hormone 1-34 vs calcitriol and calcium in the treatment of hypoparathyroidism. JAMA 1996;631–6.

4. United States Food and Drug Administration. NATPARA package insert. 2015. 435518. Available at: http://www.fda.gov/Drugs/InformationOnDrugs/ucm435518. htm. Accessed May 9, 2016.

5. Mannstadt M, Clarke BL, Vokes T, et al. Efficacy and safety of recombinant human parathyroid hormone (1-84) in hypoparathyroidism (REPLACE): a double-blind, placebo-controlled, randomised, phase 3 study. Lancet Diabetes Endocrinol 2013;1(4):275–83.

6. Rubin MR, Sliney J, McMahon DJ, et al. Therapy of hypoparathyroidism with intact parathyroid hormone. Osteoporos Int 2010;1927–34.

7. Clarke BL, Vokes TJ, Bilezikian JP, et al. Effects of parathyroid hormone rhPTH(1–84) on phosphate homeostasis and vitamin D metabolism in hypoparathyroidism: REPLACE phase 3 study. Endocrine 2017;273–82.

8. Sikjaer T, Rejnmark L, Rolighed L, et al, Hypoparathyroid Study Group. The effect of adding PTH(1-84) to conventional treatment of hypoparathyroidism: a randomized, placebo-controlled study. J Bone Miner Res 2011;26(10):2358–70.

9. Lakatos P, Bajnok L, Lagast H, et al. An open-label extension study of parathyroid hormone RHPTH(1-84) in adults with hypoparathyroidism. Endocr Pract 2016;523–32.

10. Cusano NE, Rubin MR, McMahon DJ, et al. Therapy of hypoparathyroidism with PTH(1-84): a prospective four-year investigation of efficacy and safety. J Clin Endocrinol Metab 2013;98(1):137–44.

11. Rubin MR, Cusano NE, Fan W-W, et al. Therapy of hypoparathyroidism with PTH(1–84): a prospective six year investigation of efficacy and safety. J Clin Endocrinol Metab 2016;101(7):2742–50.

12. Clarke BL, Kay Berg J, Fox J, et al. Pharmacokinetics and pharmacodynamics of subcutaneous recombinant parathyroid hormone (1-84) in patients with hypoparathyroidism: an open-label, single-dose, phase i study. Clin Ther 2014; 36(5):722–36.

13. Sikjaer T, Amstrup AK, Rolighed L, et al. PTH(1-84) replacement therapy in hypoparathyroidism: a randomized controlled trial on pharmacokinetic and dynamic effects after 6 months of treatment. J Bone Miner Res 2013;28(10):2232–43.

14. Fox J, Wells D, Garceau R. Relationships between pharmacokinetic profile of human PTH(1-84) and serum calcium response in postmenopausal women following four different methods of administration. Program of the 33rd Annual Meeting of the American Society of Bone and Mineral Research. San Diego (CA), 2011.

15. Bilezikian JP, Clarke BL, Mannstadt M, et al. Safety and efficacy of recombinant human parathyroid hormone in adults with hypoparathyroidism randomly assigned to receive fixed 25-µg or 50-µg daily doses. Clin Ther 2017;39(10):2096–102.

16. Brandi ML, Bilezikian JP, Shoback D, et al. Management of hypoparathyroidism: summary statement and guidelines. J Clin Endocrinol Metab 2016;101(6): 2273–83.

17. Abate EG, Clarke BL. Review of hypoparathyroidism. Front Endocrinol (Lausanne) 2017;7:172.

18. Bilezikian JP, Brandi ML, Cusano NE, et al. Management of hypoparathyroidism. present and future. J Clin Endocrinol Metab 2016;101(6):2313–24.

19. Sikjaer T, Rejnmark L, Thomsen JS, et al. Changes in 3-dimensional bone structure indices in hypoparathyroid patients treated with PTH(1-84): a randomized controlled study. J Bone Miner Res 2012;27(4):781–8.

20. Rubin MR, Dempster DW, Sliney J, et al. PTH(1-84) administration reverses abnormal bone-remodeling dynamics and structure in hypoparathyroidism. J Bone Miner Res 2011;26(11):2727–36.

21. Rubin MR, Zwahlen A, Dempster DW, et al. Effects of parathyroid hormone administration on bone strength in hypoparathyroidism. J Bone Miner Res 2016;31(5):1082–8.
22. Cipriani C, Abraham A, Silva BC, et al. Skeletal changes after restoration of the euparathyroid state in patients with hypoparathyroidism and primary hyperparathyroidism. Endocrine 2017;55(2):591–8.
23. Misof BM, Roschger P, Dempster DW, et al. PTH(1-84) Administration in hypoparathyroidism transiently reduces bone matrix mineralization. J Bone Miner Res 2016;31(1):180–9.
24. Winer KK, Zhang B, Shrader JA, et al. Synthetic human parathyroid hormone 1-34 replacement therapy: a randomized crossover trial comparing pump versus injections in the treatment of chronic hypoparathyroidism. J Clin Endocrinol Metab 2012;97(2):391–9.
25. Mannstadt M, Bilezikian JP, Thakker RV, et al. Hypoparathyroidism. Nat Rev Dis Primers 2017;3:17055.
26. Vokes TJ, Mannstadt M, Levine MA, et al. Recombinant human parathyroid hormone effect on health-related quality of life in adults with chronic hypoparathyroidism. J Clin Endocrinol Metab 2018;103(2):722–31.
27. Cusano NE, Rubin MR, McMahon DJ, et al. PTH(1-84) is associated with improved quality of life in hypoparathyroidism through 5 years of therapy. J Clin Endocrinol Metab 2014;99(10):3694–9.
28. Cusano NE, Rubin MR, McMahon DJ, et al. The effect of PTH(1-84) on quality of life in hypoparathyroidism. J Clin Endocrinol Metab 2013;98(6):2356–61.
29. Sikjaer T, Rolighed L, Hess A, et al. Effects of PTH(1-84) therapy on muscle function and quality of life in hypoparathyroidism: results from a randomized controlled trial. Osteoporos Int 2014;25(6):1717–26.
30. Winer KK, Yanovski JA, Sarani B, et al. A randomized, cross-over trial of once-daily versus twice-daily parathyroid hormone 1-34 in treatment of hypoparathyroidism. J Clin Endocrinol Metab 1998;83(10):3480–6.
31. Winer KK, Ko CW, Reynolds JC, et al. Long-term treatment of hypoparathyroidism: a randomized controlled study comparing parathyroid hormone-(1-34) versus calcitriol and calcium. J Clin Endocrinol Metab 2003;88(9):4214–20.
32. Winer KK, Sinaii N, Reynolds J, et al. Long-term treatment of 12 children with chronic hypoparathyroidism: a randomized trial comparing synthetic human parathyroid hormone 1-34 versus calcitriol and calcium. J Clin Endocrinol Metab 2010;95(6):2680–8.
33. Winer KK, Fulton KA, Albert PS, et al. Effects of pump versus twice-daily injection delivery of synthetic parathyroid hormone 1-34 in children with severe congenital hypoparathyroidism. J Pediatr 2014;165(3):556–63.
34. Winer KK, Sinaii N, Peterson D, et al. Effects of once *versus* twice-daily parathyroid hormone 1–34 therapy in children with hypoparathyroidism. J Clin Endocrinol Metab 2008;93(9):3389–95.
35. Santonati A, Palermo A, Maddaloni E, et al. PTH(1-34) for surgical hypoparathyroidism: a prospective, open-label investigation of efficacy and quality of life. J Clin Endocrinol Metab 2015;100(9):3590–7.
36. Palermo A, Santonati A, Tabacco G, et al. PTH(1–34) for surgical hypoparathyroidism: a 2-year prospective, open-label investigation of efficacy and quality of life. J Clin Endocrinol Metab 2018;103(1):271–80.
37. Gafni RI, Brahim JS, Andreopoulou P, et al. Daily parathyroid hormone 1-34 replacement therapy for hypoparathyroidism induces marked changes in bone turnover and structure. J Bone Miner Res 2012;27(8):1811–20.

38. Jolette J, Wilker CE, Smith SY, et al. Defining a noncarcinogenic dose of recombinant human parathyroid hormone 1-84 in a 2-year study in Fischer 344 rats. Toxicol Pathol 2006;34(7):929–40.
39. Vahle JL, Sato M, Long GG, et al. Skeletal changes in rats given daily subcutaneous injections of recombinant human parathyroid hormone (1-34) for 2 years and relevance to human safety. Toxicol Pathol 2002;30(3):312–21.
40. Capriani C, Irani D, Bilezikian JP, et al. Safety of osteoanabolic therapy: a decade of experience. J Bone Miner Res 2012;27(12):2419–28.
41. Andrews EB, Gilsenan AW, Midkiff K, et al. The US postmarketing surveillance study of adult osteosarcoma and teriparatide: study design and findings from the first 7 years. J Bone Miner Res 2012;27(12):2429–37.
42. Guo J, Khatri A, Maeda A, et al. Prolonged pharmacokinetic and pharmacodynamic actions of a pegylated parathyroid hormone (1-34) peptide fragment. J Bone Miner Res 2017;32(1):86–98.
43. Shimizu M, Joyashiki E, Noda H, et al. Pharmacodynamic actions of a long-acting PTH analog (LA-PTH) in thyroparathyroidectomized (TPTX) rats and normal monkeys. J Bone Miner Res 2016;31(7):1405–12.
44. Bi R, Fan Y, Lauter K, et al. Diphtheria toxin- and GFP-based mouse models of acquired hypoparathyroidism and treatment with a long-acting parathyroid hormone analog. J Bone Miner Res 2016;31(5):975–84.
45. Karpf DB, Mortensen E, Sprogoe K, et al. The design and preliminary results of a phase 1 TransCon PTH trial in healthy volunteers. Program of 100th Annual meeting of the Endocrine society. Endocrine Reviews. Chicago (IL), 2018.
46. Hannan FM, Babinsky VN, Thakker RV. Disorders of the calcium-sensing receptor and partner proteins: insights into the molecular basis of calcium homeostasis. J Mol Endocrinol 2016;57(3):R127–42.
47. Theman TA, Collins MT, Dempster DW, et al. PTH(1-34) replacement therapy in a child with hypoparathyroidism caused by a sporadic calcium receptor mutation. J Bone Miner Res 2009;24(5):964–73.
48. Hannan FM, Olesen MK, Thakker RV. Calcimimetic and calcilytic therapies for inherited disorders of the calcium-sensing receptor signalling pathway. Br J Pharmacol 2017;1–12. https://doi.org/10.1111/bph.14086.
49. Nemeth EF, Goodman WG. Calcimimetic and calcilytic drugs: feats, flops, and futures. Calcif Tissue Int 2016;98(4):341–58.
50. Hannan FM, Walls GV, Babinsky VN, et al. The calcilytic agent NPS 2143 rectifies hypocalcemia in a mouse model with an activating calcium-sensing receptor (CaSR) mutation: relevance to autosomal dominant hypocalcemia type 1 (ADH1). Endocrinology 2015;156(9):3114–21.
51. Gorvin CM, Hannan FM, Howles SA, et al. Gα11 mutation in mice causes hypocalcemia rectifiable by calcilytic therapy. JCI Insight 2017;2(3):e91103.
52. Roszko KL, Bi R, Gorvin CM, et al. Knockin mouse with mutant Gα11mimics human inherited hypocalcemia and is rescued by pharmacologic inhibitors. JCI Insight 2017;2(3):e91079.
53. Dong B, Endo I, Ohnishi Y, et al. Calcilytic ameliorates abnormalities of mutant Calcium-Sensing Receptor (CaSR) knock-in mice mimicking autosomal dominant hypocalcemia (ADH). J Bone Miner Res 2015;30(11):1980–93.
54. Ramnitz M, Gafni RI, Brillante B, et al. Treatment of autosomal dominant hypocalcemia with the calcilytic NPSP795. Program of the 37th Annual Meeting of the American Society of Bone and Mineral Research. Seattle (WA), 2015.

UNITED STATES POSTAL SERVICE® Statement of Ownership, Management, and Circulation (All Periodicals Publications Except Requester Publications)

1. Publication Title	2. Publication Number	3. Filing Date
ENDOCRINOLOGY AND METABOLISM CLINICS OF NORTH AMERICA	000 – 275	9/18/2018

4. Issue Frequency	5. Number of Issues Published Annually	6. Annual Subscription Price
MAR, JUN, SEP, DEC	4	$357.00

7. Complete Mailing Address of Known Office of Publication (Not printer) (Street, city, county, state, and ZIP+4®)

ELSEVIER INC.
230 Park Avenue, Suite 800
New York, NY 10169

Contact Person
STEPHEN R. BUSHING
Telephone (Include area code)
215-239-3688

8. Complete Mailing Address of Headquarters or General Business Office of Publisher (Not printer)

ELSEVIER INC.
230 Park Avenue, Suite 800
New York, NY 10169

9. Full Names and Complete Mailing Addresses of Publisher, Editor, and Managing Editor (Do not leave blank)

Publisher (Name and complete mailing address)

TAYLOR E BALL ELSEVIER INC.
1600 JOHN F KENNEDY BLVD. SUITE 1800
PHILADELPHIA, PA 19103-2899

Editor (Name and complete mailing address)

STACY EACTMAN, ELSEVIER INC.
1600 JOHN F KENNEDY BLVD. SUITE 1800
PHILADELPHIA, PA 19103-2899

Managing Editor (Name and complete mailing address)

PATRICK MANLEY, ELSEVIER INC.
1600 JOHN F KENNEDY BLVD. SUITE 1800
PHILADELPHIA, PA 19103-2899

10. Owner (Do not leave blank. If the publication is owned by a corporation, give the name and address of the corporation immediately followed by the names and addresses of all stockholders owning or holding 1 percent or more of the total amount of stock. If not owned by a corporation, give the names and addresses of the individual owners. If owned by a partnership or other unincorporated firm, give its name and address as well as those of each individual owner. If the publication is published by a nonprofit organization, give its name and address.)

Full Name	Complete Mailing Address
WHOLLY OWNED SUBSIDIARY OF REED/ELSEVIER, US HOLDINGS	1600 JOHN F KENNEDY BLVD. SUITE 1800 PHILADELPHIA, PA 19103-2899

11. Known Bondholders, Mortgagees, and Other Security Holders Owning or Holding 1 Percent or More of Total Amount of Bonds, Mortgages, or Other Securities. If none, check box ► ☐ None

Full Name	Complete Mailing Address
N/A	

12. Tax Status (For completion by nonprofit organizations authorized to mail at nonprofit rates) (Check one)
The purpose, function, and nonprofit status of this organization and the exempt status for federal income tax purposes:
☒ Has Not Changed During Preceding 12 Months
☐ Has Changed During Preceding 12 Months (Publisher must submit explanation of change with this statement)

PS Form 3626, July 2914 (Page 1 of 4 (see instructions page 4)) PSN 7530-01-000-9931 PRIVACY NOTICE: See our privacy policy on www.usps.com

---

13. Publication Title	14. Issue Date for Circulation Data Below
ENDOCRINOLOGY AND METABOLISM CLINICS OF NORTH AMERICA	JUNE 2018

15. Extent and Nature of Circulation		Average No. Copies Each Issue During Preceding 12 Months	No. Copies of Single Issue Published Nearest to Filing Date
a. Total Number of Copies (Net press run)		252	326
b. Paid Circulation (By Mail and Outside the Mail)	(1) Mailed Outside-County Paid Subscriptions Stated on PS Form 3541 (include paid distribution above nominal rate, advertiser's proof copies, and exchange copies)	116	141
	(2) Mailed In-County Paid Subscriptions Stated on PS Form 3541 (include paid distribution above nominal rate, advertiser's proof copies, and exchange copies)	0	0
	(3) Paid Distribution Outside the Mails Including Sales Through Dealers and Carriers, Street Vendors, Counter Sales, and Other Paid Distribution Outside USPS®	67	86
	(4) Paid Distribution by Other Classes of Mail Through the USPS (e.g., First-Class Mail®)	0	0
c. Total Paid Distribution (Sum of 15b (1), (2), (3), and (4))	►	183	227
d. Free or Nominal Rate Distribution (By Mail and Outside the Mail)	(1) Free or Nominal Rate Outside-County Copies included on PS Form 3541	56	82
	(2) Free or Nominal Rate In-County Copies Included on PS Form 3541	0	0
	(3) Free or Nominal Rate Copies Mailed at Other Classes Through the USPS (e.g., First-Class Mail)	0	0
	(4) Free or Nominal Rate Distribution Outside the Mail (Carriers or other means)	0	0
e. Total Free or Nominal Rate Distribution (Sum of 15d (1), (2), (3) and (4))	►	56	82
f. Total Distribution (Sum of 15c and 15e)	►	239	309
g. Copies not Distributed (See Instructions to Publishers #4 (page 4))	►	13	17
h. Total (Sum of 15f and g)	►	252	326
i. Percent Paid (15c divided by 15f times 100)		76.57%	73.46%

* If you are claiming electronic copies, go to line 16 on page 3. If you are not claiming electronic copies, skip to line 17 on page 3.

16. Electronic Copy Circulation		Average No. Copies Each Issue During Preceding 12 Months	No. Copies of Single Issue Published Nearest to Filing Date
a. Paid Electronic Copies	►	0	0
b. Total Paid Print Copies (Line 15c) + Paid Electronic Copies (Line 16a)	►	183	227
c. Total Print Distribution (Line 15f) + Paid Electronic Copies (Line 16a)	►	239	309
d. Percent Paid (Both Print & Electronic Copies) (16b divided by 16c × 100)	►	76.57%	73.46%

☒ I certify that 60% of all my distributed copies (electronic and print) are paid above a nominal price.

17. Publication of Statement of Ownership
☒ If the publication is a general publication, publication of this statement is required. Will be printed in the DECEMBER 2018 issue of this publication.   ☐ Publication not required.

18. Signature and Title of Editor, Publisher, Business Manager, or Owner

STEPHEN R. BUSHING - INVENTORY DISTRIBUTION CONTROL MANAGER

Date 9/18/2018

I certify that all information furnished on this form is true and complete. I understand that anyone who furnishes false or misleading information on this form or who omits material or information requested on the form may be subject to criminal sanctions (including fines and imprisonment) and/or civil sanctions (including civil penalties).

PS Form 3626, July 2014 (Page 3 of 4) PRIVACY NOTICE: See our privacy policy on www.usps.com

Moving?

Make sure your subscription moves with you!

To notify us of your new address, find your **Clinics Account Number** (located on your mailing label above your name), and contact customer service at:

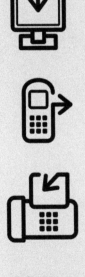

Email: journalscustomerservice-usa@elsevier.com

800-654-2452 (subscribers in the U.S. & Canada)
314-447-8871 (subscribers outside of the U.S. & Canada)

Fax number: 314-447-8029

Elsevier Health Sciences Division
Subscription Customer Service
3251 Riverport Lane
Maryland Heights, MO 63043

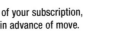

Printed and bound by CPI Group (UK) Ltd, Croydon, CR0 4YY

08/05/2025

01864735-0003